Genetics and Screening for the General Surgeon

Editor

MATHEW H. CHUNG

AF752237

SURGICAL CLINICS OF NORTH AMERICA

www.surgical.theclinics.com

Consulting Editor
PAUL J. SCHENARTS

August 2026 • Volume 106 • Number 4

ELSEVIER

1818 Market Street • Suite 3323 • Philadelphia, Pennsylvania, 19103-2899

http://www.surgical.theclinics.com

SURGICAL CLINICS OF NORTH AMERICA Volume 106, Number 4
August 2026 ISSN 0039–6109, ISBN-13: 978-0-443-42947-7

Editor: Megan Ashdown (m.ashdown@elsevier.com)
Developmental Editor: Gaurav Singh

Publishing Office: *Surgical Clinics of North America* (ISSN 0039–6109) is published bimonthly by Elsevier Inc., 1818 Market Street Philadelphia, PA 19103, United States. Periodicals postage paid at New York, NY and additional mailing offices. USA POSTMASTER: Send address changes to *Surgical Clinics of North America*, Elsevier Customer Service Department, 3251 Riverport Lane Maryland Heights, MO 63043, USA. Months of publication are February, April, June, August, October, and December. Subscription prices are $518.00 per year for US individuals, $100.00 per year for US & Canadian students and residents, $622.00 per year for Canadian individuals, $628.00 for international individuals, and $250.00 per year for foreign students/residents. For institutional access pricing please contact Customer Service via the contact information below. To receive student/resident rate, orders must be accompanied by name of affiliated institution, date of term, and the *signature* of program/residency coordinator on institution letterhead. Orders will be billed at individual rate until proof of status is received. Foreign air speed delivery is included in all *Clinics* subscription prices. All prices are subject to change without notice. Orders, claims, and journal inquiries: Please visit our Support Hub page https://service.elsevier.com for assistance.

Reprints. For copies of 100 or more, of articles in this publication, please contact the Commercial Reprints Department Elsevier Inc., 360 Park Avenue South, New York, New York 10010-1710. Tel. 212-633-3874, Fax: 212-633-3820, E-mail: reprints@elsevier.com.

Surgical Clinics of North America is also published in Spanish by McGraw-Hill Interamericana Editores S.A., P.O. Box 5-237 0650 Mexico D.F. Mexico; and in Portuguese by Interlivros Edicoes Ltda., Rua Comandante Coelho 1085, CEP 21250, Rio de Janeiro Brazil; and in Greek by Paschalidis Medical Publications, Athens Greece.

Surgical Clinics of North America is covered in *MEDLINE/PubMed (Index Medicus), EMBASE/Excerpta Medica, Current Contents/Clinical Medicine, Current Contents/Life Sciences, Science Citation Index*, and *ISI/BIOMED*.

Contributors

CONSULTING EDITOR

PAUL J. SCHENARTS, MD, FACS, MAMSE
Professor of Surgery, Associate Dean for Faculty Affairs, Homer Stryker MD School of Medicine, Western Michigan University, Kalamazoo, Michigan

EDITOR

MATHEW H. CHUNG, MD, FACS
Professor of Surgery, Division of Surgical Oncology, Lemmen Holton Cancer Pavilion, Corewell Health West Medical Group, Michigan State University College of Human Medicine, Grand Rapids, Michigan

AUTHORS

SAMI O. ABUL-KHOUDOUD, MD
General Surgery Resident, Department of Surgery, Division of Surgical Oncology, University Hospitals, Cleveland Medical Center, Cleveland, Ohio

LARITZA DIAZ, MD
General Surgery Resident, Department of Surgery, University of North Carolina, Chapel Hill, North Carolina

SARA M. GROSSI, MD
Assistant Clinical Professor, Department of Surgery, Breast Surgery Division, UC San Diego School of Medicine, San Diego, California

JEFFREY M. HARDACRE, MD, FACS
Associate Professor, Department of Surgery, Division of Surgical Oncology, University Hospitals, Cleveland Medical Center, Case Western Reserve University School of Medicine, Cleveland, Ohio

JARED R. HENDREN, MD
General Surgery Resident, Departments of General Surgery and Colorectal Surgery, Digestive Disease Institute, Sanford R. Weiss, MD Center for Hereditary Colorectal Neoplasia, Cleveland Clinic, Cleveland, Ohio

ELIZABETH M. HOGAN, MS
Licensed Genetic Counselor, Department of Genetics and Genomics, The MetroHealth System, Assistant Professor, Case Western Reserve University, School of Medicine, Cleveland, Ohio

JONATHAN HWANG, MD
Professor, Department of Urology, Georgetown University School of Medicine, Washington, DC

JULIE LE, MD, FACS
Assistant Clinical Professor, Department of Surgery, Breast Surgery Division, UC San Diego School of Medicine, San Diego, California

DAVID LISKA, MD
Chair, Department of Colorectal Surgery, Digestive Disease Institute, Sanford R. Weiss, MD Center for Hereditary Colorectal Neoplasia, Cleveland Clinic, Cleveland, Ohio

YING L. LIU, MD, MPH
Medical Oncologist and Clinical Geneticist, Department of Medicine, Gynecologic Medical Oncology Service and Clinical Genetics Service, Memorial Sloan Kettering Cancer Center, New York, New York

KARA C. LONG, MD, MSc
Associate Attending Surgeon, Department of Surgery, Gynecology Service, Memorial Sloan Kettering Cancer Center, New York, New York

LISA MADLENSKY, PhD, CGC
Professor, Department of Medicine, Division of Genomics and Precision Medicine, UC San Diego Health, San Diego, California

CHRISTOPHER R. McHENRY, MD
Vice Chairman, Professor, Department of Surgery, The MetroHealth System, Case Western Reserve University, School of Medicine, Cleveland, Ohio

MECKER G. MÖLLER, MD, FACS, MAMSE
Professor of Surgery, Section of Surgical Oncology, Director, Surgical Oncology Fellowship Program and Regional Therapies (HIPEC) Program, University of Chicago Pritzker School of Medicine, Chicago, Illinois

BELÉN MORA-GARIJO, MD
Resident, Department of Urology, MedStar Georgetown University Hospital, Washington Hospital Center, Washington, DC

CORBYN M. NCHAKO, MD
Gynecology Fellow, Department of Surgery, Gynecology Service, Memorial Sloan Kettering Cancer Center, New York, New York

JOSEPH G.R. PARTUZO, BS
Medical Student, Department of Urology, Georgetown University School of Medicine, Washington, DC

TARA A. RETSON, MD, PhD
Assistant Clinical Professor, Department of Radiology, Breast Imaging Division, UC San Diego School of Medicine, San Diego, California

PERRY SHEN, MD
Professor of Surgery, Department of Surgical Oncology and HPB Surgery, Atrium Health Wake Forest Baptist, Winston-Salem, North Carolina

SHANNON M. SMITH, MD
Resident Physician, Department of General Surgery, Corewell Health West, Michigan State University College of Human Medicine, Grand Rapids, Michigan

JOSH SOMMOVILLA, MD
Assistant Professor of Surgery, Department of Colorectal Surgery, Digestive Disease Institute, Sanford R. Weiss, MD Center for Hereditary Colorectal Neoplasia, Cleveland Clinic, Cleveland, Ohio

YUKIO SONODA, MD
Attending Surgeon, Department of Surgery, Gynecology Service, Memorial Sloan Kettering Cancer Center, New York, New York

SCOTT R. STEELE, MD, MBA
Surgeon, Department of Colorectal Surgery, Digestive Disease Institute, Sanford R. Weiss, MD Center for Hereditary Colorectal Neoplasia, Cleveland Clinic, Cleveland, Ohio

MATTHEW STEENSMA, MD
Betz Family Endowed Research Chair, Associate Professor, Section Chief, Orthopedic Oncology, Corewell Health Regional Cancer Program, Grand Rapids, Michigan

MARIE W. SU, MD
Resident, Department of Surgery, The MetroHealth System, Case Western Reserve University, School of Medicine, Cleveland, Ohio

ANGELA E. THELEN, MD, MHPE
Clinical Associate, Section of Endocrine Surgery, Integrated Surgical Institute, Cleveland Clinic Foundation, Cleveland, Ohio

ELISABETH T. TRACY, MD
Associate Professor, Division of Pediatric Surgery, UNC Children's Hospital, University of North Carolina; Member UNC Lineberger Comprehensive Cancer Center, Chapel Hill, North Carolina

SOFIA W. VIANA, MD
Research Fellow, Division of Thoracic Surgery, Department of Surgery, University of Cincinnati College of Medicine, Cincinnati, Ohio

WILLIAM WONG, DO, MPH
Physician, Section of Surgical Oncology, Department of Surgery, University of Chicago Pritzker School of Medicine, Chicago, Illinois

G. PAUL WRIGHT, MD, FACS
Assistant Professor, Division of Surgical Oncology, Corewell Health West, Michigan State University College of Human Medicine, Grand Rapids, Michigan

RUI ZHENG-PYWELL, MD
Physician and Researcher, Department of Surgical Oncology, Atrium Health Wake Forest Baptist, Winston-Salem, North Carolina

Contents

SURGICAL CLINICS OF NORTH AMERICA

FORTHCOMING ISSUES

October 2026
Advancements in Laparoscopy and Robotic Surgery
Michael Meara and Meredith Duke, *Editors*

December 2026
Pitfalls and Complications During Common Surgical Procedures
Jason Kempenich, *Editor*

February 2027
Disaster Management
Gregory Schaefer, *Editor*

RECENT ISSUES

June 2026
Social Determinants of Health, Health Disparities and Surgical Equity
Tracey Dechert and Sheina Theodore, *Editors*

April 2026
Surgical Nutrition
Jose J. Diaz, *Editor*

February 2026
Benign Colon, Rectal and Anal Disorders
Jennifer S. Beaty, *Editor*

SERIES OF RELATED INTEREST

Advances in Surgery
https://www.advancessurgery.com/
Surgical Oncology Clinics
https://www.surgonc.theclinics.com/
Thoracic Surgery Clinics
https://www.thoracic.theclinics.com/

THE CLINICS ARE AVAILABLE ONLINE!
Access your subscription at:
www.theclinics.com

Foreword

Beyond Histopathology, How Genetics Is Reshaping Surgical Oncology

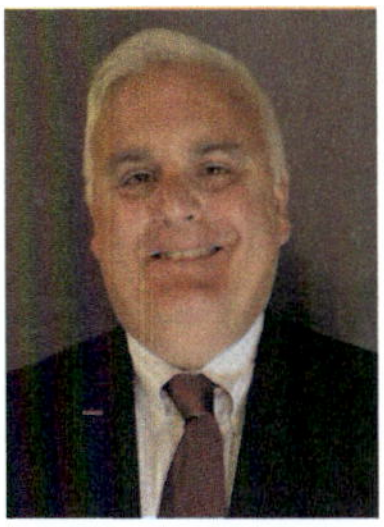

Paul J. Schenarts, MD, FACS, MAMSE
Consulting Editor

Throughout the history of *Surgical Clinics*, the battle against cancer has been the subject of many articles and issues. On page 185, of issue one, volume one, Dr Gibbon[1] of the Pennsylvania Hospital advises that a painstaking physical examination and x-ray study need to be undertaken to ensure that a cancer operation will be ultimately successful By 1944, Dr E.V. Cowdray[2] included the influence of heredity in his article, "Factors in Cancer Production." In the 1962 *Surgical Clinics* issue entitled "Cancer Management—Current Knowledge," Dr Burdette[3] states in his last sentence of his article on "Oncogenetics" that "[t]here is every indication that the gene plays an important role in oncogenesis, what it does is known in part, how it acts is much more obscure." In this issue, Dr Mathew Chung has gathered a group of outstanding authors who have clarified the important role of genetics in surgical oncology.

Historically, histopathology and anatomy alone determined our approach to cancer. Now we have a progressively greater understanding of how molecular mechanisms guide individual targeted therapy, refine prognosis, and help determine de-escalation strategies. While at present inherited cancers impact a relatively small subset of patients, understanding how molecular mechanisms drive tumor biology offers hope for future understanding of pathobiology and improved patient outcomes.

Though the reader can select the articles that address the most common cancers encountered in their practice, what was most notable to me was the crossover between the hereditary risks for multiple types of cancers. This demonstrates the future importance of polygenetic risk scoring for individual patients.

Surg Clin N Am 106 (2026) xiii–xiv
https://doi.org/10.1016/j.suc.2026.05.001
0039-6109/26/© 2026 Published by Elsevier Inc.
surgical.theclinics.com

I would like to thank each author for their meticulous approach to each article, for providing useful information to the practicing surgeon, and for providing a molecular foundation for future articles in *Surgical Clinics* on surgical oncology.

Paul J. Schenarts, MD, FACS, MAMSE
Department of Surgery
Homer Stryker MD School of Medicine
Western Michigan University
300 Portage Street
Kalamazoo, MI 49007, USA

E-mail address:
pj.schenarts@wmed.edu

REFERENCES

1. Gibbon JH. Amputation of the breast for carcinoma: the Stewart incision. Surg Clin North Am 1921;1(1):185–95.
2. Cowdray EV. Factors in cancer production. Surg Clin North Am 1944;24(5):985–93.
3. Burdette WJ. Oncogenetics. Surg Clin North Am 1962;42(2):289–303.

Preface

Genetics and Screening for the General Surgeon

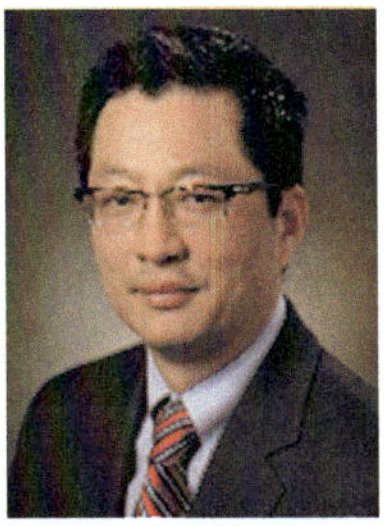

Mathew H. Chung, MD, FACS
Editor

It has been an honor to serve as a guest editor of the current issue of *Surgical Clinics* exploring the role of genetics in cancer care. I would like to express my deep and sincere gratitude to all the authors, who so generously contributed their time and efforts. In this issue, we have attempted to summarize our current understanding of genetics and its role in carcinogenesis as it relates to general surgeons.

Cancers have many contributory factors and a multitude of clinical implications. In its most basic form, however, cancer is caused by altered genes. Cancer genes that arise in the germ cells are said to be in the germline. People who inherit germline cancer genes will harbor a cancer gene in every cell, both somatic cells and germ cells alike. These individuals are known as carriers, are at increased risk of developing cancer, and can transmit that risk to their offspring. In contrast, genes that arise in somatic cells are not passed onto subsequent generations.

Germline cancer genes cause a small but significant proportion of human cancers; approximately 5% to 10% of all cancers result from a heritable predisposition. In the majority of common cancers, however, the cancer genes that underlie carcinogenesis arise spontaneously by somatic mutation. In fact, these somatic mutations lead to the development of the majority of cancers.

In this issue of *Surgical Clinics*, we have explored some of the more common cancers and their relationship to genetics. Our emerging understanding of the principles of genetics, its interplay with biological pathways, and physical manifestations have led to improved diagnosis and therapies, both preventative and therapeutic. One of the most significant intercellular interactions involves cells that mediate the immune response to pathogens.

It is an exciting time to be involved in oncologic care. Our expanding knowledge of genetics, carcinogenesis, and interplay of complex interaction of cellular pathways is leading to more effective and durable treatments for our patients.

Surg Clin N Am 106 (2026) xv–xvi
https://doi.org/10.1016/j.suc.2026.04.001
0039-6109/26/© 2026 Published by Elsevier Inc.

I hope that you enjoy reading this issue and continue to contribute to our understanding of cancer genetics, biology, and outcomes. With our combined and continued efforts in this arena, we can strive to deliver the best oncologic care possible for our patients and, quite possibly, a cure for mankind in the future.

DISCLOSURES

The author has no commercial or financial conflicts of interest.

Mathew H. Chung, MD, FACS
Division of Surgical Oncology
Lemmen Holton Cancer Pavilion
Corewell Health West Medical Group
Michigan State University
College of Human Medicine
Suite 5500
145 Michigan Street NE
Grand Rapids, MI 49503, USA

E-mail address:
mathew.chung@corewellhealth.org

Genetics, Screening, and Risk-reducing Interventions for Breast Cancer

Julie Le, MD[a,*], Lisa Madlensky, PhD, CGC[b],
Tara A. Retson, MD, PhD[c], Sara M. Grossi, MD[a]

KEYWORDS

- Genetics • High-risk screening • Risk models • Risk-reducing mastectomy
- Endocrine therapy

KEY POINTS

- Gail and Tyrer-Cuzick models can be helpful tools to estimate a patient's lifetime risk of breast cancer development that incorporates personal and familial risk factors.
- High-risk screening for patients with a lifetime risk of breast cancer greater than 20% entails alternating annual screening mammogram with one additional supplemental imaging.
- Genetic testing can be considered for women with extensive family history of cancer, diagnosis of premenopausal cancer or have high-risk heritage (ie. Ashkenazi Jewish).
- Risk-reducing mastectomies can be considered for appropriate patients with mutations in BRCA 1 and 2, CDH1, PTEN, PALB2, and TP53.

INTRODUCTION

Breast cancer (BC) affects approximately 1 in 8 women over the course of their lifetime, making it highly likely that nearly every physician will care for a patient with this disease at some point in their career. For women at increased lifetime risk of BC, targeted strategies—such as more frequent or advanced imaging and genetic testing—are essential and powerful tools in the surgeon's armamentarium for early detection and for implementing risk-reduction measures. Our article reviews current evidence-based guidelines for BC screening according to lifetime risk, approaches for assessing risk through personal and familial factors, and the indications, interpretation, and clinical implications of genetic testing.

[a] Department of Surgery, Breast Surgery Division, UC San Diego School of Medicine, San Diego, CA, USA; [b] Department of Medicine, Division of Genomics and Precision Medicine, UC San Diego Health, San Deigo, CA, USA; [c] Department of Radiology, Breast Imaging Division, UC San Diego School of Medicine, San Diego, CA, USA
* Corresponding author. UC San Diego Health Breast Surgical Oncology, 3855 Health Sciences Drive, Office 2058, San Diego, CA 92037.
E-mail address: Jul128@health.ucsd.edu

Surg Clin N Am 106 (2026) 465–479
https://doi.org/10.1016/j.suc.2026.03.003 surgical.theclinics.com
0039-6109/26/

Abbreviations

AD	autosomal dominant
AJ	Ashkenazi Jewish
AT	ataxia-telangiectasia
BC	breast cancer
CBC	contralateral breast cancer
CBEs	clinical breast examinations
CDR	cancer detection rate
CEM	contrast-enhanced mammography
CPM	contralateral prophylactic mastectomy
HDGC	hereditary diffuse gastric cancer
LBC	lobular breast cancer
MBI	molecular breast imaging
MMG	mammogram
NCCN	National Comprehensive Cancer Network
NSABP	National Surgical Adjuvant Breast and Bowel Project
PBM	prophylactic bilateral mastectomies
PDAC	pancreatic ductal adenocarcinoma
PRS	polygenic risk scores
RRSO	risk-reducing salpingo-oophorectomies
SNVs	single nucleotide variants
TC	Tyrer-Cuzick
TNBC	triple-negative breast cancer
TS	tumor suppressor
VAF	variant allele fraction

INDICATIONS FOR GENETIC TESTING

Women with Prior Diagnosis of Breast Cancer

National Comprehensive Cancer Network (NCCN) recommends genetic testing for patients with BC if diagnosed under the age of 50 years, diagnosis of triple-negative breast cancer (TNBC) and all male patients with BC.[1] For the remaining patients with BC, additional personal or family history (FH) of ovarian, pancreas, metastatic prostate cancer or Ashkenazi Jewish (AJ) heritage usually warrants testing, as well as those patients with 2 additional relatives with BC at any age. Genetic testing can also be considered if the test results will guide systemic treatment (**Fig. 1**).

Women with No Prior Diagnosis of Breast Cancer

Women without prior BC can qualify for genetic testing if any of the criteria for patients with BC was met for first-degree or second-degree relatives. Other factors that may warrant consideration for genetic testing or consultation with a genetic counselor include women who have a greater than 2.5% to 5% risk of harboring a BRCA1 or BRCA2 (BRCA1/2) pathogenic mutation based on probability models (ie, BRCAPro and CanRisk) and history of malignant phyllodes tumor.[1]

RISK ASSESSMENT AND SCREENING FOR WOMEN WITH PATHOGENIC MUTATIONS

Women diagnosed with a genetic predisposition for BC warrant earlier and more frequent screening due to higher lifetime risk compared to the average population (**Table 1**). We will review common genes that influence a woman's lifetime risk, which are categorized into high penetrance, moderate penetrance, and polygenic risk that confer greater than 50%, 20% to 50%, and variable risk, respectively.

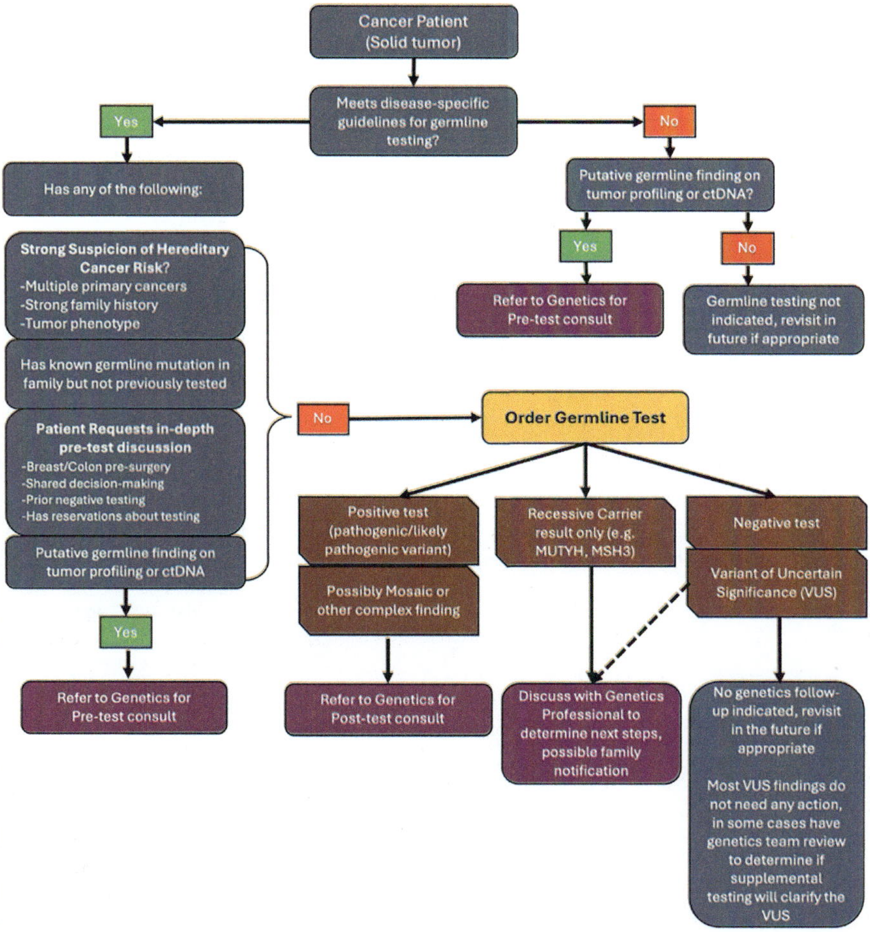

Fig. 1. Genetic testing and referral workflow schematic for patients diagnosed with breast cancer. (Used with permission from Drs. Guo and Madlensky.)

High Penetrance Genes

BRCA1 and BRCA2

The BRCA1/2 genes are tumor suppressor (TS) genes and mutations in these genes affect a cell's ability to restrict uncontrolled growth. BRCA1/2 mutations are inherited in an autosomal dominant (AD) manner with an incidence of 1 in 300 to 500 individuals of the general population.[2,3] BRCA1 and BRCA2 mutations account for 35% and 25% of hereditary BC, respectively.[2,3] BRCA1/2 mutations can be inherited or de novo. De novo BRCA1/2 mutations represent less than 5% of BRCA-positive patients.[4] Founder mutations represent those that can be traced to a specific genetic lineage in a population that was defined by a specific ancestry lineage; examples include those with AJ, Finnish, or Icelandic heritages.[3] The incidence of BRCA mutation in the AJ population is 1 in 40 individuals.[3]

BRCA1 carriers have a higher conferred lifetime risk of breast and ovarian cancers compared to BRCA2 carriers. Absolute lifetime (up to ages 70–80 years) risks of

Table 1
Breast cancer screening for women with genetic mutations

	Lifetime BC Risk	CBC Risk	Image Screening Recommendations	Role of PBM and Other Considerations
ATM	21%–24%	~4% over 10 y	Annual MRI age 30–35 y, add MMG age 40 y	• No strong evidence for PBM or CPM, can consider if other risk factors present • No contraindication for adjuvant radiation
BARD1	17%–30%	—	Annual MMG age 40 y, consider adding MRI	No strong evidence for PBM or CPM
BRCA1	50%–72%	30%–40% over 20 y	Annual MRI age 25 y, add annual MMG at age 30 y	• Consider and discuss PBM and CPM • Consider RRSO ages 45–50 y • Consider pancreatic cancer screening age 50 y if FH of PDAC
BRCA2	40%–69%	25% over 20 y	Same as BRCA1	• Consider and discuss PBM and CPM • Consider RRSO ages 45–50 y • Pancreatic cancer screening >age 50 y
CDH1	39%–55%	—	Annual MRI and MMG age 30 y	Consider and discuss PBM and CPM
CHEK2	20%–25%, higher if strong FH	—	Consider MRI age 35 y, annual MMG age 40 y	Consider PBM based on mutation type and FH
PALB2	30%–50%	5%–10% over 10 y	Annual MRI and MMG age 30 y	• Consider and discuss PBM and CPM • Consider RRSO
PTEN	40%–60%	—	Annual MRI and MMG age 30 y	Consider and discuss PBM and CPM
RAD51C/D	~20%	—	MMG age 40 y, consider MRI	• No strong evidence for PBM or CPM • Consider RRSO ages 45–50 y
TP53	>60%	18%–49% over 10 y	Annual MRI age 20 y, add annual MMG age 30 y	• Consider and discuss PBM and CPM • Toronto protocol MRI whole body surveillance

cancers in descending order for BRCA1 carriers: female BC (50%–72%), ovarian cancer (40%–60%), prostate cancer (7%–26%), pancreatic ($\leq$5%), and male BC (~1%).[1,5] The 20 year contralateral breast cancer (CBC) risk is up to 40%.[5]

BRCA2 carriers' conferred absolute lifetime risk of cancers in descending order: female BC (40%–69%), ovarian cancer (10%–29%), prostate cancer (19%–60%)

pancreatic cancer (5%–10%), and male BC (2%–7%).[1,5] The 20 year CBC risk is up to 26%.[5]

Special screening considerations for BRCA1/2 carriers include MRI breast at the age of 25 years with addition of mammogram (MMG) at the age of 30 years and pancreatic cancer screening starting at the age of 50 years for all BRCA2 carriers and in BRCA1 carriers with FH of pancreatic ductal adenocarcinoma (PDAC).[1] Prophylactic bilateral mastectomies (PBM) should be individualized with incorporation of FH, residual lifetime risk, and life expectancy. Risk-reducing salpingo-oophorectomies (RRSO) are recommended at age 35 to 40 years for BRCA1 and 40 to 45 years for BRCA2 (if childbearing is complete) with new studies suggesting that salpingectomies first with delayed oophorectomies may be an appropriate option for reducing cancer risk while preserving ovarian function longer.[1] Additionally, hereditary BC related to BRCA1/2 mutations are susceptible to PARP inhibitors that have shown to improve survival and reduce recurrence.[6]

***TP53* (Li-Fraumeni syndrome)**

TP53 is a TS gene that encodes the p53 protein, a key regulator of cellular responses to DNA damage and other cellular stress. Somatic TP53 mutations are among the most common alterations in human cancers.[7] Many germline TP53 mutations cause Li-Fraumeni syndrome, an AD hereditary cancer syndrome characterized by early onset cancers including childhood cancers, very young-onset BC, soft tissue and osteogenic sarcomas, brain tumors, leukemia, and adrenocortical carcinoma.

When a pathogenic variant in TP53 is identified on germline testing, the variant allele fraction (VAF) and tissue source are critical for interpretation. A TP53 variant detected in peripheral blood at less than 50% VAF may reflect postzygotic mosaicism or clonal hematopoiesis rather than a true germline mutation.[8,9] One important confounder is Clonal Hematopoiesis of Indeterminate Potential, an age-related expansion of hematopoietic stem cell clones carrying somatic mutations in cancer-associated genes, including TP53, which can appear on blood-based germline panels and mimic hereditary cancer syndromes.[8,10] Alternatively, a subheterozygous VAF may represent constitutional mosaicism, in which a postzygotic TP53 mutation is present in only a subset of cells across tissues.[9,11] To distinguish these possibilities when evaluating for Li-Fraumeni syndrome, testing of nonhematopoietic tissue like a skin punch biopsy with fibroblast culture or analysis of other normal tissues can help determine whether the variant is constitutional or restricted to blood cells.[9,11]

Most women with TP53 mutations have a very high lifetime risk of BC—estimated at 50% to 85%—with many cases occurring before the age of 35 years.[11–13] Early, intensive surveillance and careful avoidance of therapeutic radiation when feasible is paramount because TP53 carriers appear to have increased susceptibility to radiation-induced malignancies.[14,15] The Toronto Protocol is an MRI-based surveillance strategy for individuals with Li-Fraumeni syndrome designed to detect malignancies early while minimizing radiation exposure.[16] Core components include annual whole-body and brain MRI, breast MRI starting in early adulthood, frequent physical examinations, and selective abdominal/pelvic ultrasounds in children.[16]

***PTEN* (Cowden syndrome)**

The PTEN gene is a TS gene that helps control cell growth and division by regulating the PI3K/AKT signaling pathway. When PTEN is mutated or lost, this control is disrupted, leading to uncontrolled cell proliferation, formation of benign hamartomas. and an increased risk of cancers, particularly in the breast, thyroid, endometrium, and other organs.[17] Women with germline PTEN mutations (PTEN Hamartoma Tumor Syndrome, including Cowden syndrome) are at an increased risk for BC with lifetime risk estimates of 25% to 85% and often earlier onset than sporadic cases. Thyroid cancer, primarily follicular type, occurs in up to 35% of carriers, while endometrial cancer risk ranges from 13% to 28%.[18,19] Other associated malignancies include renal cell carcinoma, colorectal cancer, melanoma, and less frequently brain and gastrointestinal tumors.

These risks commonly manifest at younger ages than sporadic cases and are identified thorough a careful phenotypic evaluation (to identify macrocephaly, facial papules, and other noncancer features of the syndrome) coupled with genetic testing. Current surveillance strategies include annual MMG plus breast MRI beginning at age 30 to 35 years or 5 to 10 years before the earliest family BC along with clinical breast examinations (CBEs) every 6 to 12 months. Discussion of PBM should be individualized in a multidisciplinary setting, weighing personal risk, patient preferences, and reconstruction options.

CDH1 (hereditary diffuse gastric cancer syndrome)

CDH1 is a gene that encodes E-cadherin, a protein essential for cell-to-cell adhesion in epithelial tissues. Pathogenic mutations in CDH1 disrupt tissue integrity and significantly increase the risk of hereditary diffuse gastric cancer (HDGC) and lobular breast cancer (LBC) in women. Traditional estimates from consortium analyses have placed the cumulative risk of diffuse gastric cancer by the age of 80 years in women at approximately 56% to 83%, and the risk of LBC at roughly 39% to 55%.[20] However, as more individuals and families are identified with CDH1 mutations through nontargeted genetic testing, it is clear that these risk estimates may not apply to all individuals who do not have family histories of gastric or LBC, and genetic counseling to obtain personalized risk estimates is crucial for guiding management. Given the high morbidity and mortality associated with advanced diffuse gastric cancer and the known limitations of endoscopic surveillance, prophylactic total gastrectomy is the most effective risk-reducing intervention recommended for many pathogenic CDH1 carriers.[21] For women with CDH1 pathogenic variants, annual breast MRI beginning around the age of 30 years is advised because LBC can be difficult to detect with mammography alone.[21] Early involvement of multidisciplinary teams familiar with HDGC improves risk stratification and facilitates decision-making around prophylactic surgery, surveillance strategies, and long-term follow-up.

Moderate Penetrance Genes

ATM (ataxia-telangiectasia)

Ataxia-telangiectasia (AT) is a disorder characterized by cerebellar ataxia, ocular symptoms, and immunologic deficiency caused by a pathogenic mutation in the ATM gene inherited in an autosomal recessive manner.[22] The ATM protein modulates cell cycle pathways related to double DNA strand stress to reduce malignant transformation. Persons with heterozygous mutations in ATM do not display AT phenotype but do have a 2-to-3 fold increased risk of BC or lifetime risk of 21% to 24%.[1,22] Although increased lifetime risk of BC for ATM heterozygotes warrants consideration of high-risk screening, there is insufficient evidence for PBM or contralateral prophylactic mastectomy (CPM) in a setting of unilateral cancer.[1] Radiation should be offered to all ATM heterozygous mutation carriers if indicated as part of standard BC treatment without the need to adjust radiation dose; there is no increased adverse events or risk of secondary malignancies from radiation for ATM heterozygotes compared to the general population.[22] ATM mutations may also confer a modest increased lifetime risk for ovarian, pancreatic, prostate, and colorectal cancer, which warrant consideration for additional screening, in most cases dependent on the specific ATM mutation and FH.

CHEK2

The CHEK2 gene serves as a key component in cell-cycle regulation of the ATM-p53-CHEK pathway for DNA damage repair.[23] There is a wide spectrum of gene mutation penetrance that depends on the known variant and therefore leads to variable BC risk estimates. The CHEK2 c.1100del truncating variant is one that is well studied with the highest risk of BC development estimated at 2 fold risk above general population.[23] The most common missense CHEK2 variants including Ile157Thr and Ser428-Phe have lower penetrance and can likely follow average-risk women screening recommendations.[23] However, risk should be determined based on specific variant as some missense mutations may have similar impact as truncating mutations; working with a genetics specialist to understand variant-specific risks is critical to management.

Additionally, incorporation of affected first-degree and second-degree relatives with BC with type of CHEK2 mutation provides a more accurate risk assessment. Cybulski and colleagues[24] estimated lifetime risk for truncating CHEK2 mutation carriers in a setting of affected single first-degree relative, affected single second-degree relative, or both affected first-degree and second-degree relative was 34%, 28%, and 44%, respectively. NCCN recommends consideration of high-risk screening for CHEK2 mutations that have higher penetrance like truncating c1100del and avoidance of routine recommendation of PBM.[1] Risk-reducing surgery should be advised based on individualized risk incorporating FH and variant type.

PALB2

PALB2 is colloquially termed BRCA3 due to its moderate-to-high risk of BC development that is akin to BRCA2. Absolute lifetime risk of BC (up to the age of 80 years) is 30% to 50%; therefore, discussion of high-risk screening starting at the age of 30 years and/or PBM is appropriate.[1,25] The risk of CBC is less defined with 5 year cumulative risk of 10% based on a small retrospective study.[26] However, Yadav and colleagues[27] demonstrated CBC risk was elevated for those with hormone-negative disease (hazard ratio 2.9) compared to no increased risk for hormone-driven disease (hazard ratio 0.4); therefore, subsequent intensive surveillance or CPM should be individualized with inclusion of cancer biomarkers. PALB2 mutation also increases the risk for ovarian cancer (3%–5%), pancreatic cancer (2%–3%), and male BC (1%), therefore RRSO and screening for pancreatic cancer can be considered.[1]

BARD1 and RAD51C/D

RAD51C and RAD51D aid in repair of DNA double strand breaks and mutation in this gene can impair genomic stability.[28] BARD1 is a TS gene and stabilizes BRCA1 to aid in DNA damage repair.[29] RAD51C/D and BARD1 mutation carriers have approximately 20% and 17% to 30% absolute lifetime risk of BC, respectively; therefore, high-risk screening can be considered, but there is currently no role for PBM.[1,28,29] RAD51C/D confers a higher lifetime risk of ovarian cancer (10%–15%), therefore RRSO is recommended.[28] BARD1 and RAD51C/D mutation carriers have higher rates of TNBC and represent promising targets for novel agents.[28]

Polygenic Risk Scores

Separate from known pathogenic mutations, polygenic risk scores (PRS) provide estimates for genetic susceptibility for clinical conditions based on the cumulative small effects of single nucleotide variants (SNVs).[30] Genome-wide association studies identify specific loci that can be linked to a specific diagnosis (such as BC) and then it is possible to statistically combine the weight and/or effect of multiple SNVs to improve estimates of disease risk.[30] The application of PRS in BC risk assessment is still evolving but incorporation with current risk models that utilize clinical risk factors represent a promising tool to better evaluate individualized risk.

RISK ASSESSMENT AND SCREENING FOR BREAST CANCER IN WOMEN WITH NO MUTATIONS IN PREDISPOSITION GENES

Risk prediction models can be helpful in identifying women without pathogenic germline mutations who are at an increased risk for BC who may benefit from enhanced screening, chemoprevention, or referral to surgeons for consideration of PBM. The models rely on combinations of personal, reproductive, and FH factors with varying degrees of complexity and clinical applicability and the need for clinician input in interpreting these models is vital for an assessment of overall risk.

Modified Gail Model (Breast Cancer Risk Assessment Tool)

The Gail model represents the earliest widely adopted tool for individualized BC risk prediction and established the framework for nearly all subsequent BC risk models. The model was developed using data from the Breast Cancer Detection Demonstration Project and combined relative risks from reproductive and biopsy-related factors with age-specific US BC incidence and competing mortality rates, enabling estimation of both short-term and lifetime BC risk.[31] The model incorporates age, age at menarche, age at first live birth, number of prior breast biopsies, presence of atypical hyperplasia, number of affected first-degree relatives, and race/ethnicity to calculate 5 year and lifetime risk estimates.[31] The Gail model is often used as the standard risk assessment tool for chemoprevention decision-making, since it was utilized to define eligibility for the National Surgical Adjuvant Breast and Bowel Project (NSABP) P-1 Breast Cancer Prevention Trial.[32] Women with a 5 year BC risk of 1.67% or greater by the Gail model were eligible for tamoxifen chemoprevention, a threshold that subsequently became embedded in clinical practice and guideline recommendations.[32,33]

Limitations of the Gail model include inclusion of only affected first-degree relatives, without accounting for age at diagnosis, second-degree relatives, paternal FH or ovarian cancer, leading to underestimation of risk in women with complex familial patterns.[34,35] Furthermore, the model was developed primarily to estimate short-term absolute risk for chemoprevention decisions and is not well suited for determining eligibility for enhanced screening, where more comprehensive models perform better.[36]

Tyrer-Cuzick Model (International Breast Cancer Intervention Study Risk Evaluation Tool)

The Tyrer-Cuzick (TC) model, also referred to as the International Breast Cancer Intervention Study (IBIS) Risk Evaluation Tool, is among the most comprehensive BC risk models used in clinical practice. It integrates extensive multigenerational FH of breast and ovarian cancer with personal risk factors including hormone replacement therapy use, body mass index, benign breast disease, and mammographic breast density to allow for improved estimation of cumulative risk.[37] This model estimates both 10 year and lifetime BC risk and is frequently used to identify women who meet guideline thresholds (typically ≥20%–25% lifetime risk) for supplemental screening with breast MRI.[38,39]

Despite its comprehensive design and widespread use in high-risk screening pathways, the TC model has several important limitations and criticisms. Namely, this model tends to overestimate BC risk in certain populations, particularly when applied outside the cohorts on which it was developed. Accurate risk estimation is time-intensive and depends on detailed and reliable multigenerational family history. Information that is incomplete or inaccurately reported, such as limited knowledge about family members' health, recall bias or incomplete family communication, directly affect the model in clinical practice and introduce uncertainty into individual risk estimate.[40]

Screening Recommendations for Average-risk Women

Women without significant personal or familial risk factors and whose lifetime risk of BC development is less than 20% are considered average risk. For average risk women, screening MMG remains the mainstay of surveillance with frequency and starting age varying among national organizations (**Table 2**).

Screening Recommendations for High-risk Women without Pathogenic Mutations

Women who have a greater than 20% lifetime risk of developing BC based on risk calculation models or prior chest radiation exposure from ages 10 to 30 years warrant more frequent image screening.[41] NCCN recommends alternating screening MMG with 1 additional supplemental diagnostic image every 6 months to improve early detection of cancer. CBE should be performed every 6 to 12 months.

Screening MMG for high-risk individuals should start:[41]

- At the age when deemed high risk if under the age of 40 years, but not to start before the age of 30 years
- 10 years prior to youngest family member who was diagnosed with BC, but not to start before the age of 30 years
- 8 years after chest wall therapeutic radiation exposure but not before the age of 25 years

Table 2
Breast cancer screening recommendations for average-risk women[41–43]

Guideline Organization	Age (Years) to Initiate Screening	Screening Modality and Interval	Age to Stop or Continue
NCCN	40	Annual screening MMG	No specified upper age limit; continue while overall health and life expectancy support benefit
American College of Obstetricians and Gynecologists	40, no later than 50	MMG every 1 or 2 y, based on shared decision-making	Continue at least through age 75 y; beyond 75 y based on shared decision-making and health status
US Preventive Services Task Force	40	Biennial screening MMG	Through age 74 y; insufficient evidence to assess benefit beyond 75 y

IMAGING OPTIONS FOR HIGH-RISK SCREENING (LIFETIME RISK >20%)

There are several advantages and disadvantages to each type of diagnostic imaging that a surgeon should weigh when recommending supplemental imaging for a patient (**Table 3**).

Breast MRI

Breast MRI is a highly sensitive imaging modality, and the preferred method of imaging option to use alongside screening MMG for individuals with an elevated lifetime risk. Breast MRI has a sensitivity rate of 70% to 96% with a higher cancer detection rate (CDR) of 14.2 per 1000 compared to 4.9 per 1000 with MMG alone.[44] The supplemental use of MRI for high-risk patients has shown to detect cancers at an earlier stage, reduce frequency of interval cancers and reduce BC mortality in mutations carriers for ATM, CHEK2, and PALB2.[45–47]

Use of breast MRI for supplemental screening in women who solely have dense breast tissue without significant risk factors remains a controversial topic. The DENSE study (Breast Cancer Screening with MRI in Women Aged 50–75 Years with Extremely Dense Breast Tissue) demonstrated that MRI detected 16.5 per 1000 cancers, provided a 50% reduction in interval cancer rates, and cost modeling showed benefit of MRI use.[48] The European Society of Breast Imaging now recommends routine MRI surveillance in all women with dense breasts but the supplemental use in the United States for this population is still evolving.[49]

One of the main disadvantages of breast MRI is patient discomfort and claustrophobia, with the length of study averaging 45 minutes, requiring the patient to lay prone with arms extended. Additionally, there has been concern over long-term potential adverse effects of gadolinium deposition from repeated contrast administrations;

Table 3
Advantages and disadvantages of supplemental diagnostic imaging

	Advantages	Disadvantages
Breast MRI	• Better sensitivity and CDR than MMG or US • Full evaluation of lymphatic nodal basins and chest wall • Improved cancer outcomes for those with pathogenic mutation	• Costly • Unclear long-term outcome of gadolinium deposition • Patient discomfort (claustrophobia, positioning, and long test duration)
CEM	• Comparable to MRI for lesion detection • Uses existing technology and easy to interpret • Quick test (8–15 min) • Improved patient comfort	• Iodine contrast allergy reaction • Inability to assess anatomy outside breast (ie, chest wall and lymph nodes) • Limited ability for direct biopsy on CEM
MBI	Alternative imaging for those who cannot undergo MRI or CEM	Higher radiation exposure equivalent to a lifetime of annual MMG
Screening ultrasound	• No radiation exposure • Easy to use (handheld US comparable to formal US)	• Higher false-positive rate and lower positive predictive value • Operator-dependent • Incomplete evaluation of the breast or axilla for screening

however, there is no evidence at this time for clinical sequelae, and the newer contrast agents show less deposition.[39]

Contrast-enhanced Mammogram

Contrast-enhanced mammography (CEM) combines the use of MMG and iodine-based contrast to obtain images at low and high energy. Low-energy-derived images are used for morphologic evaluation akin to screening MMG whereas high-energy-derived images detect areas that have taken up an increased amount of contrast, suggesting metabolically active abnormalities.

CEM appears to have comparable performance with similar CDR as breast MRI.[50] Advantages of CEM include the use of existing technology and contrast, speed of obtaining images and interpretation (average 8–15 minutes for entire procedure), patient comfort, and reduced interpretation time.[39] Disadvantages of CEM include higher rate of possible contrast reaction (0.8%), inadequate evaluation of anatomic structures outside of the breast (ie, lymph nodes and chest wall), and limited capability for direct biopsy options.[39] Though the utility and broad application of CEM for screening continues to evolve, at this time, NCCN primarily recommends CEM as an adjunctive tool or alternative to MRI.

Molecular Breast Imaging

Molecular breast imaging (MBI) is obtained by using 99mTc-sestamibi radioactivity visualized with a gamma camera to highlight abnormal uptake in the breast. MBI is generally reserved for patients who cannot undergo MRI or CEM and is seldomly used for breast diagnostics given the radiation exposure to the whole body and high level of exposure of radiation that is nearly equivalent to a lifetime of MMG.[39]

Screening Ultrasound

Supplemental ultrasound (US) in conjunction with MMG for women with dense breasts has shown to increase CDR by 2 to 2.7 per 1000 women.[51] Cancers that were detected by US tended to be smaller and node negative.[51] Despite the ease of use and improved CDR, the improved sensitivity of US was coupled with higher recall and biopsy rates with lower positive predictive value compared to MMG.[52] Additional disadvantages include incomplete evaluation of the breast or axilla and operator-dependence for technique and interpretation remain impediments for widespread adoption of screening US.

RISK-REDUCING INTERVENTIONS

Risk-reducing Mastectomies

The role of PBM is largely dependent on a woman's residual lifetime risk, mutation status, and psychological readiness. PBM can lower incidence of BC by 90% to 95% although there is no reduction in mortality.[53] The role of PBM for women who are deemed high-risk based primarily on FH or by risk calculation is controversial and is individualized with incorporation of primary factors for patient's elevated risk and ability to proceed with screening. Incidence of occult BC discovered following PBM is 0.5% to 2.7% with most incidental cancers representing in situ disease or early stage luminal A disease.[54] The incidence of occult nodal disease at time of PBM is 0.4%, therefore, routine axillary sentinel lymph node biopsy is discouraged.[55]

Endocrine Therapy

NSABP P-1 trial evaluated the role of tamoxifen as a risk-reducing medication for BC in high-risk patients and demonstrated a 49% reduction of estrogen-driven BC incidence.[32] Follow-up NSABP Study of Tamoxifen and Raloxifene demonstrated raloxifene had comparable ability to reduce incidence of BC in high-risk patients with an improved side effect profile.[56] Tamoxifen and raloxifene represent effective options for risk-reduction in patients who have elevated lifetime risk of BC.

SUMMARY

This clinical review guides general surgeons in BC genetics, risk assessment, screening, and risk-reducing strategies, outlining evaluation and management strategies for average-risk and high-risk women using models like Gail and TC, reviews indications for genetic testing, and interpretation of results. Evidence-based screening approaches—including mammography, MRI, contrast-enhanced mammography, ultrasound, and MBI—are reviewed, highlighting benefits and limitations of supplemental diagnostic imaging. Risk-reducing interventions, such as prophylactic mastectomies and endocrine therapy, are discussed with emphasis on mutation status, family history, and individualized patient care. The review equips surgeons to integrate genetics into prevention, early detection, and tailored management strategies for BC.

CLINICS CARE POINTS

- Verify accuracy of genetic results and confirm type of mutation identified. Consult with genetics experts for evaluation of the specific mutation identified in a patient, as well as for discussion of multi-organ screening or consideration for updated, additional testing.
- BRCA1/2 carriers should be started on high-risk screening with MRI at age 25 and counseled on efficacy of PBM and RRSO. Pancreatic screening can be considered for BRCA2 carriers, and male BRCA2 carriers have specific management guidelines as well.
- Routine PBM for ATM mutation carriers is typically not indicated and there is no evidence to avoid radiation in this group.
- CHEK2 mutations have wide variability of penetrance with truncating 1100delC conferring the highest risk. Family history should be incorporated along with other risk/protective factors into a personalized risk assessment.
- Skin-sparing and nipple-sparing mastectomies are safe to perform in setting of prophylactic surgery.
- Endocrine therapy can reduce a high-risk woman's lifetime risk by 49%.

DISCLOSURE

The authors have no conflict-of-interest disclosures to report.

REFERENCES

1. Network, N.C.C. NCCN clinical practice guidelines in oncology. genetic/familia high-risk assessment: breast, ovarian, pancreatic and prostate (versior 2.2026). 2026 [cited 2026 01-16-2026]; Available at: https://www.nccn.org guidelines/guidelines-detail?category=2&id=1545.
2. Antoniou A, Pharoah PDP, Narod S, et al. Average risks of breast and ovariar cancer associated with BRCA1 or BRCA2 mutations detected in case Series un selected for family history: a combined analysis of 22 studies. Am J Hum Gene 2003;72(5):1117–30.
3. Levy-Lahad E, Catane R, Eisenberg S, et al. Founder BRCA1 and BRCA2 mutations in Ashkenazi Jews in Israel: frequency and differential penetrance in ovarian cance and in breast-ovarian cancer families. Am J Hum Genet 1997;60(5):1059–67.

4. De Leeneer K, Coene I, Crombez B, et al. Prevalence of BRCA1/2 mutations in sporadic breast/ovarian cancer patients and identification of a novel de novo BRCA1 mutation in a patient diagnosed with late onset breast and ovarian cancer: implications for genetic testing. Breast Cancer Res Treat 2012;132(1):87–95.
5. Kuchenbaecker KB, Hopper JL, Barnes DR, et al. Risks of breast, ovarian, and contralateral breast cancer for BRCA1 and BRCA2 mutation carriers. JAMA 2017;317(23):2402–16.
6. Tutt ANJ, Garber JE, Kaufman B, et al. Adjuvant olaparib for patients with BRCA1- or BRCA2-mutated breast cancer. N Engl J Med 2021;384(25):2394–405.
7. Kandoth C, McLellan MD, Vandin F, et al. Mutational landscape and significance across 12 major cancer types. Nature 2013;502(7471):333–9.
8. Bolton KL, Gillis NK, Coombs CC, et al. Managing clonal hematopoiesis in patients with solid tumors. J Clin Oncol 2019;37(1):7–11.
9. Weitzel JN, Chao EC, Nehoray B, et al. Somatic TP53 variants frequently confound germ-line testing results. Genet Med 2018;20(8):809–16.
10. Jaiswal S, Ebert BL. Clonal hematopoiesis in human aging and disease. Science 2019;366(6465).
11. Schneider K, Zelley K, Nichols KE, et al. Li-Fraumeni Syndrome. In: GeneReviews®. Seattle (WA): University of Washington, Seattle; 1999.
12. Malkin D, Li FP, Strong LC, et al. Germ line p53 mutations in a familial syndrome of breast cancer, sarcomas, and other neoplasms. Science 1990;250(4985):1233–8.
13. Mai PL, Best AF, Peters JA, et al. Risks of first and subsequent cancers among TP53 mutation carriers in the National Cancer Institute Li-Fraumeni syndrome cohort. Cancer 2016;122(23):3673–81.
14. Bougeard G, Renaux-Petel M, Flaman JM, et al. Revisiting Li-Fraumeni syndrome from TP53 mutation carriers. J Clin Oncol 2015;33(21):2345–52.
15. Kratz CP, Achatz MI, Brugières L, et al. Cancer screening recommendations for individuals with Li-Fraumeni syndrome. Clin Cancer Res 2017;23(11):e38–45.
16. Villani A, Shore A, Wasserman JD, et al. Biochemical and imaging surveillance in germline TP53 mutation carriers with Li-Fraumeni syndrome: 11 year follow-up of a prospective observational study. Lancet Oncol 2016;17(9):1295–305.
17. National Cancer Institute. Definition of PTEN gene. NCI Dictionary of Cancer Terms. Available at: https://www.cancer.gov/publications/dictionaries/cancer-terms (Accessed 8 March 2026).
18. Yehia L, Eng C. PTEN hamartoma tumor syndrome, . GeneReviews®. Seattle (WA): University of Washington, Seattle; 2001.
19. Tan MH, Mester JL, Ngeow J, et al. Lifetime cancer risks in individuals with germline PTEN mutations. Clin Cancer Res 2012;18(2):400–7.
20. Syngal S, Brand RE, Church JM, et al. ACG clinical guideline: genetic testing and management of hereditary gastrointestinal cancer syndromes. Am J Gastroenterol 2015;110(2):223–62, quiz 263.
21. van der Post RS, Vogelaar IP, Carneiro F, et al. Hereditary diffuse gastric cancer: updated clinical guidelines with an emphasis on germline CDH1 mutation carriers. J Med Genet 2015;52(6):361–74.
22. Pal T, Schon KR, Astiazaran-Symonds E, et al. Management of individuals with heterozygous germline pathogenic variants in ATM: a clinical practice resource of the American College of Medical Genetics and Genomics (ACMG). Genet Med 2025;27(1):101243.
23. Hanson H, Astiazaran-Symonds E, Amendola LM, et al. Management of individuals with germline pathogenic/likely pathogenic variants in CHEK2: a clinical practice resource of the American College of Medical Genetics and Genomics (ACMG). Genet Med 2023;25(10):100870.

24. Cybulski C, Wokołorczyk D, Jakubowska A, et al. Risk of breast cancer in women with a CHEK2 mutation with and without a family history of breast cancer. J Clin Oncol 2011;29(28):3747–52.
25. Tischkowitz M, Balmaña J, Foulkes WD, et al. Management of individuals with germline variants in PALB2: a clinical practice resource of the American College of Medical Genetics and Genomics (ACMG). Genet Med 2021;23(8):1416–23.
26. Cybulski C, Kluźniak W, Huzarski T, et al. Clinical outcomes in women with breast cancer and a PALB2 mutation: a prospective cohort analysis. Lancet Oncol 2015; 16(6):638–44.
27. Yadav S, Boddicker NJ, Na J, et al. Contralateral breast cancer risk among carriers of germline pathogenic variants in ATM, BRCA1, BRCA2, CHEK2, and PALB2. J Clin Oncol 2023;41(9):1703–13.
28. Ngeow J, Chiang J, Astiazaran-Symonds E, et al. Management of individuals with heterozygous germline pathogenic variants in RAD51C, RAD51D, and BRIP1: a clinical practice resource of the American College of Medical Genetics and Genomics (ACMG). Genet Med 2025;27(11):101557.
29. Marino E, Belloni E, Dal Molin M, et al. Characterization of a genetic variant in BARD1 in subjects undergoing germline testing for hereditary tumors. Biomedicines 2025;13(11).
30. Abu-El-Haija A, Reddi HV, Wand H, et al. The clinical application of polygenic risk scores: a points to consider statement of the American College of Medical Genetics and Genomics (ACMG). Genet Med 2023;25(5):100803.
31. Gail MH, Brinton LA, Byar DP, et al. Projecting individualized probabilities of developing breast cancer for white females who are being examined annually. J Natl Cancer Inst 1989;81(24):1879–86.
32. Fisher B, Costantino JP, Wickerham DL, et al. Tamoxifen for prevention of breast cancer: report of the National Surgical Adjuvant Breast and Bowel Project P-1 Study. J Natl Cancer Inst 1998;90(18):1371–88.
33. Visvanathan K, Hurley P, Bantug E, et al. Use of pharmacologic interventions for breast cancer risk reduction: American Society of Clinical Oncology clinical practice guideline. J Clin Oncol 2013;31(23):2942–62.
34. Amir E, Evans DG, Shenton A, et al. Evaluation of breast cancer risk assessment packages in the family history evaluation and screening programme. J Med Genet 2003;40(11):807–14.
35. Brentnall AR, Warren R, Harkness EF, et al. Mammographic density change in a cohort of premenopausal women receiving tamoxifen for breast cancer prevention over 5 years. Breast Cancer Res 2020;22(1):101.
36. Lee JM, Ichikawa LE, Wernli KJ, et al. Digital mammography and breast tomosynthesis performance in women with a personal history of breast cancer, 2007-2016. Radiology 2021;300(2):290–300.
37. Tyrer J, Duffy SW, Cuzick J. A breast cancer prediction model incorporating familial and personal risk factors. Stat Med 2004;23(7):1111–30.
38. Society AC. American Cancer Society recommendations for the early detection of breast cancer [Website] 2023 12-19-2023 [cited 2026 01-16-2026]; Available at https://www.cancer.org/cancer/types/breast-cancer/screening-tests-and-early-detection/american-cancer-society-recommendations-for-the-early-detection-of-breast-cancer.html.
39. Monticciolo DL, Newell MS, Moy L, et al. Breast cancer screening for women at higher-than-average risk: updated recommendations from the ACR. J Am Coll Radiol 2023;20(9):902–14.

40. Quante AS, Whittemore AS, Shriver T, et al. Practical problems with clinical guidelines for breast cancer prevention based on remaining lifetime risk. J Natl Cancer Inst 2015;107(7).
41. Network NCC. Breast cancer screening and diagnosis (version 2.2025). 2026 [cited 2026 01-16-2026]; Available at: https://www.nccn.org/guidelines/guidelines-detail?category=2&id=1421.
42. Gynecology ACoOa. Breast cancer risk assessment and screening in average-risk women. 2017 [cited 2026 01-16-2026]; Available at: https://www.acog.org/clinical/clinical-guidance/practice-bulletin/articles/2017/07/breast-cancer-risk-assessment-and-screening-in-average-risk-women.
43. Force USPST. Breast cancer: screening. 2024 [cited 2026 01-14-2026]; Available at: https://www.uspreventiveservicestaskforce.org/uspstf/recommendation/breast-cancer-screening.
44. Saadatmand S, Geuzinge HA, Rutgers EJT, et al. MRI versus mammography for breast cancer screening in women with familial risk (FaMRIsc): a multicentre, randomised, controlled trial. Lancet Oncol 2019;20(8):1136–47.
45. Riedl CC, Luft N, Bernhart C, et al. Triple-modality screening trial for familial breast cancer underlines the importance of magnetic resonance imaging and questions the role of mammography and ultrasound regardless of patient mutation status, age, and breast density. J Clin Oncol 2015;33(10):1128–35.
46. Sippo DA, Burk KS, Mercaldo SF, et al. Performance of screening breast MRI across women with different elevated breast cancer risk indications. Radiology 2019;292(1):51–9.
47. Lowry KP, Geuzinge HA, Stout NK, et al. Breast cancer screening strategies for women with ATM, CHEK2, and PALB2 pathogenic variants: a comparative modeling analysis. JAMA Oncol 2022;8(4):587–96.
48. Bakker MF, de Lange SV, Pijnappel RM, et al. Supplemental MRI Screening for women with extremely dense breast tissue. N Engl J Med 2019;381(22):2091–102.
49. Mann RM, Athanasiou A, Baltzer PAT, et al. Breast cancer screening in women with extremely dense breasts recommendations of the European Society of breast Imaging (EUSOBI). Eur Radiol 2022;32(6):4036–45.
50. Gelardi F, Ragaini EM, Sollini M, et al. Contrast-enhanced mammography versus breast magnetic resonance imaging: a systematic review and meta-analysis. Diagnostics 2022;12(8).
51. Berg WA, Vourtsis A. Screening breast ultrasound using handheld or automated technique in women with dense breasts. J Breast Imaging 2019;1(4):283–96.
52. Berg WA, Bandos AI, Mendelson EB, et al. Ultrasound as the primary screening test for breast cancer: analysis from ACRIN 6666. J Natl Cancer Inst 2016;108(4).
53. Ludwig KK, Neuner J, Butler A, et al. Risk reduction and survival benefit of prophylactic surgery in BRCA mutation carriers, a systematic review. Am J Surg 2016;212(4):660–9.
54. Singh P, Agnese DM, Amin M, et al. Society of surgical oncology breast disease site working group statement on bilateral risk-reducing mastectomy: indications, outcomes, and risks. Ann Surg Oncol 2025;32(2):899–911.
55. Shern TP, Holt LR, Chamberlain V, et al. Sentinel lymph node biopsy for prophylactic mastectomy: necessary precaution or unnecessary procedure? Ann Surg Oncol 2026;33(3):2316–23.
56. Vogel VG, Costantino JP, Wickerham DL, et al. Effects of tamoxifen vs raloxifene on the risk of developing invasive breast cancer and other disease outcomes: the NSABP Study of Tamoxifen and Raloxifene (STAR) P-2 trial. JAMA 2006;295(23):2727–41.

Colorectal Cancer Genetics and Hereditary Colorectal Cancer Syndromes for the Practicing General Surgeon

Jared R. Hendren, MD[a,b,c], Josh Sommovilla, MD[b,c],
Scott R. Steele, MD, MBA[b,c], David Liska, MD[b,c,*]

KEYWORDS

- Colorectal cancer • Genetics • Hereditary colorectal cancer syndromes

KEY POINTS

- All colorectal cancers should undergo universal tumor screening for mismatch repair deficiency and patients with early-onset CRC or suggestive family history should undergo germline testing.
- Cascade testing (targeted relative testing) is recommended for at-risk family members of patients diagnosed with a hereditary CRC syndrome to identify germline pathogenic variants.
- Lynch syndrome patients with CRC may undergo an extended or segmental colonic resection after shared decision-making discussions, although immunotherapy is changing surgical management.
- Familial adenomatous polyposis patients require colorectal surgery to reduce the risk of CRC, with timing and surgery type individualized based on disease and patient factors.
- Management of all hereditary CRC syndromes requires lifelong surveillance and multidisciplinary care to minimize death from cancer and to maximize quality of life preservation.

INTRODUCTION

Colorectal cancer (CRC) is the third most common cancer and is the second most common cause of cancer-related death in the United States.[1] Most CRCs arise sporadically (60%–70%), although CRC can also be familial or hereditary. Familial CRC is defined as CRC that clusters in families without a known hereditary cancer syndrome or identifiable germline pathogenic variant (PV, 25%–30%). Hereditary CRC is

[a] Department of General Surgery, Digestive Disease Institute, Cleveland Clinic, Cleveland, OH, USA; [b] Department of Colorectal Surgery, Digestive Disease Institute, Cleveland Clinic, Cleveland, OH, USA; [c] Sanford R. Weiss, MD Center for Hereditary Colorectal Neoplasia, Department of Colorectal Surgery, Digestive Disease Institute, Cleveland Clinic, Cleveland, OH, USA
* Corresponding author. Department of Colorectal Surgery, Digestive Disease Institute, 9500 Euclid Avenue/A30, Cleveland Clinic, Cleveland, OH 44195.
E-mail address: liskad@ccf.org

Surg Clin N Am 106 (2026) 481–500
https://doi.org/10.1016/j.suc.2026.03.005 surgical.theclinics.com
0039-6109/26/

Abbreviations	
APC	adenomatous polyposis coli
cCR	complete clinical response
CIMP	CpG island methylator phenotype
CIMP-H	CIMP-high
CIN	chromosomal instability
CRC	colorectal cancer
dMMR	MMR deficiency
EGAPP	Evaluation of Genomic Applications in Practice and Prevention
ER	extended resection
FAP	familial adenomatous polyposis
GI	gastrointestinal
JPS	juvenile polyposis syndrome
LARCs	locally advanced rectal cancers
LS	Lynch syndrome
MAP	MUTYH-associated polyposis
MMR	mismatch repair
MMR IHC	mismatch repair immunohistochemistry
MSI	microsatellite instability
MSI PCR	microsatellite instability polymerase chain reaction
MSI-H	MSI-high
MSI-L	MSI-low
PJS	Peutz-Jeghers syndrome
PV	pathogenic variant
SPS	serrated polyposis syndrome
SR	segmental resection
TAC/IRA	total abdominal colectomy with ileorectal anastomosis
TPC/IPAA	total proctocolectomy with ileal-pouch anal anastomosis
UTS	universal tumor screening

related to a germline PV in a known cancer-causing gene and is passed down through generations. While only about 5% of CRCs are related to a hereditary cancer syndrome, it is important to note that all CRCs are due to genetic mutations.[2,3]

Understanding CRC genetics is important for many reasons including the opportunity to prevent cancer, optimize cancer treatment, guide surgical decision-making, and inform screening and surveillance of patients and their families. This article will review CRC carcinogenesis, pathology guidelines such as universal tumor screening (UTS), genetic testing guidelines, and hereditary CRC syndrome surveillance and management.

CARCINOGENESIS

Colonocyte genetic and epigenetic mutations accumulate over time and are key drivers of colorectal tumorigenesis. Genetic mutations can either be germline or somatic. Germline mutations can be passed down from parent to child and are incorporated in every cell of the patient's body. Somatic mutations occur in tumor cells only and are the result of a complex combination of environmental and genetic risk factors.[3,4] Epigenetic modifications, such as DNA methylation, are due to alterations in gene function, which do not change the DNA sequence but can cause molecular changes.[5] Colorectal stem cell mutations accumulate over time through a process called the adenoma-carcinoma sequence, which was first described by Fearon and Vogelstein.[6] This was the first major CRC tumorigenesis molecular pathway described and is also known as the chromosomal instability (CIN) pathway. The microsatellite instability (MSI) pathway and CpG island methylator phenotype (CIMP) pathway are 2 other major CRC tumorigenesis pathways.[3]

Chromosomal Instability Pathway

CIN is the most common CRC tumorigenesis pathway (65%–70%) and is a result of the gradual accumulation of small mutations and large chromosomal alterations that typically occur somatically in colonic crypt stem cells. This process occurs over about 10 to 15 years in a stepwise manner. The initial driver of the adenoma-carcinoma sequence is loss of the *APC* tumor suppressor gene, leading to adenoma formation. The first *APC* allele in a crypt stem cell obtains a somatic or inherited mutation, but the *APC* gene is not fully inactivated until the second allele is knocked out, through a process called loss of heterozygosity, rendering the *APC* gene inactive in the crypt stem cell.[3,6,7]

Additional mutations occur in several other driver genes including *KRAS* (Kirsten rat sarcoma viral oncogene homolog), *TP53* (tumor protein p53), and *SMAD4* (Mothers against decapentaplegic homolog 4). An activating mutation in the oncogene, *KRAS*, promotes further proliferation and progression to larger adenomas with tubulovillous or villous histology. The most common late event in this sequence is the loss of tumor suppressor, *TP53*, which removes the DNA damage checkpoint and subsequently leads to high-grade dysplasia and CRC development. Of note, the CIN pathway is the typical CRC carcinogenesis pathway for familial adenomatous polyposis (FAP), which is due to a germline *APC* PV.[3,6–8]

Microsatellite Instability Pathway

The second most common CRC pathway is the MSI pathway. Normally, mismatch repair (MMR) genes encode for MMR proteins, which are involved in a system that recognizes and repairs errors that occur during DNA replication. The most important genes and protein products in this system are *MLH1*, *MSH2*, *MSH6*, and *PMS2*. These MMR proteins function as heterodimeric complexes including MLH1-PMS2, MLH1-PMS1, MSH2-MSH6, and MSH2-MSH3. Microsatellites are repetitive sequences of DNA located in coding and noncoding regions and are frequent sites for MMR errors because of their repetitive nature.[9]

These errors are typically fixed by the MMR system; however, MMR gene mutations can cause MMR system inactivation resulting in mismatches that are left unrepaired, which is called MSI. These mutations can either be germline (15%–25%), in the case of Lynch syndrome (LS), or somatic (75%–85%). A common somatic alteration is *MLH1* promoter hypermethylation, which is an epigenetic change that silences *MLH1* gene expression. This change is frequently associated with a *BRAF V600E* PV and is a sporadic form of CRC due to MSI. MSI in coding regions can inactivate tumor suppressor genes, which leads to cancer development. If 2 or more regions are unstable, then the cancer is considered to have high MSI (MSI-H), which corresponds to MMR deficiency (dMMR) and is a hallmark of LS.[9–12]

LS-associated CRC can progress via the CIN pathway; however, recent literature supports these CRCs commonly forming from dMMR crypts through a “Big Bang” pathway. Møller and colleagues hypothesize that a second hit to the wild-type MMR allele leads to dMMR crypt formation, which increases the development of driver gene mutations in these crypts. These mutations occur in a random process, which may then cause CRC with very short or absent adenoma phases. Alternatively, sporadic dMMR CRCs generally arise in sessile serrated adenomas via the CIMP pathway due to *MLH1* promoter hypermethylation.[3,9–12]

CpG Island Methylator Phenotype Pathway

About 15% to 30% of CRCs arise from the CIMP pathway. Cytosine-phosphate-guanine (CpG) islands are frequently found near gene promoter regions and cytosine methylation in these islands helps regulate gene expression.[12,13] In tumor cells, significant promoter CpG island hypermethylation can silence tumor suppressor genes and lead to tumorigenesis. When tumors have CpG island hypermethylation at multiple gene loci, they are called CIMP-high (CIMP-H). These tumors commonly have concurrent *BRAF V600E* PVs although *KRAS* variants can occasionally be seen, particularly with traditional serrated adenoma-derived cancers.[12–14] Clinically, sporadic dMMR CRCs can arise from CIMP-H sessile serrated adenomas due to MLH1 promoter hypermethylation; however, CIMP-H, proficient MMR CRCs are thought to arise from pre-existing traditional serrated adenomas. Serrated colorectal polyps include hyperplastic polyps, sessile serrated adenomas, and traditional serrated adenomas, with the latter 2 acting as cancer precursors. Importantly, the CIMP pathway is the typical carcinogenesis pathway for serrated polyposis syndrome (SPS).[13,15]

PATHOLOGY GUIDELINES FOR WORKUP OF COLORECTAL CANCER

In 2009, the Evaluation of Genomic Applications in Practice and Prevention (EGAPP) Working Group recommended all CRCs be screened for LS through microsatellite instability polymerase chain reaction (MSI PCR) or mismatch repair immunohistochemistry (MMR IHC) for evidence of dMMR.[16] This process is known as UTS, and multiple other organizations have made similar recommendations since the EGAPP Working Group's recommendation.[17–19] Prior studies have shown equal accuracy of UTS whether a preoperative, colonoscopy biopsy specimen or a surgical resection specimen are used; however, UTS should ideally be completed on a preoperative biopsy specimen to allow for a diagnosis of LS preoperatively and for consideration of neoadjuvant immunotherapy in the case of locally advanced, dMMR CRC.[20–26]

MMR IHC assesses MLH1, MSH2, MSH6, and PMS2 protein expression. If MSH2, MSH6, or PMS2 expression is absent, germline genetic testing is indicated. If MLH1 expression is absent, testing is required to determine if the dMMR is sporadic in etiology through MLH1 promoter hypermethylation or a *BRAF* V600E variant testing.[27] If the tumor tissue is positive for MLH1 promoter hypermethylation or a *BRAF* V600E variant, then the CRC is considered sporadic because MLH1 promoter hypermethylation is a somatic event and drives tumorigenesis via the CIMP pathway.[27,28] MLH1 promoter hypermethylation testing is considered first-line to distinguish sporadic from LS-associated dMMR CRC, and if this test is negative, then patients should be referred to genetic counseling to discuss germline genetic testing (**Fig. 1**).[29,30]

MSI PCR compares tumor DNA with normal DNA across a panel of microsatellite markers to assess for a change in length due to an insertion or deletion of repeating units at each respective marker. Instability, or change in microsatellite length, at 2 or more markers defines MSI-H, instability at a single marker defines MSI-low, and no instability defines microsatellite stable.[31] If tumor tissue is MSI-H, the tumor is considered MMR deficient and requires further testing to determine if the CRC etiology is sporadic, as earlier. MSI PCR testing is more expensive and less sensitive for detecting dMMR than MMR IHC; thus, MMR IHC is the preferred test for UTS.[29]

GENETIC TESTING GUIDELINES FOR WORKUP OF HEREDITARY COLORECTAL CANCER

Germline genetic testing plays an important role in the management of CRC by diagnosing nonpolyposis and polyposis-associated hereditary CRC syndromes. In general, genetic testing is indicated for all patients with early onset CRC, defined as a CRC diagnosis before the age of 50 years.[32] Patients with dMMR CRC should undergo genetic testing to assess for LS if MSH2, MSH6, or PMS2 protein expression is absent

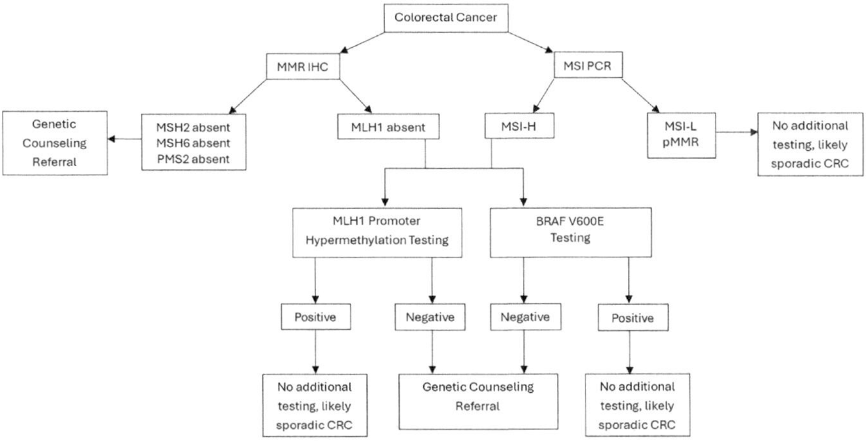

MSI-H = microsatellite instability – high; MSI-L = microsatellite instability – low; pMMR = mismatch repair proficient

Fig. 1. Universal tumor screening algorithm. MSI-H, microsatellite instability-high; MSI-L, microsatellite instability-low; pMMR, mismatch repair proficient.

or when MLH1 protein expression is absent in the setting of negative MLH1 promoter hypermethylation or *BRAF* V600E testing. Other indications to complete genetic testing for LS evaluation include a known LS PV in the family; a first-degree relative with CRC or endometrial cancer diagnosed before the age of 50 years; a first-degree relative with more than 1 LS-associated cancer, 2 or more first-degree or second-degree relatives with LS-associated cancers, with 1 diagnosed before the age of 50 years; or 3 or more relatives with an LS-associated cancers at any age (**Box 1**).[17,33,34]

For polyposis syndromes, the Collaborative Group of the Americas on Inherited Gastrointestinal Cancer recommends genetic testing for patients with 10 or greater lifetime cumulative colorectal adenomas or 3 or greater cumulative gastrointestinal (GI) hamartomatous polyps (hamartomas, ganglioneuromas, Peutz-Jeghers polyps, or Juvenile polyps).[35] Additional gene-specific indications are based on the suspected hereditary polyposis syndrome (**Box 2**).[35–39]

In general, multigene panel testing is the preferred type of genetic test compared to whole genome sequencing or single-site testing and should be obtained prior to the management of CRC when able, unless this would cause a significant delay.[32,35] Current guideline-based testing strategies can miss germline PVs in patients with CRC, which impacts management; therefore, universal germline genetic testing has emerged as a potential strategy to improve detection of hereditary CRC syndromes. This strategy may also be effective for reducing disparities in genetic testing and facilitating cascade testing for family members, although more research is needed prior to universal germline testing becoming standard of care.

MANAGEMENT OF HEREDITARY COLORECTAL CANCER SYNDROMES

Lynch Syndrome

LS is the most common hereditary CRC syndrome and is inherited in an autosomal dominant manner. LS is defined as a genetic predisposition to colorectal, endometrial, ovarian, urinary tract, gastric, duodenal, pancreatic, and other cancers due to a germline PV in the aforementioned MMR genes *MLH1*, *MSH2*, *MSH6*, *PMS2*, or *EPCAM* (epithelial cell adhesions molecule, which causes epigenetic inactivation of *MSH2*)

Box 1
Indications for genetic testing to evaluate for Lynch syndrome[17,33,34]

- Family history of known LS germline PV or likely PV
- Personal history of an LS-associated cancer with any of the following:
  - Age of diagnosis less than 50 years
  - History of at least one other LS-associated cancer
  - 1 or greater first-degree or second-degree relative with an LS-associated cancer diagnosed age less than 50 years
  - 2 or greater first-degree or second-degree relatives with LS-associated cancers diagnosed at any age
- Family history of cancer meeting the following criteria:
  - 1 or greater first-degree relative with CRC or endometrial cancer diagnosed age less than 50 years
  - 1 or greater first-degree relative with greater than 1 diagnosis of LS-associated cancer
  - 2 or greater first-degree or second-degree relatives with LS-associated cancers and 1 or greater diagnosed age less than 50 years
  - 3 or greater relatives with LS-associated cancers diagnosed at any age
- Genetic risk model score 5% or greater predicted probability of germline MMR PV or likely PV (PREMM$_5$, MMRpro)

Abbreviations: CRC, colorectal cancer; LS, Lynch syndrome; MMR, mismatch repair; PV, pathogenic variant.

resulting in MSI (**Fig. 2**). Cumulative cancer incidence is dependent upon the affected gene, organ, and patient sex (**Table 1**).[40]

Patients with LS should undergo lifelong cancer surveillance (**Table 2**). Most guidelines recommend starting surveillance colonoscopy at the age of 20 to 25 years for patients with *MLH1* or *MSH2* PVs and 30 to 35 years for patients with *MSH6* or *PMS2* PVs or 2 to 5 years prior to the youngest age of CRC diagnosis in the family before the age of 25 years (*MLH1* or *MSH2*) or the age of 35 years (*MSH6* or *PMS2*). Colonoscopy is generally repeated every 1 to 2 years, thereafter.[34,36,41–43] Importantly, studies show that patients with LS are more likely to develop CRC despite regular surveillance with possible etiologies for this including quality of colonoscopy, LS tumor biology, and types of precursor lesions. Regardless, colonoscopy remains an integral pillar of cancer prevention in LS.[44,45]

In addition to endometrial cancer surveillance, the American College of Obstetricians and Gynecology recommends risk-reducing surgery for patients with LS and should consider a patient's LS PV, childbearing potential, comorbidities, menopause status, and family history. Risk reducing total abdominal hysterectomy with bilateral salpingo-oophorectomy is generally recommended starting at the age of 40 years.[19,46]

A diagnosis of CRC in the setting of LS requires careful consideration of all available treatment options, including neoadjuvant immunotherapy and surgery with standard segmental or risk-reducing extended colectomy. Immunotherapy has demonstrated excellent efficacy for dMMR CRCs, including LS-associated CRCs, which also raises the possibility of organ-preservation for some patients with LS. Clinical trials have shown a sustained complete clinical response (cCR) for dMMR, locally advanced rectal cancers (LARCs) treated with neoadjuvant immunotherapy without surgery.[23–25] Specifically, Cercek and colleagues[23] found a 100% cCR in 12 patients after 6 months of follow-up for 12 patients treated with dostarlimab for dMMR LARC. A follow-up study showed a 100% cCR in 41 patients after treatment with dostarlimab and 20

Box 2
Indications for genetic testing to evaluate for polyposis syndromes[35–39]

Adenomatous polyposis syndromes

- FAP, MUTYH-associated polyposis
  - Family history of known *APC* germline PV or likely PV
  - Personal history of 10 or greater cumulative colorectal adenomas
  - History of colorectal adenomas and FAP-type extracolonic manifestations (gastric/duodenal adenomas, desmoid tumors, papillary thyroid cancer, congenital hypertrophy of retinal pigment epithelium, osteomas, and so forth)
  - Bilateral or multiple congenital hypertrophy of retinal pigment epithelium lesions
  - Cribriform-morular variant of papillary thyroid cancer

Hamartomatous polyposis syndromes

- PJS
  - 2 or greater histologically confirmed Peutz-Jeghers hamartomatous polyps
  - 1 or greater Peutz-Jeghers polyps with family history of PJS in close relative
  - Perioral or buccal pigmentation with family history of PJS in close relative
  - 1 or greater Peutz-Jeghers polyps with perioral or buccal pigmentation
  - Known family history of PJS
- JPS
  - Greater than 5 juvenile polyps in the colorectum
  - Juvenile polyps in other parts of the gastrointestinal tract
  - Any number of juvenile polyps and a family history of JPS
  - Known family history of JPS
- PTEN hamartoma tumor syndrome/Cowden syndrome
  - 3 or greater gastrointestinal hamartomas or ganglioneuromas
  - Known family history of PTEN hamartoma tumor syndrome
- SPS
  - Greater than 5 serrated polyps proximal to the rectum, all 5 mm or greater in size or with 2 polyps or greater 10 mm or greater in size
  - Greater than 20 serrated polyps of any size within the colorectum and at least 5 proximal to the rectum
  - Genetic testing not routinely recommended since causative pathogenic variants have not been identified

Abbreviations: APC, adenomatous polyposis coli; FAP, familial adenomatous polyposis; JPS, juvenile polyposis syndrome; PJS, Peutz-Jeghers syndrome; PV, pathogenic variant.

patients exhibited a sustained cCR over median follow-up time of 28.9 months.[24] Additionally, the NICHE trial has shown a high number of patients with a pathologic response for locally advanced colon cancer managed with neoadjuvant immunotherapy. Chalabi and colleagues[25] found 98% of 115 patients with locally advanced, dMMR colon cancer exhibited a pathologic response, 95% had a major pathologic response, and 68% had a pathologic complete response. More recent literature has found patients with stage I or II dMMR CRC may also benefit from neoadjuvant immunotherapy.[47] Immunotherapy is quickly becoming an integral component of the management of dMMR CRCs; however, the impact of immunotherapy on metachronous CRC risk and extent of surgical resection in patients with LS requires additional research.

Surgery for LS patients with CRC requires careful consideration of the PV, anatomic location (colon or rectum), and balancing the risk of metachronous CRC with quality-of-life preservation. Patients with colon cancer can undergo an extended resection (ER)—total abdominal colectomy with ileorectal anastomosis (TAC/IRA) or ileosigmoid anastomosis or a segmental resection (SR)—partial colectomy. Eikenboom and colleagues[48] retrospectively assessed 527 patients with LS and found the risk of

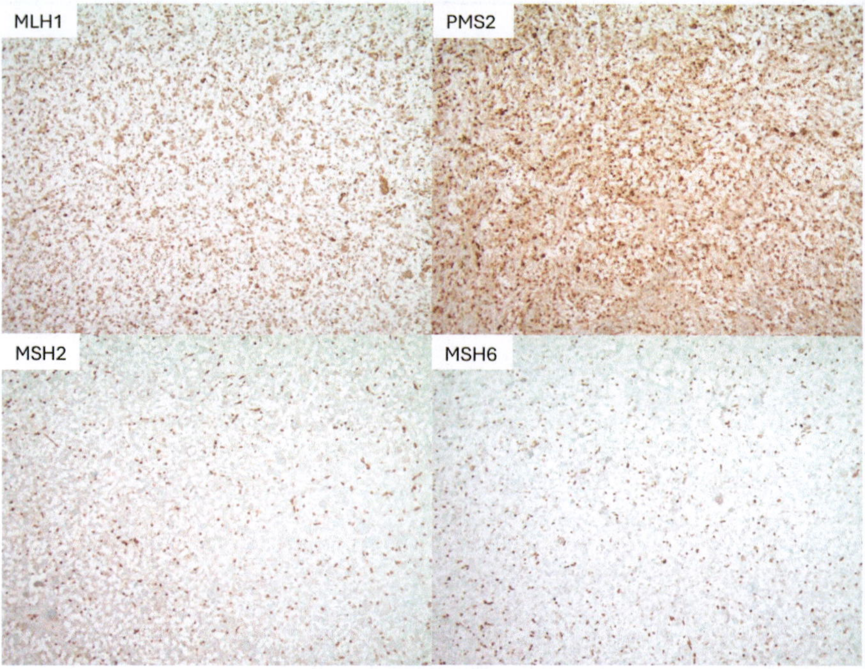

Fig. 2. Example of mismatch repair-deficient colon cancer in a patient with Lynch syndrome. Intact tumor expression for MLH1 and PMS2 and loss of tumor expression for MSH2 and MSH6 on mismatch repair immunohistochemistry for a patient with a newly diagnosed splenic flexure colon cancer. Genetic testing revealed an MSH2 pathogenic variant.

metachronous CRC to be 12% after an ER and 32% after an SR for patients with an *MLH1* or *MSH2* PV. For patients with an *MSH6* or *PMS2* PV, the risk of metachronous CRC was 0% after an ER and 16% after an SR. The study found no significant difference in metachronous CRC risk between patients with an *MLH1* or *MSH2* PV who had an ER compared to patients with an *MSH6* or *PMS2* PV who had an SR.

Other studies have similarly shown *MLH1* and *MSH2* PVs carry a higher risk of metachronous CRC following SR compared to *MSH6* or *PMS2* PVs; therefore, it is generally recommended that, within the context of shared decision-making, LS patients with *MLH1* or *MSH2* PVs have an ER and patients with *MSH6* or *PMS2* PVs have an SR.[44] There are also concerns regarding quality of life and functional outcomes for patients who have an ER compared to an SR. Studies show overall quality of life is worse and restrictions in diet, social, recreational, and travel activities are increased following ER compared to SR.[46,49] An ileosigmoid anastomosis could potentially preserve bowel function compared to an ileorectal anastomosis in patients who need an ER with similar metachronous cancer risk. Regardless, a shared decision-making discussion considering a patient's PV, goals, cancer risk, and quality of life should be completed to determine the most appropriate surgical plan.

For patients with early stage (T1/2N0) rectal cancer, upfront surgical resection remains the standard of care. In contrast, patients with LARC (T3/4 or node-positive disease) are recommended to undergo neoadjuvant immunotherapy rather than traditional TNT with chemoradiation given the high rates of cCR observed with immunotherapy and the relative resistance of dMMR tumors to chemotherapy. In patients with a complete response following neoadjuvant immunotherapy, watch and wait is

Table 1
Cumulative cancer incidence by the age of 75 y in Lynch syndrome based on organ and pathogenic variant[40]

Organ	*MLH1* PV		*MSH2* PV		*MSH6* PV		*PMS2* PV	
	Male	Female	Male	Female	Male	Female	Male	Female
Colorectal	68.5 (60.8–76.0)	80.2 (73.5–86.1)	55.8 (46.8–65.1)	42.6 (35.9–49.9)	16.4 (8.8–29.4)	17.3 (11.2–26.3)	32.8 (12.7–68.6)	8.5 (2.1–31.5)
Endometrium	—	37.2 (30.9–43.3)	—	44.1 (36.3–52.7)	—	45.7 (35.6–57.0)	—	12.7 (5.5–27.9)
Ovary	—	8.0 (5.3–12.0)	—	13.4 (8.9–20.1)	—	6.3 (2.6–15.2)	—	21.2 (8.5–46.9)
Bladder	5.6 (3.1–10.0)	4.8 (2.6–8.9)	13.1 (8.3–20.3)	9.4 (6.0–14.5)	9.0 (4.7–16.9)	2.6 (1.0–6.8)	0 (–)	0 (–)
Ureter/Kidney	4.5 (2.4–8.6)	2.9 (1.4–6.0)	15.8 (11.2–22.0)	19.5 (14.6–25.9)	3.3 (1.2–8.7)	3.9 (1.8–6.8)	5.1 (0.7–30.9)	0 (–)
Gastric	8.9 (5.5–14.4)	4.3 (2.3–7.9)	8.3 (4.8–14.2)	4.0 (2.1–7.4)	0.7 (0.1–4.9)	0.7 (0.1–4.7)	2.7 (0.4–17.5)	0 (–)
Small bowel	8.3 (5.2–13.0)	4.5 (2.6–7.8)	7.0 (4.3–11.3)	3.7 (2.1–6.4)	2.8 (0.9–8.7)	0.6 (0.1–4.0)	3.3 (0.5–21.3)	2.1 (0.3–14.0)
Pancreas	3.1 (1.4–6.9)	3.7 (1.9–7.2)	3.3 (1.5–7.1)	3.5 (1.7–7.3)	1.2 (0.2–8.1)	2.2 (0.7–6.8)	0 (–)	0 (–)
Bile duct/Gall bladder	4.0 (2.2–7.3)	1.5 (0.7–3.3)	4.6 (2.0–10.2)	2.4 (0.9–6.5)	0 (–)	0 (–)	0 (–)	0 (–)
Prostate	15.6 (10.7–22.6)	—	24.0 (17.8–32.0)	—	7.0 (3.5–13.7)	—	3.3 (0.5–21.5)	—
Brain	0.6 (0.1–3.9)	1.4 (0.5–3.4)	6.6 (3.4–12.4)	2.2 (0.8–5.7)	0.8 (0.1–5.3)	1.2 (0.3–4.6)	0 (–)	7.3 (1.1–41.6)

Data from Dominguez-Valentin M, Haupt S, Seppälä TT, et al. Mortality by age, gene and gender in carriers of pathogenic mismatch repair gene variants receiving surveillance for early cancer diagnosis and treatment: a report from the prospective Lynch syndrome database. *EClinicalMedicine* 2023;58:101909. https://doi.org/10.1016/j.eclinm.2023.101909.

Table 2
Lynch syndrome cancer surveillance by pathogenic variant[18,34,36,41–43]

Organ	Method	*MLH1*	*MSH2*	*MSH6*	*PMS2*
Colon/Rectum	Colonoscopy	Onset: 20–25 y Frequency: 1–2 y	Onset: 20–25 y Frequency: 1–2 y	Onset: 30–35 y Frequency: 1–2 y	Onset: 30–35 y Frequency: 1–2 y
Endometrium	Endometrial biopsy	Onset: 30–35 y Frequency: 1–2 y	Onset: 30–35 y Frequency: 1–2 y	Onset: 30–35 y Frequency: 1–2 y	Onset: 30–35 y Frequency: 1–2 y
Gastric/ Duodenal[a]	EGD	Onset: 30–35 y Frequency: 2–4 y	Onset: 30–35 y Frequency: 2–4 y	Onset: 30–35 y Frequency: 2–4 y	Onset: 30–35 y Frequency: 2–4 y
Pancreas[b]	MRCP and/ or EUS[c]	Onset: 50 y Frequency: 1 y	Onset: 50 y Frequency: 1 y	Onset: 50 y Frequency: 1 y	Onset: 50 y Frequency: 1 y
Skin	Skin examination	Onset: uncertain Frequency: 1–2 y	Onset: uncertain Frequency: 1–2 y	Onset: uncertain Frequency: 1–2 y	Onset: uncertain Frequency: 1–2 y

[a] Consider <30 y or frequency <2 y if family history of upper GI cancer or high-risk findings on EGD.
[b] Surveillance generally only recommended in patients with a first-degree or second-degree relative with history of pancreatic cancer.
[c] Consider onset of magnetic resonance cholangiopancreatography (MRCP) or endoscopic ultrasound (EUS) starting 10 y younger than the earliest diagnosed pancreatic cancer in the family.

an appropriate management option; however, patients with an incomplete response should undergo chemoradiation followed by surgical resection.[41,50,51]

When surgically managing LS patients with rectal cancer, European guidelines recommend standard resection with a low anterior resection or abdominoperineal resection, although if there is synchronous neoplasia or patient preference, an ER with total proctocolectomy and ileal-pouch anal anastomosis (TPC/IPAA) can be considered.[52] Alternatively, the American Society of Colon and Rectal Surgeons recommends an individualized approach when considering the extent of resection for rectal cancer. However, in the era of neoadjuvant immunotherapy with most patients being candidates for organ preservation one would very rarely recommend a TPC/IPAA.[53] Risk of metachronous CRC and quality of life are considered, similar to colon cancer, and use of neoadjuvant immunotherapy and chemoradiotherapy for LARC should also play a role in surgical decision-making.

Finally, aspirin plays an important role in CRC risk-reduction for patients with LS and the CAPP2 trial showed that patients who took 600 mg aspirin daily for at least 2 years had a 35% risk reduction at 20 years. The CAPP3 trial is nearing completion and is assessing the most ideal aspirin dose for preventing CRC.[44]

Polyposis

Familial adenomatous polyposis

FAP is inherited in an autosomal dominant pattern with 100% penetrance and is caused by germline PVs in the *APC* gene. FAP is typically characterized by the development of hundreds to thousands of adenomatous polyps throughout the colon and rectum, and nearly all patients will develop CRC if left untreated (**Fig. 3**). A severe polyposis phenotype is characterized by over 1000 colonic polyps, an intermediate polyposis phenotype is characterized by 100 to 1000 colonic polyps, and an attenuated polyposis phenotype is characterized by 10 to 100 colonic polyps.[54] In addition to colorectal polyposis, patients commonly develop extracolonic manifestations including duodenal and gastric neoplasia, thyroid nodules, desmoid tumors, benign skin and soft tissue lesions, osteomas, and brain tumors among other manifestations.[54,55]

FAP patients with a classic phenotype (intermediate or severe polyposis) should start surveillance colonoscopies between ages 12 and 14 years and patients with an attenuated phenotype should start around the age of 18 to 20 years. Surveillance should continue every 1 to 2 years based on polyp burden until colorectal surgery is indicated, and polyps 5mm or greater should be resected to prolong time to surgery and to prevent progression to advanced neoplasia or CRC.[55,56] Patients should also undergo surveillance esophagogastroduodenoscopy (EGD) for gastroduodenal polyposis starting at the age of 20 to 25 years with surveillance frequency generally dependent upon the Spigelman score, which is a classification system for duodenal

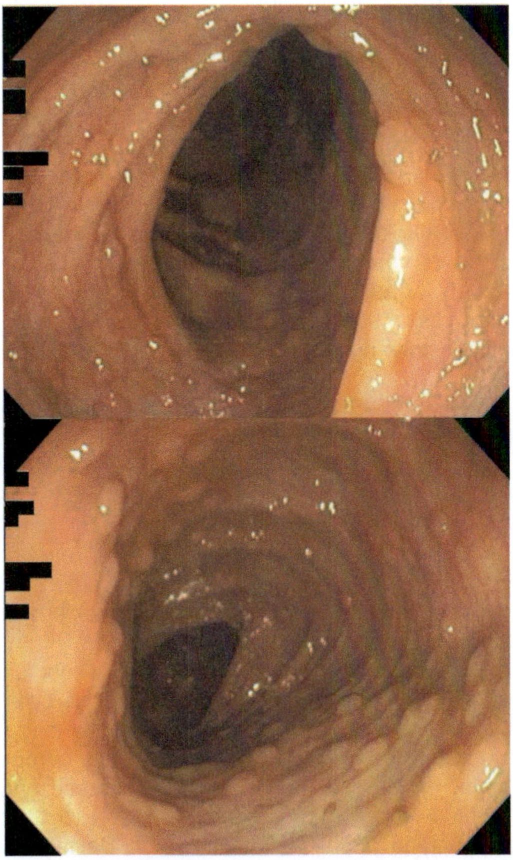

Fig. 3. Colonic polyposis in a familial adenomatous polyposis patient descending colon with approximately 140 polyps, 4 to 6 mm in size.

polyposis. However, one should ultimately consider the site with the most severe disease (stomach vs duodenum), as well as the appearance of the duodenal papilla when considering surveillance interval. Finally, annual thyroid ultrasound is recommended starting in the teenage years to monitor for thyroid cancer.[56–58]

Without colectomy, the lifetime risk of CRC in FAP approaches 100%. Although surgery is therefore inevitable, both its timing and extent should be individualized to best balance cancer risk reduction with quality-of-life implications of surgery. Timing of surgery is individualized based on many factors including the patient's polyposis phenotype, risk of polyp progression and cancer development, psychosocial needs, and risk for development of desmoid disease. Absolute indications for prompt colectomy include a cancer diagnosis and severe symptoms related to polyposis, and relative indications include adenomas with high-grade dysplasia, multiple adenomas greater than 6 mm, significant increase in polyp number between surveillance endoscopies, and inability to adequately survey the colon.[56,59,60]

Generally, the 2 main surgical options for patients with FAP that do not involve a permanent ileostomy include TAC/IRA and TPC/IPAA, and the decision of whether proctectomy is necessary involves balancing cancer prevention and quality-of-life preservation. In rare cases where restoring intestinal continuity is not desired, a TPC with end ileostomy may be considered.

Some centers favor TPC/IPAA for all patients with FAP because it provides the greatest reduction in CRC risk. However, even in high-volume centers, this approach is associated with substantial postoperative morbidity, usually requires a temporary diverting ileostomy, and carries risks including reduced female fecundity, pelvic nerve injury affecting sexual function, and an increased risk of developing intra-abdominal desmoid disease. In terms of function, a meta-analysis of 1002 patients comparing TPC/IPAA with TAC/IRA demonstrated higher rates of stool frequency, nocturnal bowel movements, and incontinence in the IPAA group. Additionally, the risk of unplanned readmission and reoperation within 30 days is higher after TPC/IPAA compared to TAC/IRA.[61] Given these considerations, TAC/IRA is a rational option for appropriately selected patients, as preservation of the rectum avoids pelvic dissection, does not require a temporary stoma, reduces the risk of fertility and sexual dysfunction, and is associated with more predictable bowel function.

Banerjee and colleagues[62] recently assessed the risk of rectal cancer development following TAC/IRA in 197 patients with FAP and reported the risk to be 3.0% overall; however, the rectal cancer risk increased to 10% in patients with 20 or greater rectal polyps at the time of TAC/IRA compared to 2.0% in patients with less than 20 rectal polyps. In comparison, the risk of small bowel or anal transition zone cancer after TPC/IPAA is reportedly less than 1% to 2%.[63,64] Thus, patients with 20 or greater rectal polyps are generally recommended to undergo a TPC/IPAA instead of a TAC/IRA; however, there are many other factors to consider when determining the surgery type.

Desmoid disease is more common in patients with FAP compared to the general population and generally occurs after surgery. Desmoids are locally aggressive fibroblastic, soft-tissue tumors that can develop in any part of the body, although they are usually located intra-abdominally (small bowel mesentery or retroperitoneum) or in the abdominal wall for patients with FAP (**Fig. 4**). Desmoid disease ranges in severity from asymptomatic to severe with complications such as bowel obstructions, bowel perforations, fistulization, bleeding, and ureteral obstruction. Desmoid disease is a leading cause of death in patients with FAP and studies have shown that desmoid disease is more common after TPC/IPAA compared to TAC/IRA. Therefore, the risk of being

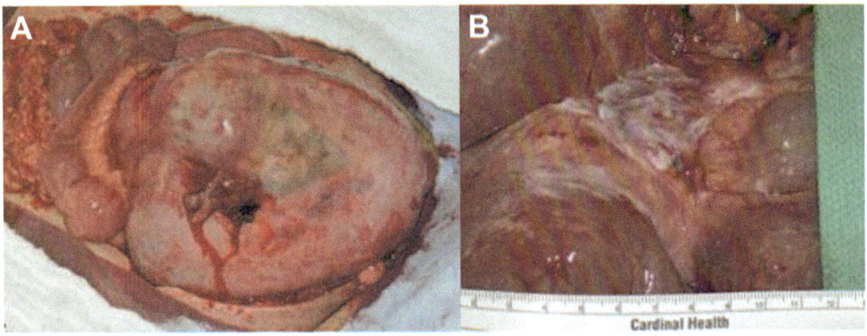

Fig. 4. (*A*, *B*) Intraoperative images of a desmoid tumor (*A*) and desmoid plaque (*B*).

diagnosed with desmoid disease should also be considered when completing shared decision-making with patients prior to their colorectal surgery.[65,66]

After colorectal surgery, patients need to continue lifelong cancer surveillance. Patients with an IRA or IPAA are typically recommended to have lower GI tract surveillance every 6 to 12 months and patients with an end ileostomy (EI) typically are recommended to have surveillance every 12 to 36 months.[55,56] Additionally, there are multiple chemoprevention medications that have been studied to prevent colorectal polyposis progression with the most common being sulindac and celecoxib, which are effective because COX-2 expression, like β-catenin, is increased by the Wnt/β-catenin signaling pathway, and overexpression of COX-2 leads to colonic adenoma progression.[67]

MUTYH-associated polyposis

MUTYH-associated polyposis (MAP) is an autosomal recessive polyposis syndrome that occurs due to PVs in the *MUTYH* base excision repair gene, which cause G>C and A>T transversions in multiple genes including *APC* and *KRAS*. Patients with MAP commonly have attenuated polyposis (10–100 adenomas); however, they may also have a classic phenotype or less than 10 adenomas. Risk of CRC is up to 48% in patients before the age of 60 years and the lifetime CRC risk is up to 80% to 90% in patients who do not complete surveillance. Therefore, colonoscopy surveillance is recommended annually starting between ages 18 and 20 years. Typically, endoscopic management of polyposis is appropriate for patients with MAP if they have an attenuated phenotype; however, surgical indications and decision-making are similar to FAP. Patients with MAP are also recommended to undergo surveillance EGD for gastroduodenal polyposis starting at the age of 35 years with frequency similar to FAP.[34,36,56]

Juvenile Polyposis syndrome

Juvenile polyposis syndrome (JPS) is an autosomal dominant hamartomatous polyposis syndrome characterized by PVs in *SMAD4* or *BMPR1A* with a reported lifetime CRC risk between 39% and 68%. The term "juvenile" refers to the histologic polyp subtype that is characterized by abundant lamina propria with elongated, cystically dilated and mucus-filled glands rather than the age of polyposis onset, which typically begins around the age of 20 years. Juvenile polyps have a risk of malignant transformation; therefore, colonoscopy surveillance is recommended starting at the age of 15 years and continuing every 1 to 3 years based on polyp burden. Surgical intervention may be considered for JPS patients with a polyp burden that is not endoscopically manageable. JPS patients with a *SMAD4* PV have a higher risk of developing gastric polyposis and gastric cancer than patients with a *BMPR1A* PV, and it is recommended that patients with a *SMAD4* PV start upper GI surveillance at the age of 18 years compared to the age of 25 years for patients with a *BMPR1A* PV and continue every 1 to 3 years. JPS is also associated with cranial abnormalities, cleft palate, polydactyly, and hereditary hemorrhagic telangiectasia. Thus, patients can also have epistaxis, mucocutaneous telangiectasias, and arteriovenous malformations.[34,36,68–70]

Peutz-Jeghers syndrome

Peutz-Jeghers syndrome (PJS) is an autosomal dominant hamartomatous polyposis syndrome due to an *STK11* PV and is characterized by the development of Peutz-Jeghers hamartomatous polyps throughout the GI tract. Polyps most commonly occur in the small bowel followed by the colorectum and the stomach, and these benign polyps can cause intussusception, obstruction, bleeding, pain, or prolapse. Surveillance of the small bowel starts between ages 8 and 10 years, or earlier if symptomatic, with video capsule endoscopy, magnetic resonance enterography, or CT enterography. If no polyps are found, then surveillance resumes at the age of 18 years and continues every 2 to 3 years.[34,36,71] Symptomatic polyps or polyps 10 mm or greater should be removed via double balloon enteroscopy. Intraoperative pan-enteroscopy or a "clean sweep" can be completed for patients with extensive, endoscopically unresectable or unreachable small bowel polyps (**Fig. 5**). This is a hybrid technique combining either laparoscopy or laparotomy with intraoperative enteroscopy to allow

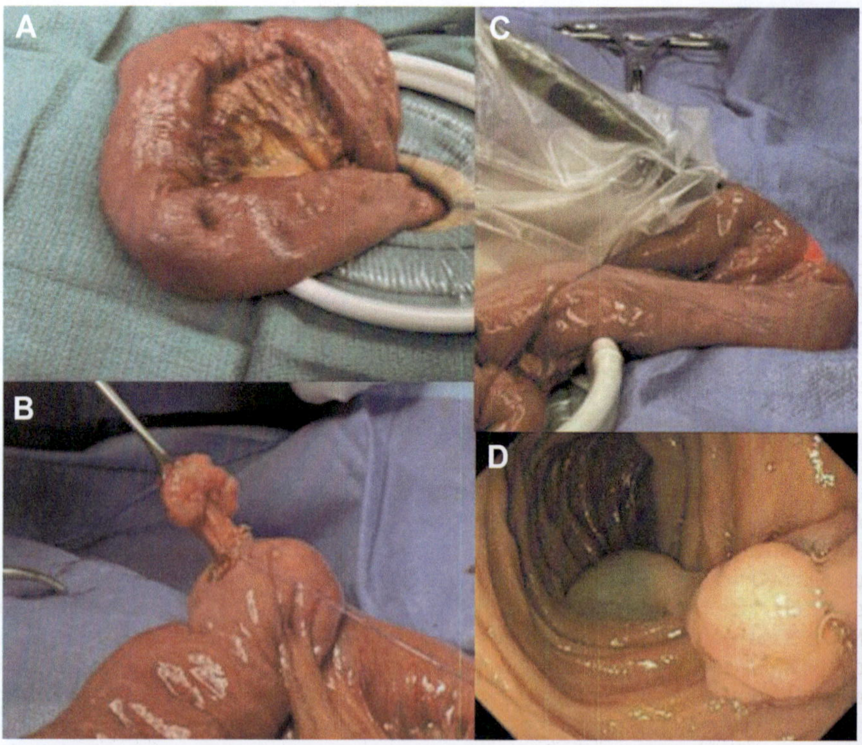

Fig. 5. (*A–D*) Clean sweep procedure for Peutz-Jeghers polyps. (*A*) Extracorporealizing the small bowel with noticeable dimpling related to Peutz-Jeghers polyp. (*B*) Creation of enterotomy and removal of small bowel polyp. (*C*) Insertion of the endoscope into the small bowel for the clean sweep. (*D*) Peutz-Jeghers polyp visualized on endoscopy during the clean sweep.

for complete removal of hamartomas from the entire small bowel.[72] Furthermore, patients should undergo surveillance EGD and colonoscopy in the same manner for gastroduodenal and colorectal polyp surveillance, respectively. Patients with PJS are at an increased risk for breast, pancreas, ovarian, testes, and lung cancer in addition to small bowel, gastric, and CRC and should additionally undergo cancer surveillance via a multidisciplinary approach.[34,36,71]

PTEN hamartomatous tumor syndrome

PTEN hamartomatous tumor syndrome, also called Cowden syndrome, is an autosomal dominant hamartomatous polyposis syndrome characterized by a PV in *PTEN* and multiple GI hamartomas or ganglioneuromas. Colorectal polyps are found in about 95% of patients and polyp types most commonly include juvenile polyps, ganglioneuromas, inflammatory polyps, and adenomas. Lifetime CRC risk for patients with Cowden syndrome is 9% to 16% and the average age of CRC diagnosis is 44 to 48 years. Therefore, surveillance colonoscopy is recommended starting at the age of 15 years and continues every 2 years depending upon findings. Patients are also at an increased risk of thyroid, breast, uterine, renal, and skin cancer (melanoma) and should undergo additional surveillance for each cancer.[34,36]

Serrated polyposis syndrome

Serrated polyps include hyperplastic polyps, traditional serrated adenomas, and sessile serrated polyps. SPS is a clinical diagnosis made for patients meeting 1 of 2 criteria including (1) more than 5 serrated polyps proximal to the rectum, all 5 mm or greater in size or with 2 or more polyps 10 mm or greater in size or (2) more than 20 serrated polyps of any size within the colorectum and at least 5 proximal to the rectum. While some patients with SPS have been shown to have genetic *RNF43* PVs, there is currently no defined monogenic basis in most cases of SPS. Patients with SPS should have an initial colonoscopy to clear all polyps which are 3 or greater to 5 mm followed by repeat colonoscopy surveillance every 1 to 3 years to decrease CRC risk. Colorectal surgery is reserved for patients who developed CRC or have an endoscopically unmanageable polyp burden. Notably, there is an association between Hodgkin's lymphoma and diagnosis of SPS. The specific etiology is unknown, although abdominal radiotherapy and/or chemotherapy with alkylating agents are thought to play a role.[34,36,73]

SUMMARY

CRC genetics carries important clinical implications for the diagnosis and management of patients with CRC and their families. All CRCs should undergo UTS, preoperatively whenever possible, to assess for dMMR due to the ability to diagnose LS preoperatively and for consideration of neoadjuvant immunotherapy in the case of locally advanced, dMMR CRC. Additionally, genetic testing plays an integral role in diagnosing polyposis and nonpolyposis hereditary CRC syndromes; therefore, understanding genetic testing criteria is critical to identify patients with these syndromes. Management of patients with hereditary CRC syndromes is complex and ultimately requires lifelong surveillance and multidisciplinary care to minimize death from cancer and to optimize quality-of-life preservation.

CLINICS CARE POINTS

- All CRCs should undergo UTS (preoperatively when possible) for MMR deficiency and patients with early onset CRC or suggestive family history should undergo germline multigene panel testing.

- Cascade testing (targeted relative testing) is recommended for at-risk family members of patients diagnosed with a hereditary CRC syndrome to identify germline PVs.
- LS patients with CRC may undergo an extended or segmental colonic resection after shared decision-making discussions, although immunotherapy is changing surgical management.
- Patients with familial adenomatous polyposis require colorectal surgery to reduce the risk of CRC, most commonly total colectomy with ileorectal anastomosis or total proctocolectomy with ileal pouch-anal anastomosis with timing and extent of surgery individualized based on polyposis severity, functional and psychosocial considerations, and desmoid risk.
- Management of all hereditary CRC syndromes requires lifelong surveillance and multidisciplinary care to minimize death from cancer and to maximize quality of life preservation.

FUNDING

J.R. Hendren was supported by the James Church, MD, and Sheetz Family Endowed Clinical Fellowship in Hereditary Colorectal Cancer Syndromes.

DISCLOSURE

D. Liska: Freenome, research support to institution.

REFERENCES

1. Siegel RL, Kratzer TB, Giaquinto AN, et al. Cancer statistics, 2025. CA Cancer J Clin 2025;75(1):10–45.
2. Kanth P, Grimmett J, Champine M, et al. Hereditary colorectal polyposis and cancer syndromes: a primer on diagnosis and management. Am J Gastroentero 2017;112(10):1509–25.
3. Fischer J, Walker LC, Robinson BA, et al. Clinical implications of the genetics o sporadic colorectal cancer. ANZ J Surg 2019;89(10):1224–9.
4. Barfield R, Qu C, Steinfelder RS, et al. Association between germline variants and somatic mutations in colorectal cancer. Sci Rep 2022;12(1):10207.
5. Goel A, Boland CR. Epigenetics of colorectal cancer. Gastroenterology 2012 143(6):1442–60.e1.
6. Vogelstein B, Fearon ER, Hamilton SR, et al. Genetic alterations during colorectal tumor development. N Engl J Med 1988;319(9):525–32.
7. Kuipers EJ, Grady WM, Lieberman D, et al. Colorectal cancer. Nat Rev Dis Primers 2015;1:15065.
8. Fang T, Liang T, Wang Y, et al. Prognostic role and clinicopathological features o SMAD4 gene mutation in colorectal cancer: a systematic review and meta-analysis. BMC Gastroenterol 2021;21(1):297.
9. Olave MC, Graham RP. Mismatch repair deficiency: the what, how and why it is important. Genes Chromosomes Cancer 2022;61(6):314–21.
10. Møller P, Haupt S, Ahadova A, et al. Incidences of colorectal adenomas and cancers under colonoscopy surveillance suggest an accelerated "Big Bang" pathway to CRC in three of the four lynch syndromes. Hered Cancer Clin Prac 2024;22(1):6.
11. Kloor M, Huth C, Voigt AY, et al. Prevalence of mismatch repair-deficient cryp foci in Lynch syndrome: a pathological study. Lancet Oncol 2012;13(6) 598–606.

12. Advani SM, Advani P, DeSantis SM, et al. Clinical, pathological, and molecular characteristics of CpG Island methylator phenotype in colorectal cancer: a systematic review and meta-analysis. Transl Oncol 2018;11(5):1188–201.
13. Rhee YY, Kim KJ, Kang GH. CpG Island methylator phenotype-high colorectal cancers and their prognostic implications and relationships with the serrated neoplasia pathway. Gut Liver 2017;11(1):38–46.
14. Zhang X, Zhang W, Cao P. Advances in CpG Island methylator phenotype colorectal cancer therapies. Front Oncol 2021;11:629390.
15. De Palma FDE, D'Argenio V, Pol J, et al. The molecular hallmarks of the serrated pathway in colorectal cancer. Cancers (Basel) 2019;11(7):1017.
16. Evaluation of Genomic Applications in Practice and Prevention (EGAPP) Working Group. Recommendations from the EGAPP working group: genetic testing strategies in newly diagnosed individuals with colorectal cancer aimed at reducing morbidity and mortality from Lynch syndrome in relatives. Genet Med 2009; 11(1):35–41. https://doi.org/10.1097/GIM.0b013e31818fa2ff.
17. Giardiello FM, Allen JI, Axilbund JE, et al. Guidelines on genetic evaluation and management of Lynch syndrome: a consensus statement by the US Multi-Society Task Force on colorectal cancer. Gastroenterology 2014;147(2):502–26.
18. Weissman SM, Burt R, Church J, et al. Identification of individuals at risk for Lynch syndrome using targeted evaluations and genetic testing: National Society of Genetic Counselors and the Collaborative Group of the Americas on Inherited Colorectal Cancer joint practice guideline. J Genet Counsel 2012;21(4):484–93.
19. ACOG practice bulletin no. 147: lynch syndrome. Obstet Gynecol 2014;124(5): 1042–54. https://doi.org/10.1097/01.AOG.0000456325.50739.72.
20. Kumarasinghe AP, de Boer B, Bateman AC, et al. DNA mismatch repair enzyme immunohistochemistry in colorectal cancer: a comparison of biopsy and resection material. Pathology 2010;42(5):414–20.
21. Shia J, Stadler Z, Weiser MR, et al. Immunohistochemical staining for DNA mismatch repair proteins in intestinal tract carcinoma: how reliable are biopsy samples? Am J Surg Pathol 2011;35(3):447–54.
22. Vazzano J, Tomlinson J, Stanich PP, et al. Universal tumor screening for Lynch syndrome on colorectal cancer biopsies impacts surgical treatment decisions. Fam Cancer 2023;22(1):71–6.
23. Cercek A, Lumish M, Sinopoli J, et al. PD-1 blockade in mismatch Repair-deficient, locally advanced rectal cancer. N Engl J Med 2022;386(25):2363–76.
24. Sinopoli JC, Shia J, Weiss JA, et al. Durable complete responses to PD-1 blockade alone in mismatch repair deficient locally advanced rectal cancer. J Clin Oncol 2024. https://doi.org/10.1200/JCO.2024.42.17_suppl.LBA3512.
25. Chalabi M, Verschoor YL, Tan PB, et al. Neoadjuvant immunotherapy in locally advanced mismatch repair-deficient Colon cancer. N Engl J Med 2024;390(21): 1949–58.
26. Hampel H, Frankel WL, Martin E, et al. Screening for the Lynch syndrome (hereditary nonpolyposis colorectal cancer). N Engl J Med 2005;352(18):1851–60.
27. Deng G, Bell I, Crawley S, et al. BRAF mutation is frequently present in sporadic colorectal cancer with methylated hMLH1, but not in hereditary nonpolyposis colorectal cancer. Clin Cancer Res 2004;10(1 Pt 1):191–5.
28. Jin M, Hampel H, Zhou X, et al. BRAF V600E mutation analysis simplifies the testing algorithm for Lynch syndrome. Am J Clin Pathol 2013;140(2):177–83.
29. Shia J. Immunohistochemistry versus microsatellite instability testing for screening colorectal cancer patients at risk for hereditary nonpolyposis colorectal

cancer syndrome. Part I. The utility of immunohistochemistry. J Mol Diagn 2008; 10(4):293–300.

30. Maloberti T, Leo AD, Sanza V, et al. BRAF and MLH1 analysis algorithm for the evaluation of Lynch syndrome risk in colorectal carcinoma patients: evidence-based data from the analysis of 100 consecutive cases. Journal of Molecular Pathology 2022;3(3):115–24.
31. Boland CR, Thibodeau SN, Hamilton SR, et al. A National Cancer Institute workshop on microsatellite instability for cancer detection and familial predisposition: development of international criteria for the determination of microsatellite instability in colorectal cancer. Cancer Res 1998;58(22):5248–57.
32. Cavestro GM, Mannucci A, Balaguer F, et al. Delphi initiative for early-onset colorectal cancer (DIRECt) International Management Guidelines. Clin Gastroenterol Hepatol 2023;21(3):581–603.e33.
33. Holter S, Hall MJ, Hampel H, et al. Risk assessment and genetic counseling for Lynch syndrome - practice resource of the National Society of Genetic Counselors and the Collaborative Group of the Americas on Inherited Gastrointestinal Cancer. J Genet Counsel 2022;31(3):568–83.
34. Syngal S, Brand RE, Church JM, et al. ACG clinical guideline: genetic testing and management of hereditary gastrointestinal cancer syndromes. Am J Gastroenterol 2015;110(2):223–62 [quiz: 263].
35. You YN, Moskowitz JB, Chang GJ, et al. Germline cancer risk profiles of patients with young-onset colorectal cancer: findings from a prospective universal Germline Testing and Telegenetics Program. Dis Colon Rectum 2023;66(4):531–42.
36. Monahan KJ, Bradshaw N, Dolwani S, et al. Guidelines for the management of hereditary colorectal cancer from the British Society of Gastroenterology (BSG)/Association of Coloproctology of Great Britain and Ireland (ACPGBI)/United Kingdom Cancer Genetics Group (UKCGG). Gut 2020;69(3):411–44.
37. Zare B, Monahan KJ. Guidelines for familial adenomatous polyposis (FAP): challenges in defining clinical management for a rare disease. Fam Cancer 2025; 24(2):35.
38. Levy RA, Hui VW, Sood R, et al. Cribriform-morular variant of papillary thyroid carcinoma: an indication to screen for occult FAP. Fam Cancer 2014;13(4):547–51.
39. Jiang W, Li L, Ke CF, et al. Universal germline testing among patients with colorectal cancer: clinical actionability and optimised panel. J Med Genet 2022;59(4): 370–6.
40. Dominguez-Valentin M, Haupt S, Seppälä TT, et al. Mortality by age, gene and gender in carriers of pathogenic mismatch repair gene variants receiving surveillance for early cancer diagnosis and treatment: a report from the prospective Lynch syndrome database. eClinicalMedicine 2023;58:101909.
41. Sinicrope FA. Lynch syndrome-associated colorectal cancer. N Engl J Med 2018; 379(8):764–73.
42. Aslanian HR, Lee JH, Canto MI. AGA clinical practice update on pancreas cancer screening in high-risk individuals: expert review. Gastroenterology 2020; 159(1):358–62.
43. Zhong CS, Horiguchi M, Uno H, et al. Clinical factors associated with skin neoplasms in individuals with Lynch syndrome in a longitudinal observational cohort. J Am Acad Dermatol 2023;88(6):1282–90.
44. Hendren JR, Sommovilla J. Segmental versus extended resection for Colon cancer in Lynch syndrome. Clin Colon Rectal Surg 2025;38(5):317–21.

45. Ahadova A, Seppälä TT, Engel C, et al. The "unnatural" history of colorectal cancer in Lynch syndrome: lessons from colonoscopy surveillance. Int J Cancer 2021;148(4):800–11.
46. Zhao S, Chen L, Zang Y, et al. Endometrial cancer in Lynch syndrome. Int J Cancer 2022;150(1):7–17.
47. Cercek A, Foote MB, Rousseau B, et al. Nonoperative management of mismatch repair-deficient tumors. N Engl J Med 2025;392(23):2297–308.
48. Eikenboom EL, Moen S, van Leerdam ME, et al. Metachronous colorectal cancer risk according to Lynch syndrome pathogenic variant after extensive versus partial colectomy in the Netherlands: a retrospective cohort study. Lancet Gastroenterol Hepatol 2023;8(12):1106–17.
49. You YN, Chua HK, Nelson H, et al. Segmental vs. extended colectomy: measurable differences in morbidity, function, and quality of life. Dis Colon Rectum 2008; 51(7):1036–43.
50. Krasnick BA, Kalady MF. Management of rectal cancer in lynch syndrome: balancing risk reduction and quality of life. Clin Colon Rectal Surg 2023;37(3): 180–4.
51. Hofheinz RD, Fokas E, Benhaim L, et al. Localised rectal cancer: ESMO Clinical Practice Guideline for diagnosis, treatment and follow-up. Ann Oncol 2025;36(9): 1007–24.
52. Seppälä TT, Latchford A, Negoi I, et al. European guidelines from the EHTG and ESCP for Lynch syndrome: an updated third edition of the Mallorca guidelines based on gene and gender. Br J Surg 2021;108(5):484–98.
53. Herzig DO, Buie WD, Weiser MR, et al. Clinical practice guidelines for the surgical treatment of patients with Lynch syndrome. Dis Colon Rectum 2017;60(02): 137–43.
54. Nieuwenhuis MH, Vasen HFA. Correlations between mutation site in APC and phenotype of familial adenomatous polyposis (FAP): a review of the literature. Crit Rev Oncol Hematol 2007;61(2):153–61.
55. Zaffaroni G, Mannucci A, Koskenvuo L, et al. Updated European guidelines for clinical management of familial adenomatous polyposis (FAP), MUTYH-associated polyposis (MAP), gastric adenocarcinoma, proximal polyposis of the stomach (GAPPS) and other rare adenomatous polyposis syndromes: a joint EHTG-ESCP revision. Br J Surg 2024;111(5):znae070.
56. Aelvoet AS, Buttitta F, Ricciardiello L, et al. Management of familial adenomatous polyposis and MUTYH-associated polyposis; new insights. Best Pract Res Clin Gastroenterol 2022;58-59:101793.
57. Poylin V, Shaffer V, Felder S, et al. The American Society of Colon and Rectal Surgeons Clinical Practice Guidelines for the management of inherited adenomatous polyposis syndromes. Dis Colon Rectum 2023. https://doi.org/10.1097/DCR.0000000000003072.
58. Galiatsatos P, Foulkes WD. Familial adenomatous polyposis. Am J Gastroenterol 2006;101(2):385–98.
59. Steinberger AE, Westfal ML, Wise PE. Surgical decision-making in familial adenomatous polyposis. Clin Colon Rectal Surg 2024;37(3):191–7.
60. Sarvepalli S, Burke CA, Monachese M, et al. Natural history of colonic polyposis in young patients with familial adenomatous polyposis. Gastrointest Endosc 2018;88(4):726–33.
61. Aziz O, Athanasiou T, Fazio VW, et al. Meta-analysis of observational studies of ileorectal versus ileal pouch-anal anastomosis for familial adenomatous polyposis. Br J Surg 2006;93(4):407–17.

62. Banerjee S, Burke CA, Sommovilla J, et al. Risk of proctectomy after ileorecta anastomosis in familial adenomatous polyposis in the modern era. Dis Colon Rectum 2024;67(3):427–34.
63. Tajika M, Niwa Y, Bhatia V, et al. Risk of ileal pouch neoplasms in patients with familial adenomatous polyposis. World J Gastroenterol 2013;19(40):6774–83.
64. Boostrom SY, Mathis KL, Pendlimari R, et al. Risk of neoplastic change in ilea pouches in familial adenomatous polyposis. J Gastrointest Surg 2013;17(10): 1804–8.
65. Bektas M, Bell T, Khan S, et al. Desmoid tumors: a comprehensive review. Adv Ther 2023;40(9):3697–722.
66. Sommovilla J, Liska D, Jia X, et al. IPAA is more "Desmoidogenic" than ileorecta anastomosis in familial adenomatous polyposis. Dis Colon Rectum 2022;65(11): 1351–61.
67. Kemp Bohan PM, Mankaney G, Vreeland TJ, et al. Chemoprevention in familia adenomatous polyposis: past, present and future. Fam Cancer 2021;20(1): 23–33.
68. Muller M, Baldysiak E, Benech N, et al. Deciphering the clinical spectrum o gastric disease in patients with juvenile polyposis syndrome. Gastrointest Endosc 2024;100(5):867–77.
69. Singh AD, Gupta A, Mehta N, et al. Occurrence of gastric cancer in patients with juvenile polyposis syndrome: a systematic review and meta-analysis. Gastrointest Endosc 2023;97(3):407–14.e1.
70. Dal Buono A, Gaiani F, Poliani L, et al. Juvenile polyposis syndrome: an overview. Best Pract Res Clin Gastroenterol 2022;58-59:101799.
71. Boland CR, Idos GE, Durno C, et al. Diagnosis and management of cancer risk in the gastrointestinal hamartomatous polyposis syndromes: recommendations from the US multi-society task force on colorectal cancer. Gastroenterology 2022;162(7):2063–85.
72. Wong J, Sommovilla J, Bhatt A, et al. How to do a laparoscopic-assisted endoscopic "clean sweep" for small bowel polyp clearance in Peutz Jeghers syndrome. ANZ J Surg 2024;94(5):952–3.
73. Mankaney G, Rouphael C, Burke CA. Serrated polyposis syndrome. Clin Gastroenterol Hepatol 2020;18(4):777–9.

The Genetics of Familial Neoplastic Thyroid Disease and Primary Hyperparathyroidism

Angela E. Thelen, MD, MHPE[a], Elizabeth M. Hogan, MS, LGC[b,c], Marie W. Su, MD[c,d], Christopher R. McHenry, MD[c,d,*]

KEYWORDS

- Familial thyroid cancer • Familial hyperparathyroidism
- Multiple endocrine neoplasia (MEN) • Genetic testing and surveillance

KEY POINTS

- Familial disease accounts for 25-30% of patients with medullary thyroid cancer (MTC), 5-15% of patients with non-MTC and 3-5% of patients with primary hyperparathyroidism (pHPT) and includes syndrome and nonsyndromic forms.
- Familial medullary thyroid cancer is associated with germline RE-arranged during transfection (RET) mutations and inherited in an autosomal dominant pattern.
- Familial nonmedullary thyroid cancer is genetically heterogeneous, often lacking a single causative mutation.
- Familial pHPT is genetically heterogeneous and occurs in Multiple endocrine neoplasia types I, IIA, and IV: HPT jaw tumor syndrome and familial isolated HPT.
- Early recognition, genetic testing, and tailored surveillance improve outcomes for patients and at-risk family members.

INTRODUCTION

Neoplastic thyroid disease and primary hyperparathyroidism (pHPT) are primarily sporadic in origin. However, familial disease occurs in 25% to 30% of patients with medullary thyroid cancer (MTC), 5% to 15% of patients with non-MTC, and 3% to 5% of patients with pHPT. Inherited thyroid and parathyroid disease can be syndromic or nonsyndromic. In general, genetic testing for familial thyroid and parathyroid disease is available via sequence analysis and deletion/duplication analysis (**Table 1**). Options for genetic testing include single-gene or multigene analyses. Diagnoses can be established by identification of a pathogenic germline variant and in some

[a] Section of Endocrine Surgery, Integrated Surgical Institute, Cleveland Clinic Foundation, Cleveland, OH, USA; [b] Department of Genetics and Genomics, The MetroHealth System, Cleveland, OH, USA; [c] Case Western Reserve University, School of Medicine, Cleveland, OH, USA; [d] Department of Surgery, The MetroHealth System, Cleveland, OH, USA
* Corresponding author. Department of Surgery, MetroHealth Medical Center, H-918, 2500 MetroHealth Drive, Cleveland, OH 44145.
E-mail address: cmchenry@metrohealth.org

Surg Clin N Am 106 (2026) 501–517
https://doi.org/10.1016/j.suc.2026.03.007 surgical.theclinics.com

Abbreviations	
AAES	American Association of Endocrine Surgeons
ATA	American Thyroid Association
CASR	calcium-sensing receptor
CDC73	Cell Division Cycle 73
CDKN1B	cyclin-dependent kinase inhibitor 1B
CI	confidence interval
CLA	cutaneous lichen amyloidosis
FAP	familial adenomatous polyposis
FIHP	familial isolated HPT
FMTC	familial MTC
FNMTC	familial nonmedullary thyroid cancer
GCM2	Glial Cells Missing Homolog 2
HD	Hirschsprung's disease
HPT-JT	hyperparathyroidism jaw tumor syndrome
IOPTH	intraoperative PTH measurement
MEN	multiple endocrine neoplasia
MEN I	multiple endocrine neoplasia type I
MEN IIA	multiple endocrine neoplasia type IIA
MEN IIB	multiple endocrine neoplasia type IIB
MEN IV	multiple endocrine neoplasia type IV
MTC	medullary thyroid cancer
pHPT	primary hyperparathyroidism
PHTS	PTEN-Hamartoma Tumor syndrome
PRKAR1A	protein kinase cAMP-dependent regulatory type I alpha
PTEN	Phosphatase and TENsin homolog
RET	RE-arranged during transfection
WRN	Werner syndrome

circumstances using clinical criteria. As a result, a negative genetic test result does not always rule out a familial syndrome.

This review focuses on syndromic and nonsyndromic forms of inherited thyroid and parathyroid disease. It will include a description of clinical elements and treatment, causative mutations, pattern of transmission, penetrance, and recommendations for genetic testing and surveillance for patients and family members.

FAMILIAL THYROID CANCER

Recognition of the phenotypical features and clinical presentation of syndromes associated with both MTC and familial nonmedullary thyroid cancer (FNMTC) are important for diagnosis, treatment, and surveillance for associated neoplasms in patients and family members. Patients with a thyroid nodule and positive family history of thyroid cancer may have a higher pretest probability of cancer; therefore, a lower threshold for fine needle aspiration biopsy is considered. In general, familial thyroid cancers present earlier, are more advanced at presentation, and are more frequently multicentric with higher recurrence rates.

Familial Medullary Thyroid Cancer

MTC accounts for 3% to 4% of all thyroid cancers and is inherited in 25% to 30% of patients as part of multiple endocrine neoplasia (MEN) IIA, MEN IIB, and isolated familial MTC (FMTC).[1] FMTC results from germline activating missense mutations in the RE-arranged during transfection (*RET*) oncogene on chromosome 10q11.2 with autosomal dominant transmission. The *RET* oncogene encodes a transmembrane tyrosine kinase receptor that is expressed in cells derived from the neural crest

Table 1
Genetic testing for familial thyroid and parathyroid disease

Syndrome	Gene	Analysis Method	Proportion of Causative Variants Detectable by Method
MEN2	*RET*	Sequencing	>98%
		Deletion/duplication	NA
FAP	*APC*	Sequencing	up to 90%
		Deletion/duplication	~8%-12%
Cowden	*PTEN*	Sequencing	up to 80% of the coding region; ~10% of the promotor region
		Deletion/duplication	~3%
Carney complex	*PRKAR1A*	Sequencing	~60%
		Deletion/duplication	~10%
Werner	*WRN*	Sequencing	~97%
		Deletion/duplication	Small percentage of cases
DICER1	*DICER1*	Sequencing	>90%
		Deletion/duplication	Small percentage of cases
CHEK2	*CHEK2*	Sequencing	83%–93%
		Deletion/duplication	up to 10%
Renal papillary neoplasia	*MET*	Sequencing	Majority of cases
		Deletion/duplication	NA
McCune Albright	*GNAS*	Sequencing	limited data
		Deletion/duplication	limited data
Li-Fraumeni	*TP53*	Sequencing	up to 95%
		Deletion/duplication	~1%
MEN1	*MEN1*	Sequencing	65% when a simplex case; 80%–90% when familial
		Deletion/duplication	1%–4%
HPT-JT	*CDC73*	Sequencing	>70%
		Deletion/duplication	up to 30%
MEN IV	*CDKN1B*	Sequencing	~95%
		Deletion/duplication	Small percentage of cases

Abbreviations: CDKN1B, cyclin-dependent kinase inhibitor 1B; FAP, familial adenomatous polyposis; HPT-JT, hyperparathyroidism jaw tumor syndrome; MEN IV, multiple endocrine neoplasia type IV syndrome; *PTEN*, Phosphatase and TENsin homolog.

branchial arches, and urogenital system.[2] Sporadic MTCs commonly harbor a somatic *RET* mutation; those that lack a *RET* mutation have somatic RAS mutations in 18% to 80% of cases: HRAS, KRAS, or rarely NRAS.[3]

Management recommendations for familial MTC are guided by strong genotype–phenotype correlations, although intrafamilial and interfamilial variability has been observed. The American Thyroid Association (ATA) divides *RET* mutations into risk categories based on phenotypical aggressiveness (**Table 2**).[4]

Table 2
American Thyroid Association risk categories for *RE-arranged during transfection* mutations

ATA Risk Category	Syndrome/Mutation
Highest risk	MEN2B, *RET* codon M918T
High risk	*RET* codon C634, codon A883F
Moderate risk	*RET* mutations without aforementioned codon mutations

All patients diagnosed with MTC should undergo genetic counseling and genetic testing. Genetic testing is recommended for family members of patients who test positive for a *RET* mutation.

Multiple endocrine neoplasia type IIA

Multiple endocrine neoplasia type IIA (MEN IIA) is the most common form of MEN II, representing 95% of cases. It is characterized by a classic triad of MTC, pheochromocytoma, and HPT. Variants of MEN IIA include associations with cutaneous lichen amyloidosis (CLA), Hirschsprung's disease (HD), and isolated FMTC.

Classic MEN IIA is the most common variant. 95% of patients with classic MEN IIA have germline *RET* mutations in codons 609, 611, 618, or 620 (exon 10), or codon 634 (exon 11).[5] Penetrance of MTC approaches 100%, while pheochromocytoma and HPT show lower and variable penetrance depending on mutation. Codon 634 mutations confer the highest incidence of pheochromocytoma with 50% to 80% penetrance. Pheochromocytoma is most often benign, multicentric, and bilateral. Penetrance of HPT varies from 2% to 12%, with the exception of codon 634 mutations which have penetrance up to 30%.[6] HPT occurs from a single adenoma (30%–50%) or diffuse hyperplasia; it is typically mild with minimal symptoms and the diagnosis is often made during follow-up after MTC has been treated. While rare, there are kindreds with the features of classic MEN IIA without an identifiable *RET* germline mutation, and diagnosis is established when one or more first-degree relatives have the appropriate clinical manifestations.

Prophylactic treatment of patients with a *RET* mutation consists of total thyroidectomy alone. Patients with clinically apparent MTC also require central neck dissection.[4] The surgical management of MEN IIA HPT is challenging due to the heterogeneity of the parathyroid glands and because most patients have already undergone total thyroidectomy and central neck dissection for MTC. American Association of Endocrine Surgeons (AAES) guidelines for the management of pHPT in patients with MEN IIA favor resecting only enlarged parathyroid glands.[7] Pheochromocytoma must be ruled out prior to thyroid or parathyroid surgery.[4]

Timing of prophylactic thyroidectomy in patients with MEN IIA is based on specific mutations and ATA risk category (see **Table 2**). ATA High Risk patients often develop MTC in the first years of life. Surveillance with annual physical examination, cervical ultrasound, and serum calcitonin should begin at 3 years, with thyroidectomy at or before 5 years.[4] Timing and extent of surgery should be guided by serum calcitonin. Children in the ATA Moderate Risk category typically develop a less aggressive MTC at a later age. These patients should have a physical examination, cervical ultrasound, and serum calcitonin monitored annually starting at 5 years. Thyroidectomy is recommended before 10 years or when calcitonin levels become elevated.[4]

Annual screening for pheochromocytoma and pHPT in MEN IIA should begin by 11 years in patients with high-risk mutations and 16 years for other mutations.[4]

Multiple endocrine neoplasia type IIA with cutaneous lichen amyloidosis
CLA is a rare disorder that is typically sporadic but can be familial in association with MEN IIA with *RET* codon 634 and 804 mutations. With a codon 634 mutation, the CLA phenotype is present in up to 34% of patients.[8] CLA in MEN IIA is characterized by hyperpigmented, pruritic skin lesions that typically occur over the scapulae corresponding to dermatomes T2 to T6, which improve with sun exposure and worsen with stress. CLA often presents at a young age, prior to the development of MTC. Detection of these lesions during adolescence should prompt genetic testing.

Multiple endocrine neoplasia type IIA with Hirschsprung's disease
HD is present in approximately 7% of patients with MEN IIA, whereas MEN IIA occurs in 2% to 5% of patients with HD.[9] Germline *RET* mutations are seen in 50% of patients with hereditary HD and 15% to 20% of patients with sporadic HD. While over 100 *RET* mutations have been identified in patients with HD, the most prevalent in MEN IIA with HD are point mutations on exon 10 codon 609, 611, 618, and 620.[10] If not previously diagnosed, HD should be excluded in older patients diagnosed with MEN IIA who have an exon 10 *RET* mutation and colonic symptoms. Similarly, HD patients with an exon 10 *RET* mutation should be evaluated for MEN IIA.

Isolated familial medullary thyroid cancer
FMTC is characterized by MTC caused by germline *RET* mutations without the development of pheochromocytoma or HPT. The most common mutations involve extracellular cystine codons in *RET* exon 10. Distinguishing FMTC from MEN IIA can be difficult, and it is now considered a subset of MEN IIA.

Multiple endocrine neoplasia type IIB
Multiple endocrine neoplasia type IIB (MEN IIB) accounts for 5% of hereditary MTC cases. Patients with MEN IIB have MTC, pheochromocytoma, and a distinct phenotypical appearance consisting of a marfanoid habitus with joint laxity, narrow, long facies with large lips and thickened, everted, and ptotic eyelids. Additional characteristics include mucosal neuromas, gastrointestinal ganglioneuromas and megacolon, ophthalmologic abnormalities including inability to make tears in infancy and medullated corneal nerve fibers, and skeletal abnormalities including pes cavus, pectus excavatum, high-arched palates, scoliosis, and slipped capital femoral epiphyses.[4,11]

Approximately 25% to 50% of MEN IIB cases are familial resulting from an inherited germline mutation in the *RET* oncogene with autosomal dominant transmission. Most patients with MEN IIB (95%) have *RET* codon M918T mutations on exon 16. Fewer than 5% harbor an exon 15 codon A883F mutation, which may be associated with a less-aggressive MTC.[12] Approximately 50% to 75% of MENIIB cases arise from de novo mutations in the *RET* oncogene.

MEN IIB-associated MTC is highly aggressive, with almost 100% penetrance. Most patients develop metastases in childhood or adolescence. Pheochromocytoma penetrance approaches 50%. Biochemical testing is recommended annually starting at 11 years and always prior to thyroidectomy.[4]

MEN IIB is often diagnosed after MTC is clinically evident and may be too advanced to be cured. Due to aggressive disease, early diagnosis of MEN IIB is imperative. MTC is rarely diagnosed through screening, as 50% to 75% of cases occur from de novo mutations.[13] Genetic testing should be done in at-risk infants soon after birth. Prophylactic total thyroidectomy is recommended within the first year of life or as soon as deemed appropriate by a multidisciplinary team. Serum calcitonin levels are of limited value in MEN IIB during infancy, as calcitonin is high in the first months of life and cannot be used to assist in timing of thyroidectomy.[4]

Familial Nonmedullary Thyroid Cancer

Approximately 5% to 15% of non-MTCs are familial, with 5% arising in the setting of inherited syndromes with well-established driver mutations.[14] Nonsyndromic FNMTC accounts for approximately 90% of all familial thyroid cancer. One or more germline pathogenic variants in cancer risk genes have been reported in 7.5% of patients with differentiated thyroid cancer, suggesting FNMTC may be an underrecognized component of cancer predisposition syndromes.[15] It is fair to say that the entirety of causative genes for hereditary thyroid cancer has not been established.

Nonsyndromic familial nonmedullary thyroid cancer

The definition of nonsyndromic FNMTC is controversial. It has been defined as 2 or more first-degree relatives with thyroid cancer in the absence of a familial syndrome or environmental risk factors, but some argue for a stricter cutoff of 3 or more first-degree relatives.[14] In a Surveillance, Epidemiology and End Results database study, families with 2 members with thyroid cancer had a 69% chance of having a sporadic cancer, while families with 3 or more affected family members had only a 6% and 4% chance of a sporadic cancer, respectively.[16]

Multiple kindreds have been identified with a clustering of thyroid cancer, however a single causative gene has not been identified, making it difficult to determine which individuals have FNMTC versus sporadic disease. Common somatic mutations found in differentiated thyroid neoplasms (eg, *BRAF*, *RAS*, *RET/PTC*, *TRK*, and *PPARγ*) have not been identified as germline mutations in nonsyndromic FNMTC kindreds. Some studies suggest nonsyndromic FNMTC follows an autosomal dominant inheritance pattern, while others consider it a polygenic disorder with a high degree of molecular heterogeneity.[17] In a pooled meta-analysis examining 12,741 patients, Wang and colleagues[18] found an increased rate of recurrence (OR 1.72, 95% confidence interval [CI] 1.34–2.20), decreased disease-free survival (HR 2.9, 95% CI 1.88–2.79), higher risk of multifocality (1.5×), bilateral tumors (1.29×), extrathyroidal extension (1.2×), and lymph node metastasis (1.18×) in FNMTC compared to sporadic disease.

Because a single mutation is lacking, genetic testing and surveillance strategies vary. Total thyroidectomy should be considered as the initial surgical approach given higher rates of multifocality, bilaterality, and recurrence. NCCN and ATA guidelines recommend completion thyroidectomy in patients with macroscopic multifocal disease.[19,20] There is no evidence to support prophylactic thyroidectomy in family members of patients with nonsyndromic FNMTC.

Screening family members is controversial. In a prospective study, Klubo-Gwiezdzinska and colleagues[21] found the prevalence of thyroid cancer detected by screening in at-risk patients with 2 first-degree relatives was the same as the general population (4.6% vs 4.5%). With 3 or more first-degree relatives, the prevalence of thyroid cancer was 22.7%. The 2025 ATA guidelines recommended individuals with a family history of thyroid cancer undergo careful history and physical examination as part of their regular health maintenance. They do not recommend for or against ultrasound screening of families with nonsyndromic FNMTC, as there is no evidence this would affect outcomes.[19] AAES suggests screening ultrasound beginning 5 years before the youngest adult relative was diagnosed.[22]

Syndromic familial nonmedullary thyroid cancer

Syndromic FNMTC constitutes less than 3% of all familial cases. The most common associated syndromes are familial adenomatous polyposis (FAP), Cowden syndrome (Phosphatase and TENsin homolog [PTEN]-Hamartoma syndrome), Carney complex, Werner syndrome, and DICER1 syndrome. Other rare inherited cancer syndromes with an increased prevalence of thyroid cancer include CHEK2, papillary renal neoplasia, McCune-Albright syndrome, and Li-Fraumeni syndrome.

Familial adenomatous polyposis

FAP is an autosomal dominant syndrome caused by germline mutations in the adenomatous polyposis coli tumor suppressor gene on chromosome 5q21. De novo mutations are responsible for 10% to 30% of cases. FAP is characterized by adenomatous polyps of the colon and rectum, most often in the hundreds, with a near 100% lifetime risk of colorectal cancer. Patients may also have upper gastrointestinal polyps with an increased risk of periampullary and duodenal cancer. Gardner syndrome is a variant of FAP associated with extraintestinal tumors such as osteomas of the skull, fibromas, epithelial cysts, and desmoid tumors.

FAP and Gardner syndrome carry an increased risk of thyroid cancer. Benign thyroid disease is also associated, including hypothyroidism, goiter, thyroiditis, and nodules. In one meta-analysis of patients with FAP screened with ultrasound, the prevalence of thyroid cancer, benign structural thyroid disease, and functional thyroid disease was 2.6%, 48.8%, and 6.9%, respectively.[23]

Thyroid cancer is the third most common neoplasm in FAP, with an incidence of 1% to 7.3%.[24] There is a 10 fold increase in frequency of thyroid cancer in FAP compared to the general population.[25] Patients with FAP who develop thyroid cancer are most often female and diagnosed between 18 and 35 years of age. Thyroid cancer is commonly papillary, with 20% to 40% of patients having the cribriform-morular variant.[23] FAP should be considered in any patient with the cribriform-morular variant of PTC. In up to a third of patients with FAP, thyroid cancer precedes the diagnosis of FAP.[25] Total thyroidectomy is recommended for patients with FAP-related thyroid cancer given a high risk of multifocal and bilateral cancers.

Current guidelines suggest annual screening ultrasound beginning in adolescence. A recent study of 267 patients with FAP undergoing screening ultrasound reported 63.3% had a normal thyroid gland, 27.7% had low-risk nodules, and 9.0% had high-risk nodules on initial examination. Over an almost 5 year follow-up period, no patients with normal thyroid glands on initial ultrasound developed thyroid cancer or new nodules.[24] Surveillance strategy may be able to be individually tailored based on the presence of structural thyroid disease on initial examination.

Cowden syndrome

Cowden syndrome is a phenotype of the PTEN-Hamartoma Tumor syndrome (PHTS) caused by pathogenic germline variants in the tumor suppressor gene *PTEN* on chromosome 10q22 to 23.[26] Cowden syndrome is a rare (prevalence 1 in 200,000) autosomal dominant disease characterized by benign hamartomas and mucocutaneous lesions with an increased risk of breast, thyroid, kidney, colon, and endometrial cancer. The hallmark features include macrocephaly and neurodevelopmental disorders.[26] Diagnosis is based on clinical criteria in conjunction with genetic testing for *PTEN* mutations.

The lifetime risk of thyroid cancer is 35% to 38% and patients present at a younger age compared to sporadic differentiated thyroid cancer.[27] Papillary is the most common subtype, but cases of follicular and anaplastic thyroid cancer have been described. Metastatic disease and mortality rates from thyroid cancer are low due to screening, early detection, and treatment.[27] Multinodular goiter is also prevalent, affecting up to three-quarters of patients with Cowden syndrome.

Screening guidelines recommend yearly ultrasound starting at 18 years.[26] Given the high risk of thyroid cancer and difficulties performing fine needle aspiration biopsy on patients with concomitant developmental disorders, prophylactic thyroidectomy has been considered.[28] Childhood thyroid cancer has been described, with the youngest reported at 7 years old. Some therefore advocate for screening ultrasound starting at 7 years and continuing every 2 years throughout childhood.[29]

Carney complex

Carney complex is an autosomal dominant disease caused by mutations in the protein kinase cAMP-dependent regulatory type I alpha (*PRKAR1A*) tumor suppressor gene on chromosome 17q22 to 24.[30] It is inherited in 70% of cases and develops from a de novo mutation in 30% of cases. It is characterized by cardiac and soft tissue myxomas, atypical skin and mucus membrane pigmentation, schwannomas, and various endocrine tumors including nodular adrenocortical disease with manifestations of Cushing syndrome, pituitary tumor leading to acromegaly, and thyroid disease. Thyroid disease is present in 75% of Carney complex patients; 25% have thyroid neoplasm, most commonly follicular adenoma, and 2.5% develop thyroid cancer, most commonly follicular.[31] Thyroid nodules are often diagnosed during the first 10 years of life and as early as 2 years.[32]

Carney complex can be diagnosed based on clinical criteria. Therefore, a negative genetic test result does not rule out the disease. There are no screening guidelines for thyroid cancer in Carney complex.

Werner syndrome

Werner syndrome (WRN) is an autosomal recessive disorder characterized by premature aging beginning after puberty. Clinical characteristics include graying of the hair, cataracts, osteoporosis, atherosclerosis, loss of fertility, and a predisposition to neoplasms, notably melanoma, meningioma, and soft tissue sarcomas.[33] Thyroid tumors develop in 17% to 18% of patients including follicular (48%), papillary (35%), and anaplastic cancers (13%).[34]

WRN is caused by caused by mutations in the *WRN* gene on chromosome 8p11 to 21 that impair the function of telomere maintenance. Genotype/phenotype correlations have been observed. N-terminal variants are associated with PTC and C-terminal variants are commonly associated with follicular carcinoma.[33,34] Due to the rarity of WRN, no defined screening guidelines exist, but routine screening ultrasound is recommended.

DICER1 syndrome

DICER1 syndrome is a rare autosomal dominant disease caused by a loss-of-function mutation in the *DICER1* gene on chromosome 14q32.13, which aids in cleaving N-precursors to functional miRNA. Most individuals with DICER1 syndrome inherit it from an affected parent; however, approximately 20% of individuals with certain phenotypes have a de novo variant. An estimated 1:2500–1:10,600 people carry a pathogenic *DICER1* mutation, with penetrance estimated at 15%.

DICER1 syndrome is characterized by pleuropulmonary blastoma, Sertoli-Leydig ovarian tumors, pineoblastoma, and other rare tumors. Follicular nodular thyroid disease and multinodular goiter are the most common thyroid manifestations. Follicular nodular thyroid disease occurring in childhood or adolescence is suspicious for an underlying germline *DICER1* variant.[35] There is a 16 to 24 fold increased risk of differentiated thyroid cancer, most commonly papillary cancer.[36] Individuals with germline *DICER1* variants and differentiated thyroid carcinoma are commonly diagnosed between ages 10 and 20 years, with affected individuals reported from 5 to 40 years.[37] There are no specific screening guidelines for DICER1 syndrome. It has been suggested to obtain a screening ultrasound at 8 years old with follow-up every 3 years as 13% to 32% of individuals will have multinodular goiter and 16% will have differentiated thyroid cancer.[36]

Other syndromes. Other rare inherited syndromes have been associated with an increased prevalence of thyroid disease, including CHEK2, papillary renal neoplasia, McCune-Albright syndrome, and Li-Fraumeni syndrome. These syndromes and their thyroid manifestations are summarized in **Table 3**.

Molecular testing in thyroid disease

Molecular testing in thyroid cancer has grown exponentially over the past several years. Molecular testing serves two primary clinical roles: (1) refining the diagnosis of cytologically indeterminate nodules, and (2) identfying actionable theraapeutic targets in advanced thyroid cancer. Using cellular material collected during fine needle aspiration biopsy, DNA or RNA is extracted depending on the brand of test being used. Specific genetic alterations are interrogated that are known to oncogenic mutations and fusions in thyroid cancer. These mutations are mostly somatic, rather than germline, mutations and can have important implications for management. For any cytologically indeterminate nodule, the NCCN recommends pursuing molecular testing for more precise diagnostic informtation.[20] The 2025 ATA guidelines do not recommend the use of routine genomic evaluation prior to surgery in known differentiated thyroid cancers at this time.[19] However, if the molecular profile is known, it can be considered alongside clinical, radiographic, and cytopaathologic data to inform extent of surgery. Some relevant mutations commonly seen on molecular profiling include: *BRAF V600E, RAS, RET/PTC* fusions, *NTRK* fusions, *PAX8-PPAR*γ, *DICER1*, nd the *TERT* promoter mutation.

BRAF V600E. *BRAF V600E* is the most common driver mutation, found in approximately 60% of PTCs. It causes a robust activation of the MAPK pathway which suppresses thyroid differentiation genes including the sodium-iodide symporter.[38] This renders *BRAF* positive cancers less responsive to radioactive iodine. *BRAF* mutations are most commonly associated with classic/conventional type PTC and tall-cell variant PTC histology.[39] *BRAF* mutations alone are not an independent poor prognostic factor in small PTCs, however when found in combintation with a *TERT* promoter mutation there is a high rate of lymph node metastases and recurrence. There are targeted therapies available for *BRAF* mutated advanced or aggressive thyroid cancer.[19,20]

RAS. *RAS* mutations are associated with follicular-patterned neoplasms including the folicullar variant of PTC, FTC, follicular adenomas, and non-invasive follicular thyroid neoplasms with papillary-like nuclear features (NIFTP).[39] *RAS* mutations including *NRAS*, *HRAS*, and *KRAS* are found in about 13% of PTCs and 25-50% of FTCs. *RAS* mutated tumors tend to retain radioactive iodine avidity. Tumors with *RAS* mutations co-occuring with *TERT* promoter mutations or *EIF1AX* mutations tend to exhibit more aggressive behavior.[19]

RET/PTC fusions. *RET* fusions are the most common chromosomal fuions in PTC representing about 7% of adult PTCs.[38] *RET* fusions are strongly associated with radiation-related thyroid cancer such as patients exposed during the Chernobyl disaster.[40] There are targetable therapies including selective *RET* inhibitors for patients with radioactive iodine refractory *RET/PTC* fusion-positive disease.[20]

NTRK fusions. *NTRK* fusions are found in approximately 2-7% of adult PTC.[19] Tumors with *NTRK* fusions tend to exhibit a multinodular invasive growth pattern with mixed

Table 3
Rare inherited neoplastic thyroid syndromes and their associated genetic and clinical features

Syndrome	Gene	Inheritance Pattern	Characteristics	Thyroid Findings	Genetic Testing	Thyroid Screening
CHEK2[44]	*CHEK2*	Autosomal dominant	Predisposition to breast and prostate cancer	Potential increased risk of NMTC in c.1100del and c.470T>C/p.I157T variants	Sequence analysis and del/dup analysis; single-gene or panel	Not recommended
Papillary renal neoplasia[45]	*MET*	Autosomal dominant	Hereditary papillary renal carcinoma	Limited data, possible correlation with papillary and medullary thyroid cancer	Sequence analysis; single-gene or panel	Not recommended
McCune Albright[46]	*GNAS*	Not inherited, spontaneous somatic variants occurring in a mosaic manner	Precocious puberty, fibrous dysplasia of bone, and café-au-lait skin macules	Thyroid nodules or multinodular goiter (31%); thyroid cancer; and hyperthyroidism (40%)	Limited due to mosaic and somatic variants; targeted testing of affected tissue	Not recommended
Li-Fraumeni[47]	*TP53*	Autosomal dominant	Cancer predisposition syndrome; commonly CNS tumors, sarcomas, adrenocortical, and breast carcinomas	NMTC (6%–9%)	Sequence analysis and del/dup analysis; single-gene or panel	Not recommended

papillary and follicular architecture. Extensive lymphovascular invasion is common and there is a high rate of lymph node metastases at presentation. NTRK fuusions are associated with a background of Hashimoto's thyroiditis.[41] Targeted TRK inhibitorss are highly effective and recommended as first-line therapy for NTRK fusion positive radioactive iodine refractory differentiated thyroid cancer.[19]

PAX8-PPARγ. *PAX8-PPARγ* fusions are classified as a *RAS*-like alteration producing follicular-patterned neoplasms. This fusions is found in approximately 25-50% of FTC, 38% of follicular variant PTC, and 2-13% of follicular adenomas.[19,40] Tumors tend to present at a younger age, be smaller, and show vascular or capsular invasion. Most tumors are clinically indolent.[42]

DICER1. *DICER1* mutations can occur as somatic or germline mutations, as in *DICER1* syndrome. Any patient with a positive *DICER1* mutation on molecular profiling should be considered for germline genetic testing. Tumors are typically follicular-patterened, RAS-like neoplasms. While patients with germline *DICER1*-related PTC generally develop low risk tumors for recurrence or metastasis, somatic *DICER1* mutations demonstrate a broader histologic spectrum.[43]

FAMILIAL PRIMARY HYPERPARATHYROIDISM

Familial pHPT is genetically heterogeneous and occurs in MEN I, MEN IIA, MEN IV, HPT jaw tumor syndrome (HPT-JT) and familial isolated HPT (FIHP).

Compared with sporadic pHPT, familial disease presents earlier, more frequently involves multiglandular disease, and has higher recurrence rates (17%–46% in MEN I, 6%–11% in MEN IIA, 15%–20% in HPT–JT, and 11% in FIHP).[7] Lifelong follow-up is required due to high recurrence rates.

All patients with pHPT should be evaluated for a family history of HPT, thyroid cancer, other endocrinopathies associated with syndromic HPT, nephrolithiasis, and prior neck surgery. Genetic counseling and testing are recommended for patients younger than 40 years with multiglandular disease, all patients with parathyroid carcinoma, and those with clinical manifestations or family history consistent with a hereditary syndrome.[7] Identification of causative genetic mutations has important implications for management and surveillance for associated tumors and identifying or excluding asymptomatic carriers of mutations in relatives.

Multiple Endocrine Neoplasia Type I

Multiple endocrine neoplasia type (MEN I) is a rare autosomal dominant syndrome (prevalence of 1–10 per 100,000) and is the most common familial cause of pHPT, accounting for 2% to 4% of cases. Patients typically develop pHPT between ages 20 and 25 years, and almost all patients develop HPT by the age of 50 years.[48] HPT is the initial manifestation in over 90% of patients. HPT occurs in association with gastro-entero-pancreatic neuroendocrine tumors (~40%–70%) and anterior pituitary adenomas (~30%–40%), most commonly prolactinomas. Less common features include adrenocortical and thyroid tumors, neuroendocrine (carcinoid) tumors of the thymus, bronchus and lung, facial angiofibromas, skin hamartomas, multiple lipomas, and central nervous system tumors (meningioma, ependymoma, and neuroblastoma). MEN I can be diagnosed when 2 of the 3 MEN I-associated endocrine tumors affecting the parathyroid, pituitary, and pancreas occur in an individual, when one MEN I-associated endocrine tumor occurs in a first-degree relative of an individual with MEN I, or identification of a pathologic MEN I mutation.[49]

MEN I results from germline inactivating mutations in the *MEN1* tumor suppressor gene on chromosome 11q13, which encodes for the nuclear protein menin. Somatic loss of the remaining functional copy of the gene results in nonfunctional menin, leading to dysregulated cellular proliferation, with penetrance reaching 95% by the age of 40 years.[7] MEN I is inherited in 90% of individuals and occurs from a de novo mutation in 10% of individuals.[50]

Genetic testing can identify pathogenic germline variants in the *MEN1* gene in 70% to 90% of affected individuals and cascade testing is recommended for relatives of affected family members. Guidelines recommend annual screening for HPT with serum calcium and parathyroid hormone in early childhood for mutation carriers and lifelong surveillance for associated tumors starting in adolescence.

All 4 parathyroid glands are typically affected in an asynchronous and asymmetric pattern.[48] MEN I-associated HPT is generally treated with a bilateral neck exploration with subtotal parathyroidectomy and transcervical thymectomy or total parathyroidectomy, transcervical thymectomy, and parathyroid autotransplantation. Even with more extensive parathyroidectomy, recurrence rates are high (17%–46%).[7] Parathyroid carcinoma rarely occurs.

Hyperparathyroidism Jaw Tumor Syndrome

Hyperparathyroidism jaw tumor syndrome (HPT–JT) is a rare autosomal dominant disorder characterized by pHPT, ossifying fibromas of the mandible or maxilla, renal abnormalities including cysts, hamartomas, Wilms tumor, and adenocarcinoma and uterine tumors. HPT–JT is caused by germline inactivating mutations of the Cell Division Cycle 73 (*CDC73*) gene on chromosome 1q31.2, which codes for parafibromin, a tumor suppressor protein that regulates transcription. Genotype/phenotype correlations have been suggested for different *CDC73* mutations; however, clinical variation has been observed among and within variants.[51] The proportion of variants that are inherited versus de novo has not been well established.

pHPT is the most common manifestation, occurring in 80% to 95% of individuals, with a median age of diagnosis between 23 and 38 years. In contrast to other familial pHPT, single gland disease is more common, occurring in up to 90% of patients, although asynchronous involvement of additional glands may occur.[52] Patients with single gland involvement are treated with resection of the enlarged gland and intraoperative PTH measurement (IOPTH) to ensure there is no residual hyperfunctioning parathyroid tissue.[53]

Patients with HPT-JT have much higher frequency of parathyroid carcinoma compared to other forms of HPT (15%–30%). Parathyroid cancer is resected en bloc with all tissue it is invading. Loss of parafibromin expression on nuclear immunostaining is a distinctive pathologic feature of the disease. Outcomes are largely determined by the presence or absence of carcinoma and the completeness of initial resection. Long-term follow-up is required due to malignancy risk and a 25% recurrence rate in another gland.

Jaw tumors have been reported in only 27% of patients with HPT-JT, thus the term CDC73-related familial pHPT may be more appropriate to ensure a degree of clinical suspicion even in the absence of jaw tumors.[54] Genetic testing is recommended for relatives of affected individuals. Mutation carriers should undergo annual biochemical screening for HPT starting at the age of 10 years, regular dental and maxillofacial evaluation for jaw tumors, renal imaging, and gynecologic examination with pelvic ultrasound for women of reproductive age.[55]

Familial Isolated Hyperparathyroidism

FIHP is defined by pHPT in 2 or more first-degree relatives without other syndromic features. FIHP may represent incomplete expression of MEN1, HPT-JT, and familial hypocalciuric hypercalcemia from mutations in the *MEN1*, *CDC73*, and calcium-sensing receptor (*CASR*) or the Glial Cells Missing Homolog 2 (*GCM2*) genes.[56] Clinical presentation varies by genotype. Multiglandular disease is more common in *MEN1* or *GCM2* mutations compared to *CDC73* or *CASR* mutations.[56] *CDC73* and *GCM2*-related FIHP has higher risk of parathyroid carcinoma.[57] Bilateral neck exploration is recommended for patients with FIHP because of the increased frequency of multiglandular disease. It is our preference to resect only enlarged parathyroid glands and use IOPTH to help determine when to conclude the operation. Screening and surveillance should be tailored to the specific gene involved, with ongoing reassessment if other syndromic features emerge.

Multiple Endocrine Neoplasia Type IV Syndrome

Multiple endocrine neoplasia type IV syndrome (MEN IV) is a rare autosomal dominant syndrome with MEN I–like features in the absence of *MEN1* mutations. Parathyroid disease is the most common manifestation, with a prevalence of 70% to 80%, typically presenting later than MEN I (median age 51 years), with milder biochemical abnormalities and more commonly from single-gland disease (70%).[56,58] Pituitary adenoma is the second most common manifestation (~30%). Patients with MEN IV are less likely to have gastro-entero-pancreatic neuroendocrine tumors (~9%).

MEN IV results from germline inactivating mutations in the cyclin-dependent kinase inhibitor 1Bgene on chromosome 12p13.1, which encodes the cell cycle inhibitor p27Kip1.[58] Most individuals with MEN IV inherit the condition from an affected parent. De novo inheritance rates are unknown.

The prevalence of MEN IV is low, accounting for 0.07% of suspected patients with MEN I. As a result, there are limited long-term data and no established treatment or screening protocols. Genetic testing should be considered in individuals with MEN I-like features who test negative for *MEN1* mutations. Our preference for treatment of MEN IV HPT is bilateral neck exploration, resection of enlarged parathyroid glands, and adjunctive IOPTH. Surveillance strategies are extrapolated from MEN I guidelines and should include periodic biochemical screening for HPT starting at 15 years and assessment for pituitary tumors.[59]

CLINICS CARE POINTS

- Always evaluate for hereditary MTC. Up to 25-30% of MTC is familial, and all patients with MTC require genetic counseling and RET testing. Missing a hereditary diagnosis is a critical pitfall as it affects treatment, surveillance for associated conditions, and screening of at-risk relatives.
- Have a lower threshold for biopsy and more aggressive surgical planning in FNMTC. Patients with a family history have higher malignancy risk and tend to present with multifocal, bilateral, and more aggressive disease, favoring consideration of total thyroidectomy as the initial operation rather than lobectomy.
- Recognize syndromic features that change management beyond the thyroid. Syndromes such as MEN2, FAP, and Cowden require screening for associated malignancies. Failure to identify these features can lead to incomplete care and missed life-threatening comorbidities.
- Familial pHPT often means multigland disease—plan the operation accordingly. Compared with sporadic disease, familial hyperparathyroidism more commonly involves multiple

glands and higher recurrence rates, making bilateral neck exploration and use of intraoperative PTH monitoring essential. Focal exploration is a common pitfall.

- Consider hereditary syndromes early in atypical or high-risk pHPT presentations Genetic evaluation is recommended in patients <40 years with multigland disease, parathyroid carcinoma, syndromic features, or a consistent family history. Identifying a mutation directly impacts operative strategy, surveillance, and family screening.

DISCLOSURE

The authors have no disclosures to declare.

REFERENCES

1. Medullary thyroid cancer (MTC). NIH National Cancer Institute. 2019. Available at: https://www.cancer.gov/pediatric-adult-rare-tumor/rare-tumors/rare-endocrine-tumor/medullary-thyroid-cancer. Accessed November 17, 2025.
2. Pachnis V, Mankoo B, Costantini F. Expression of the *c-ret* proto-oncogene during mouse embryogenesis. Development 1993;119(4):1005–17.
3. Moura MM, Cavaco BM, Pinto AE, et al. High prevalence of *RAS* mutations in *RET* -Negative sporadic medullary thyroid carcinomas. J Clin Endocrinol Metabol 2011;96(5):E863–8.
4. Wells SA, Asa SL, Dralle H, et al. Revised American Thyroid Association Guidelines for the management of medullary thyroid carcinoma: the American thyroid Association Guidelines task force on medullary thyroid carcinoma. Thyroid 2015;25(6):567–610.
5. Raue F, Frank-Raue K. Genotype-phenotype correlation in multiple endocrine neoplasia type 2. Clinics 2012;67:69–75.
6. Imai T, Uchino S, Okamoto T, et al. High penetrance of pheochromocytoma in multiple endocrine neoplasia 2 caused by germ line RET codon 634 mutation in Japanese patients. Eur J Endocrinol 2013;168(5):683–7.
7. Wilhelm SM, Wang TS, Ruan DT, et al. The American Association of Endocrine Surgeons Guidelines for definitive management of primary hyperparathyroidism. JAMA Surg 2016;151(10):959.
8. Verga U, Fugazzola L, Cambiaghi S, et al. Frequent association between MEN 2A and cutaneous lichen amyloidosis. Clin Endocrinol 2003;59(2):156–61.
9. Decker RA, Peacock ML. Occurrence of MEN 2a in familial hirschsprung's disease: a new indication for genetic testing of the RET proto-oncogene. J Pediatr Surg 1998;33(2):207–14.
10. Attié T, Pelet A, Edery P, et al. Diversity of *RET* proto-oncogene mutations in familial and sporadic hirschsprung disease. Hum Mol Genet 1995;4(8):1381–6.
11. Cohen MS, Phay JE, Albinson C, et al. Gastrointestinal manifestations of multiple Endocrine Neoplasia type 2. Ann Surg 2002;235(5):648–55.
12. Jasim S, Ying AK, Waguespack SG, et al. Multiple endocrine neoplasia type 2B with a *RET* proto-oncogene A883F mutation displays a more indolent form of medullary thyroid carcinoma compared with a *RET* M918T mutation. Thyroid 2011;21(2):189–92.
13. Waguespack SG, Rich TA, Perrier ND, et al. Management of medullary thyroid carcinoma and MEN2 syndromes in childhood. Nat Rev Endocrinol 2011;7(10) 596–607.
14. Capezzone M, Robenshtok E, Cantara S, et al. Familial non-medullary thyroid cancer: a critical review. J Endocrinol Investig 2021;44(5):943–50.

15. Kamihara J, Zhou J, LaDuca H, et al. Germline pathogenic variants in cancer risk genes among patients with thyroid cancer and suspected predisposition. Cancer Med 2022;11(8):1745–52.
16. Charkes ND. On the prevalence of familial nonmedullary thyroid cancer in multiply affected kindreds. Thyroid 2006;16(2):181–6.
17. Hińcza K, Kowalik A, Kowalska A. Current knowledge of germline genetic risk factors for the development of non-medullary thyroid cancer. Genes 2019; 10(7):482.
18. Wang X, Cheng W, Li J, et al. Endocrine tumours: familial nonmedullary thyroid carcinoma is a more aggressive disease: a systematic review and meta-analysis. Eur J Endocrinol 2015;172(6):R253–62.
19. Ringel MD, Sosa JA, Baloch Z, et al. American Thyroid Association Management Guidelines for adult patients with differentiated thyroid cancer. Thyroid 2025; 35(8):841–985.
20. National Comprehensive Cancer Network. Thyroid carcinoma (version 1.2025). 2025. Available at: https://www.nccn.org/guidelines.
21. Klubo-Gwiezdzinska J, Yang L, Merkel R, et al. Results of screening in familial non-medullary thyroid cancer. Thyroid 2017;27(8):1017–24.
22. Patel KN, Yip L, Lubitz CC, et al. The American Association of Endocrine Surgeons Guidelines for the definitive surgical management of thyroid disease in adults. Ann Surg 2020;271(3):e21–93.
23. Chenbhanich J, Atsawarungruangkit A, Korpaisarn S, et al. Prevalence of thyroid diseases in familial adenomatous polyposis: a systematic review and meta-analysis. Fam Cancer 2019;18(1):53–62.
24. Monachese M, Mankaney G, Lopez R, et al. Outcome of thyroid ultrasound screening in FAP patients with a normal baseline exam. Fam Cancer 2019; 18(1):75–82.
25. Dinarvand P, Davaro EP, Doan JV, et al. Familial adenomatous polyposis syndrome: an update and review of extraintestinal manifestations. Arch Pathol Lab Med 2019;143(11):1382–98.
26. Macken WL, Tischkowitz M, Lachlan KL. PTEN hamartoma tumor syndrome in childhood: a review of the clinical literature. Am J Med Genet C Semin Med Genet 2019;181(4):591–610.
27. Szabo Yamashita T, Baky FJ, McKenzie TJ, et al. Occurrence and natural history of thyroid cancer in patients with Cowden syndrome. Eur Thyroid J 2020;9(5): 243–6.
28. Milas M, Mester J, Metzger R, et al. Should patients with Cowden syndrome undergo prophylactic thyroidectomy? Surgery 2012;152(6):1201–10.
29. Schultz KAP, Rednam SP, Kamihara J, et al. PTEN, DICER1, FH, and their associated tumor susceptibility syndromes: clinical features, genetics, and surveillance recommendations in childhood. Clin Cancer Res 2017;23(12):e76–82.
30. Bouys L, Bertherat J. Management of endocrine disease: carney complex: clinical and genetic update 20 years after the identification of the CNC1 (PRKAR1A) gene. Eur J Endocrinol 2021;184(3):R99–109.
31. Bertherat J, Horvath A, Groussin L, et al. Mutations in regulatory subunit type 1A of cyclic adenosine 5′-Monophosphate-Dependent protein kinase (*PRKAR1A*): phenotype analysis in 353 patients and 80 different genotypes. J Clin Endocrinol Metabol 2009;94(6):2085–91.
32. Stratakis CA, Kirschner LS, Carney JA. Clinical and molecular features of the carney complex: diagnostic criteria and recommendations for patient evaluation. J Clin Endocrinol Metabol 2001;86(9):4041–6.

33. Oshima J, Martin GM, Hisama FM. Werner syndrome. In: Adam MP, Feldman J, Mirzaa GM, et al, editors. GeneReviews®. Seattle (WA): University of Washington 1993. Available at: http://www.ncbi.nlm.nih.gov/books/NBK1514/. Accessed Jul 23, 2025.
34. Ishikawa Y, Sugano H, Matsumoto T, et al. Unusual features of thyroid carcinoma in Japanese patients with Werner syndrome and possible genotype-phenotyp relations to cell type and race. Cancer 1999;85(6):1345–52.
35. Riascos MC, Huynh A, Faquin WC, et al. Expanding our knowledge of DICER gene alterations and their role in thyroid diseases. Cancers 2024;16(2):347.
36. Schultz KAP, Williams GM, Kamihara J, et al. DICER1 and associated conditions identification of At-risk individuals and recommended surveillance strategies. Cli Cancer Res 2018;24(10):2251–61.
37. Caroleo AM, De Ioris MA, Boccuto L, et al. DICER1 syndrome and cancer predis position: from a rare pediatric tumor to lifetime risk. Front Oncol 2020;10:61454
38. Fagin JA, Wells SA Jr. Biologic and clinical perspectives on thyroid cancer. N Engl J Med 2016;375(11):1054–67.
39. Kakarmath S, Heller HT, Alexander CA, et al. Clinical, sonographic, and patholog ical characteristics of RAS-positive versus BRAF-positive thyroid carcinoma. Clin Endocrinol Metab 2016;101(12):4938–44.
40. Durante C, Grani G, Lamartina L, et al. The diagnosis and management of thyroi nodules: a review. JAMA 2018;319(9):914–24.
41. Chu YH, Dias-Santagata D, Farahani AA, et al. Clinicopathologic and molecula characterization of NTRK-rearranged thyroid carcinoma (NRTC). Mod Patho 2020;33(11):2186–97.
42. Armstrong MJ, Yang H, Yip L, et al. PAX8/PPARγ rearrangement in thyroid nod ules predicts follicular-pattern carcinomas, in particular the encapsulated follic ular variant of papillary carcinoma. Thyroid 2014;24(9):1369–74.
43. Ghossein CA, Dogan S, Farhat N, et al. Expanding the spectrum of thyroid car cinoma with somatic DICER1 mutation: a survey of 829 thyroid carcinomas using MSK-IMPACT next-generation sequencing platform. Virchows Arch 2022;480(2) 293–302.
44. Brock P, Liynarachchi S, Nieminen TT, et al. *CHEK2* founder variants and thyroi cancer risk. Thyroid 2024;34(4):477–83.
45. Johansson K, Stenman A, Paulsson JO, et al. Development of metastatic poorl differentiated thyroid cancer from a sub-centimeter papillary thyroid carcinoma i a young patient with a germline MET mutation - association or random chance Thyroid Res 2021;14(1):19.
46. Tessaris D, Corrias A, Matarazzo P, et al. Thyroid abnormalities in children and adolescents with McCune-Albright syndrome. Horm Res Paediatr 2012;78(3) 151–7.
47. Le AN, Delaney T, McWilliams T, et al. Increased risk for thyroid carcinoma in pa tients with Li-Fraumeni syndrome. J Clin Orthod 2024;42(16_suppl):10612.
48. Del Rivero J, Gangi A, Annes JP, et al. American Association of Clinical Endocri nology Consensus statement on management of multiple Endocrine Neoplasia type 1. Endocr Pract 2025;31(4):403–18.
49. Brandi ML, Agarwal SK, Perrier ND, et al. Multiple endocrine neoplasia type 1 latest insights. Endocr Rev 2021;42(2):133–70.
50. Thakker RV. Multiple endocrine neoplasia type 1 (MEN1). Best Pract Res Clin En docrinol Metabol 2010;24(3):355–70.
51. Simonds WF, Li Y, Jha S. Genotype-phenotype correlations in the hyperparathyroidism jaw tumor syndrome. J Clin Endocrinol Metabol 2025;110(4):931–9.

52. Skefos CM, Waguespack SG, Perrier ND, et al. CDC73-Related disorders. In: Adam MP, Bick S, Mirzaa GM, et al, editors. GeneReviews®. Seattle (WA): University of Washington; 1993. Available at: http://www.ncbi.nlm.nih.gov/books/NBK3789/. Accessed January 23, 2026.
53. Cristina EV, Alberto F. Management of familial hyperparathyroidism syndromes: MEN1, MEN2, MEN4, HPT-Jaw tumour, Familial isolated hyperparathyroidism, FHH, and neonatal severe hyperparathyroidism. Best Pract Res Clin Endocrinol Metabol 2018;32(6):861–75.
54. Iacobone M, Camozzi V, Mian C, et al. Long-term outcomes of parathyroidectomy in hyperparathyroidism-jaw tumor syndrome: analysis of five families with *CDC73* mutations. World J Surg 2020;44(2):508–16.
55. Tora R, Welch J, Sun J, et al. Phenotypic profiling and molecular mechanisms in hyperparathyroidism-jaw tumor syndrome. J Clin Endocrinol Metabol 2023;108(12):3165–77.
56. Cetani F, Dinoi E, Pierotti L, et al. Familial states of primary hyperparathyroidism: an update. J Endocrinol Investig 2024;47(9):2157–76.
57. Figueiredo AA, Saramago A, Cavaco BM, et al. Familial parathyroid tumours—comparison of clinical profiles between syndromes. J Endocrinol Investig 2023;46(9):1799–806.
58. Singeisen H, Melanie Renzulli M, Pavlicek V, et al. Multiple endocrine neoplasia type 4: a new member of the MEN family. Endocrine Connections 2023;12(2):e220411.
59. Brock P, Kirschner L. Multiple endocrine neoplasia type 4. In: Adam MP, Bick S, Mirzaa GM, et al, editors. GeneReviews®. Seattle (WA): University of Washington; 1993. Available at: http://www.ncbi.nlm.nih.gov/books/NBK594826/. Accessed January 23, 2026.

Role of Genetics in Gastric Malignancy

Screening, Prevention and Treatment

Rui Zheng-Pywell, MD[a], Perry Shen, MD[b,*]

KEYWORDS

• Hereditary gastric cancer • Heritable genetic syndromes • Screening

KEY POINTS

- Prophylactic total gastrectomy is only recommended in pathogenic *CDH1* mutations with familial history of diffuse gastric cancer. All cases should be discussed at a multidisciplinary tumor board with input from genetics, endoscopy, and surgical oncology with subsequent shared decision making with the patient.
- Frequent, high-quality esophagogastroduodenoscopies at high-volume centers are necessary for all patients with increased lifetime risk of gastric cancer as a result of hereditary gastric cancer or any other hereditary cancer syndromes. Total gastrectomy should be pursued with any evidence suggestive of underlying malignancy.
- Germline genetic testing should be pursued in patients with qualifying personal or family history of malignancies for early detection of high-risk mutations for gastric adenocarcinoma. Recent data on multi-gene panel analysis of known gastric malignancies have identified germline DNA damage repair gene mutations to potentially play a role in the pathogenesis of gastric adenocarcinoma.

BACKGROUND

Gastric cancer is ranked fifth for incidence and cancer-related deaths worldwide.[1] The incidence of gastric malignancy is highest in East Asian countries with over half of global cases occurring in China.[2] The majority of gastric malignancies is sporadic though approximately 10% are found to have familial clustering. However, only 1% to 3% of cases are attributed to hereditary gastric cancer syndromes: hereditary diffuse gastric cancer (HDGC), gastric adenocarcinoma and proximal polyposis of the stomach (GAPPS), and familial intestinal gastric cancer (FIGC).[3]

[a] Department of Surgical Oncology, Atrium Health Wake Forest Baptist, Winston-Salem, NC, USA; [b] Department of Surgical Oncology kand HPB Surgery, Atrium Health Wake Forest Baptist, Winston-Salem, NC, USA
* Corresponding author.
E-mail address: Perry.Shen@wfusm.edu

Surg Clin N Am 106 (2026) 519–531
https://doi.org/10.1016/j.suc.2026.03.006 surgical.theclinics.com
0039-6109/26/

Abbreviations	
DDR	DNA damage repair
DGC	diffuse gastric cancer
FAP	familial adenomatous polyposis
FDP	fundic gland polyp
FIGC	familial intestinal gastric cancer
GA	gastric adenoma
HDGC	hereditary diffuse gastric cancer
GAPPS	gastric adenocarcinoma and proximal polyposis of the stomach
JPS	juvenile polyposis syndrome
NCCN	The National Comprehensive Cancer Network
PGA	pyloric gland adenoma

DISCUSSION

Hereditary Gastric Cancer Syndromes

Hereditary diffuse gastric cancer

HDGC was first identified in the Māori population due to familial clustering of disease. Further studies identified pathogenic mutations of the E-cadherin (*CDH1*) and alpha-E-catenin (*CTNNA1*) genes, contributing to extremely high risks of gastric cancer at a young age.[4–6] Patients with HDGC are estimated to have a cumulative risk of gastric cancer by age 80 years of 37.2% to 70.0%. Percentages vary by sex: 24.7% to 33.0% for females and 37.2% to 42.0% for males. Simultaneously, patients were at increased cumulative risk of lobular breast cancer (42.9%–56.0%), with similar familial patterns of inheritance.[7–9] *CDH1* mutations are also associated with increased incidence of congenital cleft lip and palate malformations, which are utilized as separate identifying risk factors for genetic screening (**Table 1**).[3,10] Per recent consensus guidelines, patients with identified risk factors for HDGC should first be screened for pathologic mutations in *CDH1*, but in the absence of germline mutation, it is recommended to proceed to *CTNNA1* screening (**Fig. 1**).

There is a limited role for surgical treatment outside of confirmed malignancy. The only indication for prophylactic gastrectomy is if the patient is a known carrier of a pathogenic variant of *CDH1* mutation with known family history of diffuse gastric cancer (DGC).[6] The 2015 American College of Gastroenterology guidelines had recommended pursuit of prophylactic gastrectomy in pathogenic *CDH1* carriers after age 20 years, but the 2020 updated clinical practice guidelines for HDGC did not recommend a specific age for surgical intervention.[6,11] Shared decision making to pursue a prophylactic total gastrectomy should be made after patient presentation at multidisciplinary team of experts (including genetics, endoscopy, and surgical oncology) with consideration for familial incidence of gastric cancer and patient preference.[9] A 2024 systemic review of quality of life post-gastrectomy reported a 19.2% major complication rate with a 0.3% mortality risk.[12] The NIH study found 42% of their patients with post-prophylactic total gastrectomy expressed regret, often as a result of postoperative complications and/or negative pathology for underlying malignancy.[13] In direct contrast, a study from the Columbia University found that all patients who underwent a total prophylactic gastrectomy would make the same decision, rating on long-term follow-up that they have a good quality of life despite ongoing difficulties with oral intake.[14]

Discussion of prophylactic surgery can be considered for patients with pathogenic *CTNNA1* mutations in the setting of family history or concerning endoscopic findings. Otherwise, gastrectomy is only favored in the setting of positive biopsy or suspected underlying malignancy based on signs, symptoms, or tissue characteristics on

Table 1
Clinical criteria and recommended screening and treatment of gastric adenocarcinoma syndromes

	Genetic Testing Criteria	Prevention and Treatment
Hereditary diffuse gastric cancer[6,9]	Family criteria: • ≥ 2 cases of gastric cancer in family regardless of age with at least 1 DGC • ≥ 1 case of DGC at any age and ≥ 1 case of lobular breast cancer at age <70 y in different family members • ≥2 cases lobular breast cancer in family member <50 y of age Individual Criteria • DGC age <50 y • DGC at any age for individuals of Māori ethnicity • DGC at any age in individuals with personal or first-degree relative with cleft lip or palate • History of DGC and lobular breast cancer, both diagnosed at age <70 y • Bilateral lobular breast cancer, diagnosed at age <70 y Endoscopic findings of gastric in situ signet ring cells or pagetoid spread of signet ring cells in individuals <50 y of age If *CDH1* testing is negative in those who qualify for genetic screening, then proceed to *CTNNA1* analysis	Known pathologic *CDH1* variant carriers with known familial DGC • Prophylactic total gastrectomy vs annual surveillance • Annual breast surveillance • Consider bilateral risk-reducing mastectomy with or without reconstruction Known pathologic *CDH1* variant carriers without known DGC with hereditary lobular breast cancer • Annual gastric surveillance • Consideration of prophylactic total gastrectomy • Annual breast surveillance • Consider bilateral risk-reducing mastectomy with or without reconstruction Known pathologic *CDH1* variant carriers without known DGC or breast cancer • Annual gastric surveillance • Consideration of prophylactic total gastrectomy • Annual breast surveillance *CHD1* variant of unknown significance or strong family history of gastric cancer • Consideration of annual gastric surveillance for at least 2 y • Prophylactic gastrectomy is not advised • Breast surveillance based on individual assessment

(*continued on next page*)

Table 1
(*continued*)

	Genetic Testing Criteria	Prevention and Treatment
		Known pathologic *CTNNA1* variant carriers without family history DGC or breast cancer • Consideration of annual gastric surveillance • Consideration of prophylactic total gastrectomy with positive family history or positive endoscopic biopsies • Breast surveillance based on individual assessment Gastrectomy is recommended for persistent signs, symptoms, or endoscopic findings associated with underlying malignancy
Gastric adenocarcinoma and proximal polyposis of the stomach[16]	Exclude use of proton pump inhibitors and presence of polyposis elsewhere in gastrointestinal tract prior to consideration of diagnosis Clinical criteria (both): • Phenotypical features: ◦ Proximal (body and fundus) gastric polyposis with antral sparing ◦ No evidence of colorectal or duodenal polyposis ◦ >100 polyps carpeting the proximal stomach in the index patient or >30 polyps in a first-degree relative ◦ Predominantly fundic gland polyps and/or fundic gland-like polyps • Family member with either dysplastic fundic gland polyps or gastric adenocarcinoma Supportive criteria (any): • Spectrum of histologic lesions: ◦ Hyperproliferative aberrant pits ◦ Hyperplastic polyps ◦ Gastric-type adenomas • Family history (autosomal dominance pattern of inheritance)	Endoscopic surveillance for GAPPS families is recommended by frequency and age of initiation should be decided on case-by-case basis. Colorectal surveillance should be considered in GAPPS families in the event there is family history of colon cancer. Prophylactic total gastrectomy should be considered in cases of high-grade dysplasia and progressive gastric polyposis though age for risk-reducing prophylactic gastrectomy should be decided on case-by-case basis.
Familial intestinal gastric cancer[25]	Any family with $\geq$2 gastric cancer cases with $\geq$1 intestinal histology of any age	No current standard

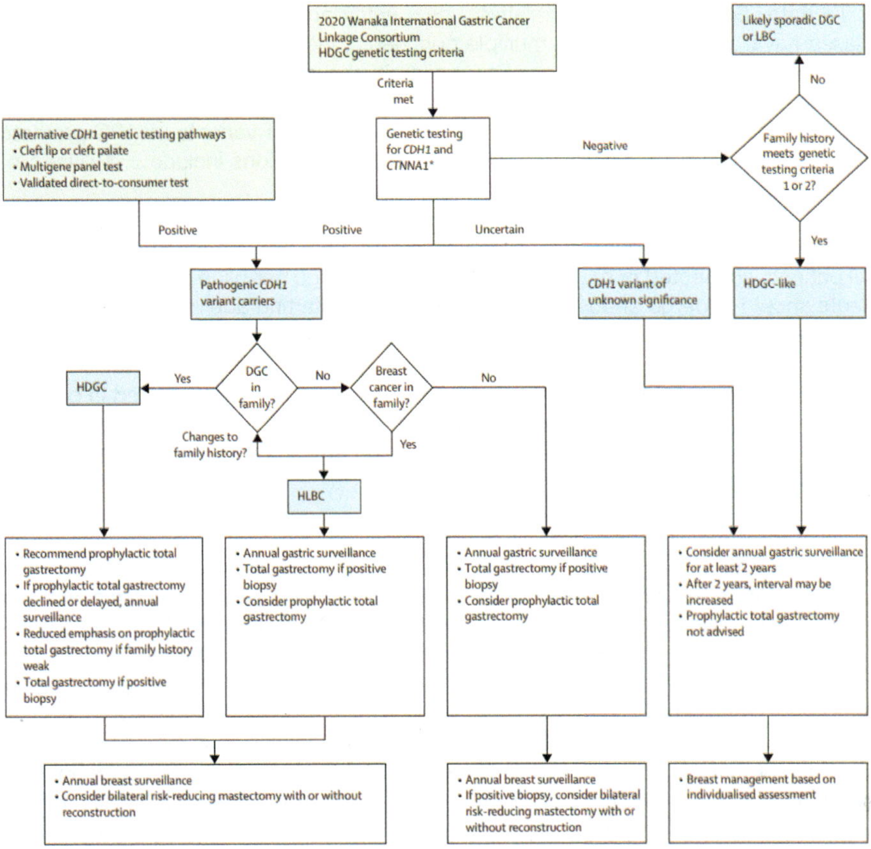

Fig. 1. 2020 Consensus guidelines regarding screening and treatment of Hereditary Diffuse Gastric Cancer (HDGC). *See **Table 1** for CTNNA1 pathway. (*Data from* Updated Clinical Practice Guidelines.[6]) [Reprinted with permission from Elsevier. The Lancet Oncology, 2020;21(8): e386-e97.]

endoscopy.[6,9] In the absence of known family history of DGC, annual endoscopic surveillance is the only recommendation (see **Fig. 1**). Surveillance can be tapered in the context of *CDH1* mutations of unknown significance. Patients can be followed annually for at least 2 years before decreasing frequency in the absence of significant findings. Endoscopic screenings in the setting of HDGC should composed of both targeted and random biopsies. A total of 28 to 30 random biopsies are recommended: 3 to 5 of the cardia, 5 of the fundus, 10 of the body, 5 involving the transition zone, and 5 of the antrum.[6]

Gastric adenocarcinoma and proximal polyposis of the stomach

GAPPS differs from HDGC in that penetrance is usually incomplete, and patients symptomatic from autosomal dominant transmission are found to have fundic gland polyposis restricted to the proximal stomach with no evidence of colorectal or duodenal polyposis in the absence of other hereditary cancer syndromes.[3] Endoscopic findings of hyperproliferative aberrant pits are unique to GAPPs and is considered the earliest marker of dysplasia.[15] The presence of duodenal adenomas should raise suspicion of attenuated familial adenomatous polyposis (FAP) instead of GAPPS.[16]

To date, GAPPS remains a relatively new entity and additional study is required. Cases have been identified on multiple continents, including North America, Europe, Australia, and Asia. The incidence of adenocarcinoma is 12% to 15% with age of onset varying between 22 and 75 years.[17–21] Genetic analysis from a familial case series revealed there may be a pathogenic role for heterozygous variants of *APC* promoter 1B on chromosome 5. Specific putative pathogenic mutations include c.-191T>C, c.-192A>G, and c.-195A>C.[9,17,21–24]

The 2024 European guidelines for clinical management of polyposis syndromes have basic recommendations for the clinical screening and management of GAPPS. All patients suspected of having GAPPS should undergo germline genetic testing. Patients should undergo endoscopic surveillance with starting age dependent on youngest age of gastric cancer within the family (intervals not yet determined). In the setting of additional colorectal cancer history within the family, colorectal surveillance should also be considered. Prophylactic gastrectomy should only be considered in cases of high-grade dysplasia and progressive polyposis though evidence is lacking regarding appropriate timing or patient age. All decisions on endoscopic and surgical interventions should be made on a case-by-case basis.[16]

Familial intestinal gastric cancer

FIGC is similar to GAPPS in that both are autosomal dominant, though the genetic origin of FIGC remains unclear despite being identified as a syndromic entity in 1999.[25] It is associated with increased risk of intestinal-type gastric cancer in the absence of gastric polyposis, often occurring 10 years earlier than in patients with sporadic disease with increased incidence of up to 18 different associated malignancies. It is currently hypothesized to be polygenic on both germline and somatic levels, distinct from sporadic cases.[26] Two culprits identified thus far include heterozygous mutations found in *IL12RB1* as well as *TP53*.[26,27] No strong recommendations currently exist for screening, surveillance, or intervention in patients with FIGC, though a Spanish group recently evaluated the role of surveillance endoscopy noting an incidence of 4.9% (2 patients out of 41) of precancerous lesions within their cohort of initially healthy individuals from 31 families. Only one case was found to have progression to gastric cancer over 9 years. Of note, the authors identified *Helicobacter pylori* to be a strong independent predictor of dysplasia with an odds ratio of 6.4 (1.3–30.6, P=.02), which may be confounding their surveillance findings.[28]

Other Hereditary Cancer Syndromes Associated with Gastric Cancer

In addition to the 3 hereditary gastric cancer syndromes, gastric malignancies are on the spectrum of several other hereditary syndromes (**Table 2**).

Hereditary nonpolyposis colorectal cancer (Lynch syndrome)

Lynch syndrome, otherwise known as hereditary nonpolyposis colorectal cancer, is caused by germline mutations in mismatch repair genes (*MLH1*, *MSH2*, *MSH6*, *PMS2*, and *EPCAM*). However, only select mutations were found to increase lifetime risk of gastric cancer (see **Table 2**).[29] The average age of diagnosis is 52 years old with a cumulative risk of gastric cancer through age 80 years of 0.2% to 9%. The highest rates are seen with *MSH2* and *MLH1* mutations with lifetime risks of 9% and 4.8% respectively.[30–33] Aside from primary gastrointestinal malignancies, Lynch also predisposes toward endometrial, ovarian, urothelial, prostate, sarcoma, and central nervous system malignancies.[9] In patients with Lynch, there is no recommendation for prophylactic gastrectomy, however, taking a daily aspirin is advised to reduce risk of colorectal malignancies.

Table 2
Other hereditary cancer syndromes with increased spectrum of gastric cancer

Syndrome	Gene Mutations	Absolute Risk	Gastric Cancer Screening and Treatment[9]
Lynch	*MLH1* *MSH2* *MSH6* *EPCAM*	0.2%–9.0%	High-quality esophagoduodenoscopy with extended duodenal examination starting at age 30–40 y and repeating every 2–4 y • Consideration for earlier surveillance or more frequent interval on case-by-case basis based on family history or high-risk endoscopic findings • Random biopsies of *H pylori*, autoimmune gastritis, and intestinal metaplasia
FAP	*APC*	0.1%-7.1%	High-quality esophagoduodenoscopy starting at age 20–25 y with surveillance timing pending endoscopic findings of polyp size, type, and dysplasia

Peutz-Jeghers	*STK11*	29%	Pediatric surveillance
			• Esophagoduodenoscopy with polypectomy starting between ages 8 and 10 y
			  ○ If polyps are found, repeat every 2–3 y (shorter intervals may be indicated based on polyp size, number, and pathology)
			  ○ If no polyps, resume surveillance at age 18
			  ○ Initiation of endoscopy sooner than age 8 or after initial screening endoscopy if having signs of iron deficiency anemia or gastrointestinal bleeding
			Adult surveillance
			• Esophagoduodenoscopy every 2–3 y (shorter intervals may be indicated based on polyp size, number, and pathology)

Li-Fraumeni	*TP53*	10.7%	High-quality esophagoduodenoscopy every 2–5 y starting at 20–25 y old • Initiation of endoscopy 5 y earlier than earliest known gastric cancer in the family in patients with known family history of gastric cancer earlier than 20 y old
Juvenile Polyposis Syndrome	*SMAD4*	≤ 21%	Pediatric surveillance • Esophagoduodenoscopy starting between ages 12–15 y old ○ Initiation of endoscopy sooner than age 12 y if having signs of iron deficiency anemia or gastrointestinal bleeding Adult surveillance • Esophagoduodenoscopy every 1–3 y (shorter intervals may be indicated based on polyp size, number, and pathology) • Gastrectomy should be considered if polyp burden or symptoms are unable to be managed endoscopically

Familial adenomatous polyposis

FAP involves an *APC* mutation that can lead to a large volume of polyps within the gastrointestinal tract including the gastric fundus, antrum, and duodenum. Approximately 5% of untreated upper gastrointestinal tract adenomas can progress onto malignancy.[3] The cumulative risk for diagnosis of gastric cancer in patients with FAP through age 80 years ranges from 0.1% to 7.1%, but there is a notable difference in incidence between Western and Asian populations. Prior studies noted that Western patient populations with FAP had no difference in incidence of gastric cancer compared to the general population (0.1%–0.8%) while Asian populations had an increased frequency ranging between 4% and 7%.[25,34,35] Despite that, surveillance of the duodenum results in gastric evaluation, and frequency is determined by a variant of Spigelman criteria as seen in the National Comprehensive Cancer Network (NCCN) guidelines.[9]

FAP can result in gastric polyps of multiple premalignant histologies: fundic gland polyps (FDPs), gastric adenomas (GAs), pyloric gland adenomas (PGAs), or proximal polypoid mounds. Should any of the above subtypes demonstrate high-grade dysplasia, 3 to 6 month surveillance at an expert center is recommended and surgical evaluation for gastrectomy candidacy should be considered, especially in the setting of multifocal disease. Otherwise, surveillance strategies differ depending on the histology. Proximal polypoid mounds without high-grade dysplasia should be surveilled every 3 to 6 months regardless of size. In contrast, patients with GAs or PGAs of any size can be screened on a yearly basis unless a piecemeal extraction is needed or a degree of polyposis requiring multiple procedures for resection is found. Then frequency of screening is increased to every 6 months. Finally, in patients with FDPs, surveillance is titrated according to size. Polyps less than 1 cm without dysplasia can be surveyed ever 3 years. In FDPs 1 cm or greater in size without high-grade dysplasia, yearly endoscopic surveillance is recommended with increased frequency to every 6 months should endoscopy find a polyp requiring piecemeal extraction or a degree of polyposis requiring multiple procedures for resection.[9]

Peutz-Jeghers

Peutz-Jeghers is a syndrome resulting from STK11 mutations leading to hamartomatous polyp formation in the gastrointestinal tract along with increased risk of predominantly gastrointestinal and breast cancer. Lifetime risk for gastric cancer is high at 29%. Screening recommendations vary by age (see **Table 2**). Children are at higher risk of reproductive organ malignancies and screening for abnormalities should begin at time of diagnosis. Additional organs with increased risk include pancreas, cervix, uterus, and lung. Gastrointestinal screening begins in childhood but in the absence of abnormal symptoms or findings, serial surveillance should resume at the age of 18 years per adult criteria (see **Table 2**).[9]

Li-Fraumeni

Li-Fraumeni syndrome is an autosomal dominant condition that can be inherited or arise de novo without family history. Additionally, within individuals with germline *TP53* mutations, there can be post-zygotic mosaicism that limits the tissues predisposed to malignant transformation.[36] The classic spectrum of associated malignancies includes breast, soft tissue sarcoma, osteosarcoma, central nervous system, adrenocortical carcinoma, melanoma, and prostate. Disease onset tends to occur at a young age with the initial malignancy before the age of 45 years and second primary prior to the age of 55 years.[9] In the setting of screening for upper gastrointestinal cancers, these patients are found to have high grade dysplasia by the age of 25 years, and most malignancies were of epithelial origin.[37] Thus far, no relationship has been identified between the locus of mutation with predictable malignancies (ie, age of onset and familial patterns of organs involved).[38]

Juvenile polyposis syndrome

Similar to Peutz-Jeghers, juvenile polyposis syndrome (JPS) is an autosomal dominant disorder involving *SMAD4* or *BMPR1A* mutations leading to pathologic hamartomatous polyp formation.[9,39] Of the two associated mutations, only *SMAD4* is associated with increased lifetime risk of gastric cancer.[39,40] A clinical diagnosis of JPS can be considered in any patient with any one of the following: 5 or greater juvenile polyps of the colon, multiple juvenile polyps throughout gastrointestinal tract, or any number of juvenile polyps in an individual with positive family history. In addition to gastric cancer, JPS is associated with increased risk of colorectal cancer.[9] Screening surveillance practices, like in Peutz-Jeghers, is split into pediatric and adult practices. Initial gastrointestinal screening begins in adolescence (ages 12–15 years) but in the absence of abnormal symptoms or findings, serial surveillance should resume at the age of 18 years per adult criteria (see **Table 2**).

FUTURE CONSIDERATIONS

Genetic Screening Criteria and Implications Moving Forward

The NCCN criteria for genetic testing for the hereditary cancer syndromes with increased incidence of gastrointestinal malignancy are strict on qualifications for screening and limited by patient knowledge of family history. A prospective multicenter study led by Mayo noted that 80% of patients with upper gastrointestinal malignancies (esophageal, gastroesophageal junction, and gastric cancer) found to have pathologic germline variants identified via universal multi-gene panel would not have been tested by standard screening guidelines.[41] Pathologic germline variants were noted in 17.6% of patients with gastric cancer. These patients had a high penetrance of mutations in DNA damage repair (DDR) genes associated with hereditary cancer syndromes not thought of as associated with increased spectrum of gastric malignancies (such as *BRCA1*, *BRCA2*, *ATM*, and *PALB2*).[36,41] This was similarly replicated by a separate international, collaborative group when looking at gastric malignancy alone. Patients with gastric cancer were screened for germline mutations, and 6% were found to have variants in *BRCA1*, *BRCA 2*, *ATM*, *PALB2*, *CHEK2*, *RAD51C*, *RAD51D*, *MLH1*, and *PMS2*.[42]

These genetic findings have practical implications on the treatment of the underlying upper gastrointestinal malignancies. A group looking into the presence of DNA damage repair germline mutations in gastroesophageal adenocarcinoma notes that ex vivo testing of tumors from patients harboring *BRCA2* germline mutations (even variants classified as benign) had improved response to platinum-based agents and the PARP inhibitor olaparib. Clinical features of patients from which the xenografts were derived also suggested the *BRCA2* mutation was clinically significant in observed aggressiveness and treatment response of the malignancy.[43] However, data are still limited in what this may mean for future guidelines on genetic testing for upper gastrointestinal malignancies, though these findings may explain the gap between the percentage of familial gastric cancers and the incidence of known hereditary gastric cancers.

SUMMARY

Gastric cancer is a leading cause of cancer-related deaths worldwide. The incidence of disease has improved since the advent of *H pylori* testing and treatment. However, information about genetics of gastric malignancies remains limited. While most gastric cancer is sporadic in nature, approximately 10% of cases are clustered in families of which only 1% to 3% can be attributed to hereditary gastric cancer syndromes. Criteria for germline genetic testing for both hereditary gastric cancer syndromes and other hereditary genetic syndromes with increased risk of gastric cancer remain strict. However, ongoing work using multi-gene panels to identify high-risk mutations in gastric cancer has identified new relationships between germline DNA damage repair mutations and disease behavior with implications for future genetic screening processes and therapeutic modalities.

CLINICS CARE POINTS

- Prophylactic total gastrectomy is only recommended in pathogenic *CDH1* mutations with familial history of DGC. All cases should be discussed at a multidisciplinary tumor board with input from genetics, endoscopy, and surgical oncology with subsequent shared decision making with the patient.
- Frequent, high-quality esophagogastroduodenoscopies at high-volume centers are necessary for all patients with increased lifetime risk of gastric cancer as a result of hereditary gastric cancer or any other hereditary cancer syndromes. Total gastrectomy should be pursued with any evidence suggestive of underlying malignancy.
- Germline genetic testing should be pursued in patients with qualifying personal or family history of malignancies for early detection of high risk mutations for gastric adenocarcinoma. Recent data on multi-gene panel analysis of known gastric malignancies have identified germline DNA damage repair gene mutations to potentially play a role in the pathogenesis of gastric adenocarcinoma.

REFERENCES

1. Bray F, Laversanne M, Sung H, et al. Global cancer statistics 2022: GLOBOCAN estimates of incidence and mortality worldwide for 36 cancers in 185 countries. CA Cancer J Clin 2024;74(3):229–63 [published Online First: 20240404].
2. Global Burden of Diseases I, and Risk Factors Study 2017 Stomach Cancer Collaborators. The global, regional, and national burden of stomach cancer in 195 countries, 1990-2017: a systematic analysis for the Global Burden of Disease study 2017. Lancet Gastroenterol Hepatol 2020;5(1):42–54. https://doi.org/10.1016/s2468-1253(19)30328-0 [published Online First: 20191021].
3. Oliveira C, Pinheiro H, Figueiredo J, et al. Familial gastric cancer: genetic susceptibility, pathology, and implications for management. Lancet Oncol 2015;16(2): e60–70.
4. Majewski IJ, Kluijt I, Cats A, et al. An α-E-catenin (CTNNA1) mutation in hereditary diffuse gastric cancer. J Pathol 2013;229(4):621–9.
5. Guilford P, Hopkins J, Harraway J, et al. E-cadherin germline mutations in familial gastric cancer. Nature 1998;392(6674):402–5.
6. Blair VR, McLeod M, Carneiro F, et al. Hereditary diffuse gastric cancer: updated clinical practice guidelines. Lancet Oncol 2020;21(8):e386–97.
7. Xicola RM, Li S, Rodriguez N, et al. Clinical features and cancer risk in families with pathogenic CDH1 variants irrespective of clinical criteria. J Med Genet 2019;56(12):838–43 [published Online First: 20190711].
8. Hansford S, Kaurah P, Li-Chang H, et al. Hereditary diffuse gastric cancer syndrome: CDH1 mutations and beyond. JAMA Oncol 2015;1(1):23–32.

9. Network NCC. Genetic/Familial High-Risk Assessment: Colorectal, endometrial, and gastric (version 1.2025). Secondary Genetic/Familial High-Risk Assessment: Colorectal, Endometrial, and Gastric (Version 1.2025. 2025. Available at: https://www.nccn.org/professionals/physician_gls/pdf/genetics_ceg.pdf.
10. Frebourg T, Oliveira C, Hochain P, et al. Cleft lip/palate and CDH1/E-cadherin mutations in families with hereditary diffuse gastric cancer. J Med Genet 2006;43(2): 138–42 [published Online First: 20050414].
11. Syngal S, Brand RE, Church JM, et al, American College of Gastroenterology. ACG clinical guideline: genetic testing and management of hereditary gastrointestinal cancer syndromes. Am J Gastroenterol 2015;110(2):223, 62; quiz 63 [published Online First: 20150203].
12. Lim HJ, di Pietro M, O'Neill JR. A systematic review on clinical and health-related quality of life outcomes following total gastrectomy in patients with hereditary diffuse gastric cancer. Cancers (Basel) 2024;16(3). https://doi.org/10.3390/cancers16030473 [published Online First: 20240123].
13. Gamble LA, Grant RRC, Samaranayake SG, et al. Decision-making and regret in patients with germline CDH1 variants undergoing prophylactic total gastrectomy. J Med Genet 2023;60(3):241–6 [published Online First: 20220711].
14. Stillman MD, Kusche N, Toledano S, et al. Short and long-term outcomes of prophylactic total gastrectomy in 54 consecutive individuals with germline pathogenic mutations in the CDH1 gene. J Surg Oncol 2022;126(8):1413–22 [published Online First: 20220905].
15. de Boer WB, Ee H, Kumarasinghe MP. Neoplastic lesions of gastric adenocarcinoma and proximal polyposis syndrome (GAPPS) are gastric phenotype. Am J Surg Pathol 2018;42(1):1–8.
16. Zaffaroni G, Mannucci A, Koskenvuo L, et al. Updated European guidelines for clinical management of familial adenomatous polyposis (FAP), MUTYH-associated polyposis (MAP), gastric adenocarcinoma, proximal polyposis of the stomach (GAPPS) and other rare adenomatous polyposis syndromes: a joint EHTG-ESCP revision. Br J Surg 2024;111(5). https://doi.org/10.1093/bjs/znae070.
17. Worthley DL, Phillips KD, Wayte N, et al. Gastric adenocarcinoma and proximal polyposis of the stomach (GAPPS): a new autosomal dominant syndrome. Gut 2012;61(5):774–9 [published Online First: 20110803].
18. Beer A, Streubel B, Asari R, et al. Gastric adenocarcinoma and proximal polyposis of the stomach (GAPPS) - a rare recently described gastric polyposis syndrome - report of a case. Z Gastroenterol 2017;55(11):1131–4 [published Online First: 20171115].
19. Repak R, Kohoutova D, Podhola M, et al. The first European family with gastric adenocarcinoma and proximal polyposis of the stomach: case report and review of the literature. Gastrointest Endosc 2016;84(4):718–25 [published Online First: 20160623].
20. Yanaru-Fujisawa R, Nakamura S, Moriyama T, et al. Familial fundic gland polyposis with gastric cancer. Gut 2012;61(7):1103–4 [published Online First: 20111025].
21. Foretová L, Navrátilová M, Svoboda M, et al. GAPPS - Gastric adenocarcinoma and proximal polyposis of the stomach syndrome in 8 families tested at Masaryk Memorial Cancer Institute - Prevention and prophylactic gastrectomies. Klin Onkol 2019;32(Supplementum2):109–17.

22. Dixon K, Senz J, Kaurah P, et al. Rare APC promoter 1B variants in gastric cancer kindreds unselected for fundic gland polyposis. Gut 2021;70(7):1415–6 [published Online First: 20200907].
23. Sakuma T, Sera T, Aoyama R, et al. Two families with gastric adenocarcinoma and proximal polyposis of the stomach (GAPPS): case reports and literature review. J Gastrointest Oncol 2023;14(6):2650–7 [published Online First: 20231102].
24. Li J, Woods SL, Healey S, et al. Point mutations in exon 1B of APC reveal gastric adenocarcinoma and proximal polyposis of the stomach as a familial adenomatous polyposis variant. Am J Hum Genet 2016;98(5):830–42 [published Online First: 20160414].
25. Carneiro F. Familial and hereditary gastric cancer, an overview. Best Pract Res Clin Gastroenterol 2022;58-59:101800. https://doi.org/10.1016/j.bpg.2022.101800 [published Online First: 20220504].
26. Carvalho J, Oliveira P, Senz J, et al. Redefinition of familial intestinal gastric cancer: clinical and genetic perspectives. J Med Genet 2021;58(1):1–11 [published Online First: 20200217].
27. Vogelaar IP, van der Post RS, van de Vosse E, et al. Gastric cancer in three relatives of a patient with a biallelic IL12RB1 mutation. Fam Cancer 2015;14(1):89–94.
28. Llach J, Salces I, Guerra A, et al. Endoscopic surveillance for familial intestinal gastric cancer in low-incidence areas: an effective strategy. Int J Cancer 2024;154(1):124–32 [published Online First: 20230907].
29. Capelle LG, Van Grieken NC, Lingsma HF, et al. Risk and epidemiological time trends of gastric cancer in Lynch syndrome carriers in the Netherlands. Gastroenterology 2010;138(2):487–92 [published Online First: 20091110].
30. Møller P, Seppälä TT, Bernstein I, et al. Cancer risk and survival in path_MMR carriers by gene and gender up to 75 years of age: a report from the prospective Lynch syndrome database. Gut 2018;67(7):1306–16 [published Online First: 20170728].
31. Bonadona V, Bonaïti B, Olschwang S, et al. Cancer risks associated with germline mutations in MLH1, MSH2, and MSH6 genes in Lynch syndrome. JAMA 2011;305(22):2304–10.
32. Engel C, Loeffler M, Steinke V, et al. Risks of less common cancers in proven mutation carriers with Lynch syndrome. J Clin Oncol 2012;30(35):4409–15 [published Online First: 20121022].
33. Watson P, Vasen HFA, Mecklin JP, et al. The risk of extra-colonic, extra-endometrial cancer in the Lynch syndrome. Int J Cancer 2008;123(2):444–9.
34. Offerhaus GJ, Giardiello FM, Krush AJ, et al. The risk of upper gastrointestinal cancer in familial adenomatous polyposis. Gastroenterology 1992;102(6):1980–2.
35. Shibata C, Ogawa H, Miura K, et al. Clinical characteristics of gastric cancer in patients with familial adenomatous polyposis. Tohoku J Exp Med 2013;229(2):143–6.
36. Network NCC. Genetic/Familial High-Risk Assessment: Breast, Ovarian, pancreatic, and Prostate (Version 2.2026). Secondary Genetic/Familial High-Risk Assessment: Breast, Ovarian, pancreatic, and Prostate (Version 2.2026). 2026. Available at: https://www.nccn.org/professionals/physician_gls/pdf/genetics_bopp.pdf#page=59&zoom=100,0,0.
37. Hatton JN, de Andrade KC, Frone MN, et al. Spectrum and excess risk of gastrointestinal tumors in Li-Fraumeni syndrome. Clin Gastroenterol Hepatol 2024;22(3):662–5.e1 [published Online First: 20230914].

38. Masciari S, Dewanwala A, Stoffel EM, et al. Gastric cancer in individuals with Li-Fraumeni syndrome. Genet Med 2011;13(7):651–7.
39. Muller M, Baldysiak E, Benech N, et al. Deciphering the clinical spectrum of gastric disease in patients with juvenile polyposis syndrome. Gastrointest Endosc 2024;100(5):867–77 [published Online First: 20240520].
40. Singh AD, Gupta A, Mehta N, et al. Occurrence of gastric cancer in patients with juvenile polyposis syndrome: a systematic review and meta-analysis. Gastrointest Endosc 2023;97(3):407–14.e1 [published Online First: 20221018].
41. Uson PLS Jr, Kunze KL, Golafshar MA, et al. Germline cancer testing in unselected patients with gastric and esophageal cancers: a multi-center prospective study. Dig Dis Sci 2022;67(11):5107–15 [published Online First: 20220205].
42. Guerra J, Estrada-Florez AP, Lott PC, et al. The role of multi-organ cancer predisposition genes in the risk of inherited and histologically diverse gastric cancer. EBioMedicine 2025;116:105759. https://doi.org/10.1016/j.ebiom.2025.105759 [published Online First: 20250529].
43. Petrelli A, Rizzolio S, Pietrantonio F, et al. BRCA2 germline mutations identify gastric cancers responsive to PARP inhibitors. Cancer Res 2023;83(10):1699–710.

Pancreatic Cancer

Genetics, Screening, Prevention, and Treatment

Sami O. Abul-Khoudoud, MD[a,*], Jeffrey M. Hardacre, MD[a,b,*]

KEYWORDS

• Pancreatic cancer • Genetics • Targeted therapy • Familial pancreatic cancer
• Screening

KEY POINTS

- Pancreatic cancer (PC), particularly pancreatic ductal adenocarcinoma (PDAC), is among the deadliest malignancies, largely due to late-stage presentation.
- Core driver mutations include *KRAS*, *CDKN2A*, *TP53*, and *SMAD4*; these alterations are present in the majority of sporadic pancreatic ductal adenocarcinoma cases.
- Pathogenic germline variants (eg, BRCA1/2, PALB2, and STK11) underlie hereditary pancreatic cancer syndromes; familial pancreatic cancer also occurs in the absence of an identifiable mutation.
- Advances in molecular profiling and targeted therapy have allowed for the development of precision medicine regimens for small subsets of patients with PC.
- Screening is currently recommended only for high-risk populations due to PC's low incidence and a lack of validated early biomarkers in the general population.

INTRODUCTION

Despite substantial advances in molecular characterization and targeted therapeutics, pancreatic cancer remains among the most lethal malignancies in the United States, with pancreatic ductal adenocarcinoma (PDAC) being the sixth leading cause of cumulative mortality despite being the 12th most common malignancy.[1] The prognosis of patients diagnosed with PC remains poor, with a 5-year survival of approximately 13% for all types of pancreatic cancer, and is even worse for PDAC, the most common histologic subtype, accounting for approximately 90% of all pancreatic malignancies, with a 5-year survival rate of approximately 8%.[1–3] This reflects, in part, complex genetic, epigenetic, and tumor microenvironment alterations that confer proliferative and

[a] Department of Surgery, Division of Surgical Oncology, University Hospitals, Cleveland Medical Center, 11100 Euclid Avenue, Cleveland, OH 44106, USA; [b] Case Western Reserve University School of Medicine, Cleveland, OH, USA
* Corresponding authors.
E-mail addresses: Sami.Abul-Khoudoud@UHhospitals.org (S.O.A.-K.); Jeffrey.Hardacre@uhhospitals.org (J.M.H.)

Surg Clin N Am 106 (2026) 533–553
http://dx.doi.org/10.1016/j.suc.2026.03.009 surgical.theclinics.com
0039-6109/26/

Abbreviations	
AGA	American Gastroenterological Association
ASGE	American Society for Gastrointestinal Endoscopy
CDKN2A	cyclin-dependent kinase inhibitor 2A
CI	confidence interval
DDR	DNA damage response
EMT	epithelial-to-mesenchymal transition
FAMMM	familial atypical multiple mole melanoma
FPC	familial pancreatic cancer
HP	hereditary pancreatitis
HRR	homologous recombination repair
KRAS	Kirsten rat sarcoma
MMR	mismatch repair
NCCN	National Comprehensive Cancer Network
PanIN	pancreatic intraepithelial neoplasia
PC	pancreatic cancer
PDAC	pancreatic ductal adenocarcinoma
PJS	Peutz–Jeghers syndrome
Rb	Retinoblastoma
RTKs	receptor tyrosine kinases
SPINK1	serine protease inhibitor Kazal-type 1
TGF-β	transforming growth factor-beta

survival advantages for neoplasms in an otherwise hostile growth environment. While sporadic and familial forms of PDAC may share similar molecular features at their core, the mechanisms underlying their tumorigenesis may cause differences within their risk profiles and present unique susceptibilities. Recent advances in high-throughput sequencing, multiomic integration, and single-cell technologies have substantially improved our understanding of PDAC biology, including identification of driver mutations, new genetic alterations, and the prognostic and therapeutic significance of molecular subtypes. This article reviews the molecular genetics of sporadic and familial pancreatic cancer (PC) and their management implications.

SPORADIC PANCREATIC DUCTAL ADENOCARCINOMA: MOLECULAR GENETICS AND PATHOGENESIS

PDAC develops through stepwise genetic and epigenetic alterations, progressing from precursor lesions such as pancreatic intraepithelial neoplasia (PanIN) to invasive carcinoma.[4–6] Many factors, genetic and otherwise, drive this progression. Among the most frequently mutated genes are Kirsten rat sarcoma *(KRAS)*, cyclin-dependent kinase inhibitor 2A (*CDKN2A)*, tumor protein p53 (*TP53)*, and SMAD family member 4 (Mothers against decapentaplegic homolog 4) *(SMAD4)*. These 4 genes are considered the core driver mutations and are present in most sporadic PDAC.[5,6] These core driver mutations promote PDAC pathogenesis through chromosomal, metabolic, and epigenetic remodeling, thereby driving genomic instability, transcriptional reprogramming, and the progressive accumulation of additional oncogenic alterations. **Fig. 1** illustrates the key pathways involved in the development of PDAC from premalignant lesion to invasive adenocarcinoma.

Among risk factors for sporadic PC, smoking is the strongest modifiable risk factor, with an OR of 1.74 (95% confidence interval [CI] 1.61–1.87) for current smokers when compared to never smokers.[6,7] In population attributable fraction analyses, smoking accounts for an estimated approximately 19% to 24% of sporadic PDAC.[8] Other factors include chronic pancreatitis, which has a pooled relative risk (RR) of 13.3

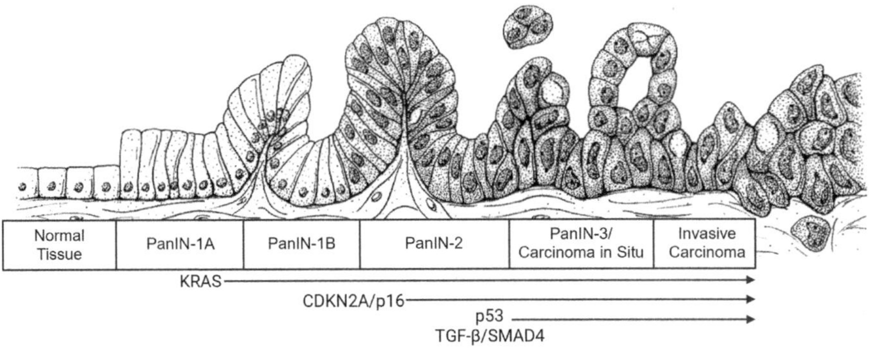

Fig. 1. Progression of pancreatic ductal adenocarcinoma, the PanINgram. (Anirban Maitra et al., Multicomponent Analysis of the Pancreatic Adenocarcinoma Progression Model Using a Pancreatic Intraepithelial Neoplasia Tissue Microarray, Modern Pathology, 16 (9), 2003, 902-912, https://doi.org/10.1097/01.MP.0000086072.56290.FB.[50])

(CI 6.1–28.9), obesity with an RR of 1.54 (CI 1.04–2.29) for individuals in the highest body mass index quintile, and type 2 diabetes mellitus, both new-onset and long-standing (odds ratio [OR] 1.57–1.80).[4,7] Heavy alcohol consumption, male sex, Black race, and exposure to heavy metals and chemicals are also correlated with higher incidence.[2]

Kirsten Rat Sarcoma Signaling Pathway

The *KRAS* gene (12p) is a proto-oncogene that has been identified as mutated in approximately 88% to 95% of PDAC.[9,10] *KRAS* mutations occur early in PDAC tumorigenesis, as they are present in the vast majority of PanIN lesions.[6,11] *KRAS* encodes a small GTPase that functions as a molecular switch in the Rat sarcoma virus (as in KRAS)/Mitogen-activated protein kinase *(RAS/MAPK)* signaling pathway. Mutation of *KRAS* results in constitutive activation of downstream signaling pathways, including the *MAPK* (Rapidly accelerated fibrosarcoma/Mitogen-activated protein kinase kinase/extracellular signal-regulated kinase [*RAF-MEK-ERK*]) and Phosphoinositide 3-kinase/Protein kinase B (*PI3K-AKT*) cascades, promoting uncontrolled proliferation, survival, metabolic reprogramming, and a tumorigenic microenvironment (**Fig. 2**). *KRAS* activity also supports desmoplasia and immune evasion with the recruitment of suppressive myeloid cells and stromal activation (eg, sonic hedgehog [*SHH*] and transforming growth factor-beta [*TGF-β*]).[9] Mutations most often occur at codon 12 (90%–98%), and less often occur at codons 13 (~5%–7%) and 61 (~4%–7%), with G12D mutation being most common.[12]

Its central role in the development of PDAC has made *KRAS* a primary target in the development of therapeutics. While KRAS has long been considered a difficult therapeutic target, emerging allele-specific inhibitors (eg, sotorasib for *KRAS* G12C and MRTX1133 for *KRAS* G12D) have shown promising preclinical activity and are being assessed in early phase clinical studies.[13] Resistance to monotherapy in preclinical studies with *KRAS* inhibitors has been shown to emerge via downstream reactivation, parallel signaling, or adaptations within the tumor microenvironment.[2,9,12] Combination strategies pairing *KRAS* inhibitors with Src homology region 2 domain-containing phosphatase-2 (*SHP2*), son of sevenless homolog 1 (*SOS1*), or B-cell lymphoma-extra large (*BCL-XL)* degraders are currently in preclinical or early phase clinical trials. More recently, RMC-6236 a pan-RAS(ON) multiselective inhibitor that targets active,

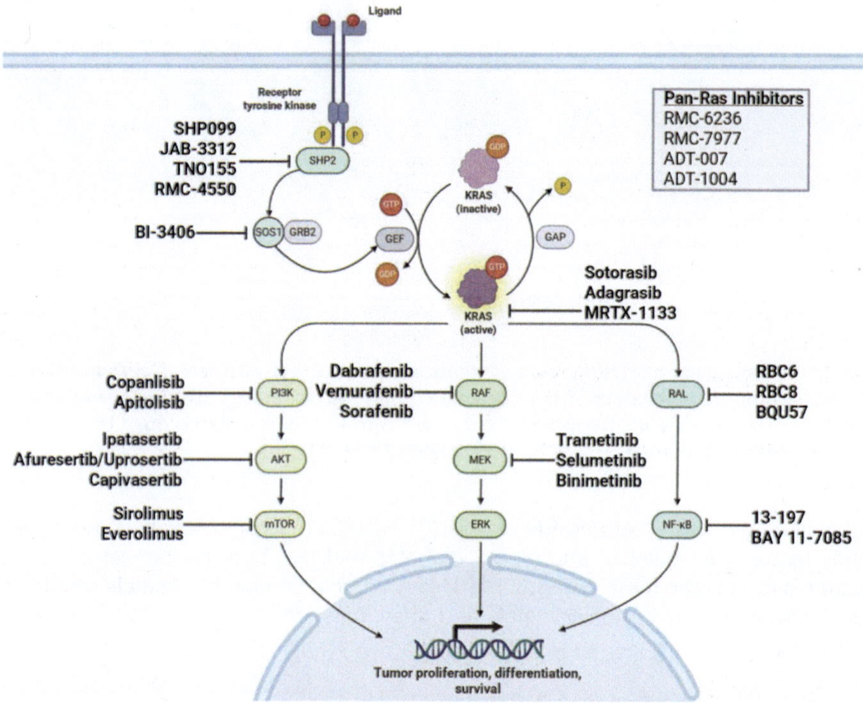

Fig. 2. Representation of the KRAS signaling cascade, with nonexhaustive list of existing targeted inhibitors. (*Created in* BioRender. Abul-Khoudoud, S. (2026) BioRender.com/asgquyl.)

GTP-bound RAS across multiple mutant alleles common in PDAC, has demonstrated early clinical activity, further expanding strategies for direct RAS inhibition.[14]

Cyclin-dependent Kinase Inhibitor 2A and Its Role in Cell Cycle Regulation

The cyclin-dependent kinase inhibitor 2A (*CDKN2A*) gene (9p21) is inactivated in approximately 90% to 95% of PDAC tumors by deletion, mutation, or promoter hypermethylation.[15] Through alternative reading frames, *CDKN2A* encodes 2 tumor suppressors: p16(INK4a) and p14(ARF). The tumor suppressor p16(INK4a) restrains the G1 to S transition via the inhibition of *CDK4/6*-mediated phosphorylation of the retinoblastoma (*Rb*) protein. Alternatively, p14(ARF) triggers a p53-mediated checkpoint response, inducing cell cycle arrest in both G1 and G2/M. Loss of *CDKN2A* function results in impaired activity of its encoded tumor suppressors, p16(INK4a) and p14(ARF). This deactivation corresponds to unchecked *CDK4/6* activity, which leads to *Rb* hyperphosphorylation, resulting in uncontrolled cellular proliferation.[16] The loss of *CDKN2A* is nearly universal in PDAC and is considered a rate-limiting step in carcinogenesis, driving the transition from precursor lesion (PanIN-2/3) into an invasive carcinoma.[4]

Therapeutic strategies focusing on downstream targets of the *CDKN2A* cascade, such as *CDK4/6* (eg, palbociclib), or multi-*CDK* inhibitors (eg, dinaciclib) have been studied in PC in the context of *CDKN2A* loss or inactivation. These inhibitors have demonstrated limited efficacy in preclinical models; while they have been able to induce G1 cell cycle arrest, these models have demonstrated limited response to single-agent therapy, developing resistance early, including through the loss of the

Rb protein.[17] Combination strategies, such as *CDK4/6* inhibitors with taxanes or *MEK* inhibitors have been demonstrated to enhance antitumor effects while also preventing recovery from chemotherapy-induced damage in preclinical models.[3,17] Biomarker-driven approaches, such as in *Rb*-deficient tumors, may help identify appropriate patients for these therapies, though this research is ongoing.

TP53: Maintaining Genomic Stability

TP53 (17p) encodes the p53 tumor suppressor and is mutated in approximately 50% to 75% of PDAC.[2,4] Unlike *KRAS* and *CDKN2A*, which are commonly altered early in PanIN development and contribute to tumor initiation, *TP53* mutations are typically acquired later and contribute primarily to malignant transformation and disease progression. Accordingly, they are more frequently detected in advanced precursor lesions and invasive disease. In its wild-type state, it acts as a central tumor suppressor via several mechanisms that collectively maintain genomic stability. It has been shown to limit acinar-to-ductal metaplasia, suppress proliferation of PanIN cells, and dampen oncogenic *KRAS* signaling, preventing progression to PDAC.[18] Inactivation of p53 allows premalignant cells to evade cell-cycle checkpoints, ultimately allowing for unchecked proliferation. Beyond loss of tumor-suppressive functionality, mutant p53 may acquire protumorigenic gain-of-function properties, promoting metastasis, enhancing metabolic adaptation, and facilitating establishment of a tumor microenvironment that promotes malignant proliferation and survival.[19]

Pharmacologic restoration of wild-type *TP53* functionality has not been achieved clinically in PC.[20,21] Small molecule therapies, such as p53 reactivation and induction of massive apoptosis (PRIMA-1) and reactivation of p53 and induction of tumor cell apoptosis (RITA), have been able to restore wild-type p53 function in vitro and in preclinical models, though these have not been approved for clinical use in PC to date. Early clinical trials of p53-reactivating agents have not demonstrated efficacy in PC and have had variable efficacy in broader oncologic trials, presumably due to the diverse functions encompassed by p53 as well as tumor stromal factors.[20,21] Study surrounding appropriate patient selection and optimization of these therapeutics is still ongoing.

The Transforming Growth Factor-beta Pathway: Transforming Growth Factor-beta/SMAD4

TGF-β signaling has context-dependent tumor-suppressive and protumorigenic roles in PDAC. Under normal physiologic conditions, *TGF-β* functions as a context-dependent, tumor-suppressive cytokine that inhibits epithelial cell proliferation and induces apoptosis through *SMAD*-dependent pathways.[22] Alterations in the *TGF-β* pathway include mutations in *TGFBR2* (3p; ~4%–7%), as well as frequent inactivation of downstream mediators, particularly *SMAD4* (~50%–60%). As PDAC progresses through carcinogenesis, cancer cells typically develop mutations along the *SMAD*-dependent pathways, causing *TGF-β* to shift into a protumorigenic role.[23,24] Once the transition to invasive carcinoma has been established, overexpression of this pathway continues to promote the survival of the tumor by inducing the epithelial-to-mesenchymal transition (EMT). EMT allows the tumor to increase its motility, invasiveness, and ability to disseminate from the primary tumor; further, this leads to intratumoral heterogeneity and cancer stem cell-like properties, driving resistance to therapies and disease recurrence.[25,26] This transition leads to perineural and lymphovascular invasion as well as angiogenesis within the tumor. Consequently, PC tends to metastasize early in its course, further contributing to its poor prognosis.[26]

As a central mediator of the *TGF-β* signaling cascade, *SMAD4* (18q) serves as a tumor suppressor, as well as a transcription factor. Under normal physiologic conditions, following *TGF-β* activation, *SMAD4* interacts with receptor-activated *SMADs* (such as *SMAD2/3*), ultimately regulating transcription of genes that regulate cell growth, apoptosis, and differentiation.[22,23] It is inactivated in approximately 50% to 60% of PC cases, usually due to inactivating mutation or deletion. While the loss of *SMAD4* is not typically one which precipitates early tumorigenesis, it does facilitate tumor progression, particularly following other oncogenic mutations such as those discussed previously. Removing this last barrier to malignant proliferation, the loss of *SMAD4* enables rapid progression from PanIN into invasive carcinoma. Its loss, similar to the loss of *TGF-β*, also drives EMT, increasing the tumor's metastatic capacity and therapeutic resistance.[22,23]

TGF-β pathway inhibitors are currently under development, with the goal of modulating the immunosuppressive stroma found within PDAC, as well as modulating tumor-stroma interactions. Recent preclinical studies have demonstrated that *SMAD4*-deficient PC may be susceptible to *TGF-β* inhibition.[24,25,27,28] In animal models, inhibition with neutralizing antibodies has demonstrated decreased tumor burden and improved survival in these *SMAD4*-deficient tumors. There is currently interest in coinhibition of *SMAD4* with *TGF-β*, or *TGF-β* inhibitors with immunotherapy or chemotherapy, though no *TGF-β* pathway inhibitor has received regulatory approval for PDAC currently.[24,28]

Other Key Molecular Pathways and Their Therapeutic Implications

Additional pathways (epigenetic regulation, DNA damage response [DDR], Wingless-related integration site/neurogenic locus notch homolog protein [WNT/NOTCH], axon guidance, and receptor tyrosine kinases [RTKs]) contribute to PDAC progression and treatment resistance and may offer targeted opportunities. **Table 1** summarizes more common genetic and epigenetic alterations involved in the pathogenesis of PDAC, but a detailed discussion is beyond the scope of this article.[2,6]

FAMILIAL SYNDROMES ASSOCIATED WITH PANCREATIC CANCER

Familial syndromes and predispositions account for approximately 5% to 10% of PDAC cases. These syndromes are defined by pathogenic germline variants in genes that increase predisposition to malignancy, conferring risk for PDAC as well as other malignancies.[29] These are broadly known as hereditary cancer syndromes, such that patients have a genetically increased susceptibility to multiple types of malignancy, versus familial pancreatic cancer (FPC), in which individuals have at least 2 first-degree relatives who have had PC in the absence of a known hereditary cancer syndrome. The genetic etiology of these cancers may help us better target our therapies toward their underlying pathways. The familial syndromes associated with PC can be found in **Table 2**.

Per National Comprehensive Cancer Network (NCCN) Hereditary Cancer Testing Criteria (version 1.2026), testing for hereditary cancer is generally recommended in individuals who (1) have a blood relative with a known pathologic or likely pathologic variant in a cancer susceptibility gene; (2) have a pathologic/likely pathologic gene variant on tumor genomic testing with clinical implications if also identified in the germline; (3) may benefit from systemic therapy or to aid surgical decision-making; (4) individuals meeting prior criteria but testing negative with prior limited testing; (5) meet Li-Fraumeni syndrome testing criteria, Cowden syndrome/Phosphatase and tensin homology (PTEN) hamartoma tumor syndrome testing criteria, or Lynch

Table 1
Key molecular pathways and therapeutic targets in pancreatic cancer

Pathway/ Category	Mechanism	Key Genes	Physiologic Function	Function in Pancreatic Cancer	Clinical Implications	Targeted Therapies
Core driver mutations	*KRAS/RAS-MAPK* and *PI3K*	*KRAS*[5,9,11,12]	Functions as a "switch" for growth signaling	Becomes constitutively activated, promoting growth, survival, and metabolism pathways	Present in ~90%–95% of PDAC; occurs early in PanIN progression. Drives resistance to many therapies	Allele-specific *KRAS* inhibitors (eg, MRTX1133 and sotorasib); combination therapies with *SHP2*, *SOS1*, and *BCL-XL*
	Cell-cycle regulator (G1 -> S transition)	*CDKN2A*, *CDK4/6*, and *RB1*[5,11,16,27]	G1/S transition checkpoint	Inactivation results in unchecked *CDK4/6* activity, causing *RB1* hyperphosphorylation and unmitigated proliferation	Inactivated in ~90%–95% of PDAC tumors; drives PanIN2/3 transition, results in invasive adenocarcinoma	*CDK4/6* inhibitors (eg, palbociclib); used in combination with taxanes, *MEK* inhibitors
	Genomic stability (TP53 checkpoint)	*TP53*[5,11,21]	DNA damage sensing, arrest/ apoptosis of cells with significant DNA damage	Loss/gain-of-function mutations yield progression of premalignant lesions, protumorigenic tumor microenvironment	Mutated in 50%–75% of PDAC, later in PanIN progression	p53 reactivators (PRIMA-1, RITA) in preclinical/early trials; no approved therapeutics to date

(*continued on next page*)

Table 1
(continued)

Pathway/ Category	Mechanism	Key Genes	Physiologic Function	Function in Pancreatic Cancer	Clinical Implications	Targeted Therapies
	TGF-β signaling/ EMT regulation	*TGFBR2* and *SMAD4*[22–25,28]	Regulates epithelial growth inhibition and differentiation via *SMAD*-mediated transcription	Context-dependent shift toward EMT, invasion, stromal remodeling, and immune suppression; loss of *SMAD4* accelerates progression and metastatic potential	Loss of function in ~50%–60% of tumors; associated with tumor progression and metastatic potential	*TGF-β* inhibitors (preclinical); no approved use in PDAC
Epigenetic regulation	Chromatin remodeling	PBRM1, KDM6A, ARID1A, and SWI/SNF complex[5,11,51–53]	Regulate DNA accessibility, gene expression, and cell differentiation	Epigenetic dysregulation results in altered gene expression, early PanIN progression, and therapy resistance	Associated with aggressive disease; reversible nature offers biomarker and therapeutic potential	DNMT/G9a dual inhibitor CM272; HDAC inhibitors (eg, panobinostat); other chromatin-modifying enzyme inhibitors
	DNA/histone modification	DNMT1, G9a, and UHRF1[54,55]				
DNA damage repair	Homologous recombination repair (HRR)	BRCA1, BRCA2, PALB2, ATM, and CHEK2[3,30–32]	Maintain genomic stability and repair double-strand breaks	Loss of normal DNA repair pathways yield genomic instability, and tumor progression	HRR-deficient tumors sensitive to platinum chemo; germline testing recommended per ESDO/NCCN	PARP inhibitors (eg, olaparib); PARP + ATR/ATM/CHEK inhibitor combination therapy (investigational)
	MMR	MLH1, MSH2, MSH6, and PMS2[3,27,34,56–58]				

Developmental signaling	WNT/β-catenin	RNF43 and WNT ligands (eg, WNT7B)[59,60]	Pancreatic development and stem cell maintenance	Aberrant activation, especially in KRAS WT tumors → proliferation, EMT, and chemoresistance	Predictor of aggressive biology; often mutually exclusive with KRAS mutations	PORCN inhibitors (ETC-159, LGK-974), WNT-pathway inhibitors (early trials)
	NOTCH	NOTCH1 and NOTCH2[61,62]	Regulates differentiation in pancreatic development	Upregulated in PanIN/PDAC → increased proliferation, angiogenesis; mixed oncogenic/tumor-suppressive roles depending on receptor	Potential biomarker for aggressive subtypes	Gamma-secretase inhibitors (MRK-003, PF-03084014); combination therapy with JAK/STAT or mTOR inhibitors
Axon guidance pathways	Axon guidance and perineural invasion pathways	ROBO/SLIT family, EPH/EPHRIN, semaphorins, and netrins[63–65]	Guide axonal pathfinding during neural development	Promote tumor migration, perineural invasion, stromal remodeling → increased pain and recurrence	Strong link to PNI, aggressive growth, and metastatic spread	EPH/ephrin inhibitors (antibodies, ligand traps, and small molecules); inhibitors of semaphorins/netrins (preclinical)
RTKs	Growth factor receptor pathways	EGFR, MET, ERBB3, PDGFRA, AXL, and MerTK[3,9,66,67]	Cell growth, differentiation, and survival signaling	Overexpression/activation → MAPK and PI3K pathway activation, EMT, stromal fibrosis, and immune suppression	EGFR inhibition is minimally effective in unselected PDAC; rare RTK fusions are actionable	Erlotinib (EGFR); NTRK fusions → larotrectinib/entrectinib; ALK → crizotinib/ensartinib; NRG1 fusions → afatinib, zenocutuzumab

(*continued on next page*)

Table 1
(*continued*)

Pathway/ Category	Mechanism	Key Genes	Physiologic Function	Function in Pancreatic Cancer	Clinical Implications	Targeted Therapies
Classic/ Actionable genes	HER2/ERBB2	HER2/ERBB2[68,69]	RTK involved in growth signaling	Amplification drives tumorigenesis, esp. KRAS WT	Seen in 2%–8% of PDAC; benefit mostly in KRAS wild-type	Trastuzumab, HER2-directed combinations (investigational)
	BRAF pathway	BRAF V600E[70,71]	MAPK pathway activation	Oncogenic driver in KRAS WT tumors	Present in ~1%–3%; potentially targetable	BRAF/MEK inhibitors (eg, vemurafenib, trametinib, and selumetinib)
Metabolic Vulnerabilities	Mitochondrial metabolism	HOGA1[72]	Hydroxyproline metabolism in mitochondria, producing pyruvate and glyoxylate[73–75]	Role not yet well-established; presumed to play intermediary role in metabolism and redox homeostasis	HOGA1 loss promotes tumor growth via LARP7-CDK1 pathway	No inhibitors developed thus far
Novel gene targets	Cell-cycle regulation	ADAM9[76,77]	Regulates cell adhesion	Overexpression increases metastatic potential	Overexpression in PDAC is correlated with poor differentiation and significantly shorter overall survival	Multiple targeted therapeutic approaches in preclinical and early clinical development
		CDK1[78]	Regulates G2/M transition of cell cycle	Promotes cell division and survival in PC		Early investigation; inhibition may chemosensitize and radiosensitize PC

Abbreviations: AXL, AXL receptor tyrosine kinase; BRAF, B-raf proto-oncogEne, serine/threonine kinase; EGFR, epidermal growth factor receptor; EPH, erythropoietin-producing hepatocellular; ERBB3, erb-b2 receptor tyrosine kinase 3; EPHRIN, eph family receptor interacting protein; HER2/ERBB2, human epidermal growth factor receptor 2/erb-b2 receptor tyrosine kinase 2; JAK/STAT, janus kinase/signal transducer and activator of transcription; MET, mesenchymal-epithelial transition factor; MerTK, MER tyrosine kinase; mTOR, mechanistic target of rapamycin; PDGFRA, platelet-derived growth factor alpha; PNI, perineural invasion; PORCN, por-

Table 2
Familial pancreatic cancer syndromes and their associated genetics, risks, clinical implications

Syndrome/Category	Gene(s)	Physiologic Function	Pancreatic Cancer Risk/ Behavior	Additional Cancer Risks	Clinical Implications
Hereditary breast and ovarian cancer syndrome	BRCA1, BRCA2, and PALB2[31–33]	Homologous recombination DNA repair	BRCA1: RR 1.6–2.4; BRCA2: RR 2.5–6.6; PALB2: RR 3.5–6.2. Lifetime PDAC risk: BRCA2 ~2.7%, BRCA1 ~2.2%	Breast, ovarian, and prostate cancers	Higher sensitivity to platinum-based chemotherapeutics and PARP inhibitors
Lynch syndrome	MLH1, MSH2, MSH6, PMS2, and EPCAM[34,38]	MMR	8.6 fold increased risk; ~3.7% lifetime risk by age 70 y	Colorectal, endometrial, ovarian, gastric, small bowel, urinary tract, and skin cancers	Strong response to checkpoint inhibitors
FAMMM	CDKN2A (p16INK4A)[16,35]	Cell-cycle regulation (G1/S checkpoint)	RR 13–39; lifetime risk 5%–24%	Melanoma, nonmelanoma skin cancers, and pancreatic neuroendocrine tumors	High-risk families require early pancreatic screening
PJS	STK11[37,38]	Tumor suppression, cellular metabolism and polarity	RR 132; lifetime PDAC risk 11%–36%; average onset 41–52 y	Breast, colon, gastric, ovarian, lung, and small bowel	Requires intensive multiorgan surveillance
HP	PRSS1 and SPINK1[39–41]	PRSS1: trypsinogen activation; SPINK1: trypsin inhibition	RR 53–87; lifetime risk 7.2%–40%; mean PDAC diagnosis ~55 y	No established increase in nonpancreatic cancers	Early onset chronic pancreatitis with cumulative damage Screening recommended in adulthood

(*continued on next page*)

Table 2
(*continued*)

Syndrome/Category	Gene(s)	Physiologic Function	Pancreatic Cancer Risk/ Behavior	Additional Cancer Risks	Clinical Implications
Ataxia-telangiectasia	ATM[42]	DDR and cell-cycle checkpoint control	3–9 fold increased PDAC risk; lifetime risk ~6.3% by age 70 y	Lymphoid cancers (leukemia, lymphoma), breast, prostate, and gastric cancers	May respond to DDR-targeted therapeutics
FPC	Unknown/ polygenic (autosomal dominant pattern suspected)[29,43]	N/A	Lifetime risk 8%–12% (6.4 fold increase) Accounts for 4%–10% of PDAC	Not routinely associated with other cancers	Unexplained inherited susceptibility

syndrome. Specific to PC, the NCCN further recommends testing in individuals with exocrine PCs, including acinar cell carcinoma, as well as first-degree relatives of individuals diagnosed with exocrine PC.[30]

Hereditary Breast and Ovarian Cancer Syndrome

Mutations to breast cancer type 1 susceptibility protein (*BRCA*)*1/2* and *PALB2* are found in 5% to 17% of familial PDACs. *BRCA1* mutation confers the lowest risk of PDAC with an RR of 1.6 to 2.4. *BRCA2* confers a higher risk, with RR of 2.5 to 6.6, and some standardized incidence ratios as high as 5.8. *BRCA2* carriers are estimated to have an approximately 2.7% lifetime risk of PC compared to 2.2% for *BRCA1* carriers. *PALB2* mutations are less extensively studied, but confer a risk like that of *BRCA2,* with an OR of approximately 3.1 and RR of 3.5 to 6.2. Patients with these germline mutations are also at an increased risk for breast, ovarian, and prostate cancers.[31–33] These PDAC subtypes are more susceptible to poly(ADP-ribose) polymerase (PARP) inhibitors as well as platinum-based chemotherapeutics.[3,6,27]

Lynch Syndrome

Germline mutations to DNA mismatch repair (MMR) genes (MutL homolog 1 [*MLH1*], MutS homolog 2 [*MSH2*], MutS homolog 6 [*MSH6*], PMS1 homolog 2, mismatch repair system component [*PMS2*]), and Epithelial cellular adhesion molecule [*EPCAM*] have been found to have an 8.6 fold increased risk of PC compared to the general population, with a lifetime cumulative risk of 3.7% by the age of 70 years. This risk may be further increased in individuals who have a family history of PC or dependent on the specific MMR gene affected. Other malignancies associated with Lynch syndrome include colorectal, endometrial, ovarian, gastric, small bowel, urinary tract, and skin cancer, with variable risks dependent on a multitude of factors. PC associated with these mutations tends to display more responsiveness to immune checkpoint blockade due to microsatellite instability, with response rates ranging from 18% to 50% in recent studies.[34] As a result, assessment of MMR and microsatellite instability status should be used to guide therapy in patients with Lynch syndrome.

Familial Atypical Multiple Mole Melanoma Syndrome

Familial atypical multiple mole melanoma (FAMMM) syndrome, defined as germline mutation to *CDKN2A*, confers a relative risk of 13 to 39 times higher than the general population of PC. This risk is associated with pathogenic mutations causing impaired *p16INK4* protein function; kindreds without this impairment do not demonstrate an increased risk of PC. Unlike patients with wild-type germline *CDKN2A*, in whom progression from PanIN to invasive cancer requires sequential accumulation of multiple mutations, those with germline *CDKN2A* mutations rapidly progress into invasive PC following oncogenic *KRAS* mutation.[35] Patients with these mutations have a lifetime risk estimated between 5% and 24% by the age of 75 years, more pronounced in families with p16-Leiden mutation.[36] This syndrome is also strongly associated with multiple nevi causing a substantially increased risk of melanoma, as well as nonmelanoma skin cancers and, less commonly, pancreatic neuroendocrine tumors.

Peutz–Jeghers Syndrome

Peutz–Jeghers syndrome (PJS) is an autosomal dominant syndrome, defined by germline mutations of the *STK11* gene. Patients with this syndrome have a 15 to 18 fold increased lifetime risk of malignancy. This syndrome confers a relative risk of 132 (CI 44–261) compared to the general population of developing PC, with a lifetime risk between 11% and 36% and a mean age of diagnosis between 41 and

52 years.[37] This syndrome is also associated with substantially increased risk for other malignancies: from highest to lowest risk, these include breast (54% lifetime), colon (39%), gastric (29%), ovarian (21%), lung (15%), and small intestinal (13%).[38]

Hereditary Pancreatitis

Hereditary pancreatitis (HP) is an autosomal dominant disorder, most often characterized by mutation to serine protease 1 (*PRSS1*), which encodes cationic trypsinogen. This disorder demonstrates incomplete penetrance, with studies on penetrance varying by mutation but estimated to be about 80% overall.[5,36,39] Serine protease inhibitor Kazal-type 1 (*SPINK1*) mutation is also associated with HP, acting as a modulator of the disease, conferring increased risk in patients with HP. *SPINK1* mutations alone are not usually sufficient enough to drive the disease but have been associated with a lower threshold for the development of pancreatitis in the presence of additional genetic and environmental factors.[30,36,40] Patients with HP demonstrate a significantly increased risk of PC compared to the background population (RR 53–87), with cumulative lifetime risk ranging from 7.2% to 40% depending on the specific mutation.[29,39] The average age at diagnosis of PDAC in patients with HP is approximately 55 years.[39] The presence of modifiable risk factors synergistically increases the risk of these patients developing PC.[41] Unlike other hereditary cancer syndromes previously described, HP does not confer an increased risk for nonpancreatic malignancies.[39,41]

Ataxia-telangiectasia

Ataxia-telangiectasia is an autosomal recessive syndrome, characterized by germline pathogenic mutations to the DDR gene, *ATM*. Patients with ataxia-telangiectasia have an increased risk of PC, with a risk approximately 3-to-9 fold increase over the general population, and a lifetime risk of 6.3% by the age of 70 years.[42] This syndrome is associated with a broad spectrum of malignancies, including lymphoid cancers (Hodgkin/non-Hodgkin lymphoma and acute leukemias), as well as breast, prostate, and gastric malignancies.[30,42]

Familial Pancreatic Cancer and Emerging Genetic Associations

In addition to the more established genetic associations previously described, FPC is defined as a genetic predisposition to PC, identified as having 2 or more first-degree relatives with PDAC, not meeting criteria for other hereditary cancer syndromes. The lifetime risk for developing PC in individuals with FPC is 8% to 12%, a 6.4 fold increase, when 2 first-degree relatives are affected; this increases to 40% (32 fold increase) with 3 or greater affected relatives.[29] FPC accounts for about 4% to 10% of all PDAC cases.[29] Segregation analyses suggest an autosomal dominant inheritance pattern in FPC, with heritability estimates as high as 51% despite no known mutation.[29] Ultimately, FPC likely represents an aberrant genetic pathway or pathways that have yet to be described. Given the absence of a known mutation-driving FPC, genetic testing is not currently possible, and risk assessment relies on family history.

SCREENING AND EARLY DETECTION OF PANCREATIC CANCER

Given PC cannot reliably be prevented, the most appropriate treatment strategy relies on early detection during stages in which PC is potentially curable. The goal of current screening and surveillance plans is oriented toward identifying early malignant or premalignant lesions and curatively resecting them.[30,36,43]

Screening in Average-risk (Sporadic) Individuals

Population-based screening for PC in average-risk individuals is not currently recommended, due to its low incidence, lack of proven mortality benefit with screening, and the potential for false positives to cause harm.[43] However, several ongoing studies are investigating targeted screening approaches in individuals who may have transiently increased risk. The Early Detection Initiative is a large randomized controlled trial oriented toward evaluating algorithm-based screening in patients aged over 50 years with new-onset diabetes, using the enriching new-onset diabetes for pancreatic cancer (ENDPAC) risk scoring system to select individuals for CT screening, with the goal of detecting PDAC at earlier, more treatable stages.[44] Another study, the Pancreatic Cancer Early Detection in New-Onset Diabetes (PANDOME) study, is prospectively enrolling patients aged over 50 years with new-onset or worsening diabetes for MRI-based screening.[45] The recently published Multimetabolite signature for Pancreatic Cancer (METAPAC) study also identified plasma-based metabolic signatures, in conjunction with CA 19-9, for noninvasive exclusion of PDAC in patients with newly discovered pancreatic lesions or new-onset diabetes, noting 2 plasma-based metabolic signatures demonstrated significant improvement in exclusion of PDAC when compared to CA 19-9 alone.[46]

Screening of High-risk (Familial/Hereditary) Individuals

Selective surveillance has been deemed to be appropriate for individuals at significantly increased risk due to their genetic susceptibility or strong family history. Per the NCCN, American Society for Gastrointestinal Endoscopy (ASGE), and the American Gastroenterological Association (AGA), surveillance is recommended for high-risk individuals with pathogenic germline variants in genes associated with an increased risk of PC. Per these guidelines, the screening should be managed by experienced, high-volume PC centers within research protocols when feasible.[29,30,47]

Screening Modalities and Intervals

The NCCN, ASGE, and AGA recommend initiation of screening in high-risk populations beginning at the age of 50 years, or 10 years younger than the earliest diagnosed PC in the family. The exception to this is PJS, in which screening should begin as early as 35 years of age. Annual surveillance with EUS and/or MRI/Magnetic resonance cholangiopancreatography (MRCP) is the current standard screening regimen for high-risk patients. There is no consensus on the superiority of endoscopic ultrasound (EUS) when compared to MRI, with both modalities demonstrating similar performance in the detection of early stage PDAC and high-risk precursor lesions.[30,47]

Efficacy and Harms of Current Screening Regimens

Observational studies, prospective cohorts, and meta-analyses have demonstrated earlier detection of PDAC in high-risk individuals, with a higher proportion diagnosed at surgically resectable stages when compared to unscreened cohorts, with an associated survival advantage.[48] The Multicenter Cancer of Pancreas Screening-5 Study reported that 77.8% of PDACs detected during surveillance within their cohort were detected at stage I, with a significant improvement in 5 year survival rate for screen-detected cases compared to the unscreened cohort (73.3% 5 year survival, median OS 9.8 years versus 1.5 year median OS).[49] Importantly, however, the NCCN, ASGE, and AGA have emphasized that current screening regimens do not demonstrate a clear benefit in reducing mortality from PC, and may instead bring harm to the patient, such as with false positives, unnecessary procedures, psychological distress, and procedural complications.[29,30,43] Despite the overall safety of these screening regimens in the detection of PC, these modalities detect high-risk lesions at a low frequency, predicted at about 0.8%, with most identified lesions being low-risk or intermediate-risk lesions such as branch-duct intraductal papillary mucinous neoplasms. Reported complication rates are low in experienced centers, and both EUS and MRI are generally well tolerated within structured surveillance programs, with most risk attributable to sedation or invasive sampling rather than diagnostic imaging itself.[43,47] Per cost-effectiveness analyses by the ASGE, screening may demonstrate cost efficacy in individuals with lifetime risk exceeding 5%, but this is dependent on the prevalence of actionable lesions, the specificity of available imaging modalities, and the cost of surveillance and downstream interventions as indicated.[47]

Limitations of Screening and Ongoing Research

Currently, no randomized controlled trial evidence has demonstrated reduction in PDAC-specific mortality despite advances in the sensitivity of surveillance technology; further, optimal screening intervals, modalities, and duration are not yet well-described. These screening regimens are costly, with lack of access to specialized programs, and surveillance may have a psychosocial impact on patients' well-being. There are no consensus guidelines for the management of indeterminate or intermediate-risk pancreatic lesions, and this remains a clinical uncertainty.[43]

The lack of validated biomarkers for early detection of PDAC remains one of the most significant limitations of current screening regimens. Ongoing research focusing on validating novel biomarkers, as well as refining risk prediction models and integrating multiomic approaches may help improve the sensitivity and specificity of early detection. Ultimately, with a paucity of clear evidence guiding our decision-making, a shared decision-making model as well as substantial counseling regarding the risks and benefits of screening are recommended in the navigation of these disease processes.[30,43]

CONTROVERSIES AND KNOWLEDGE GAPS

Despite significant ongoing advances in our understanding of PC, several unresolved knowledge gaps as well as some controversies regarding the molecular genetics and targeted therapy for PDAC persist. These include

- Limited clinical efficacy in targeted therapies for most patients, including for common driver mutations (*KRAS* and *TP53*).
- Rapidly evolving resistance to targeted therapies driven by pathway redundancy, compensatory signaling, and the tumor microenvironment.
- Inadequate preclinical models with limited translatability of preclinical success.
- Limited benefit of immunotherapies except for rare molecular subgroups.
- Lack of validated biomarkers for patient selection, response monitoring, and early detection in sporadic disease.

SUMMARY

PDAC is a complex disease process, driven by genetic alterations that promote tumor initiation, progression, and therapeutic resistance. A core set of driver genes and pathways have been identified by foundational research, and recent studies have continued to build upon our understanding of the additional genetic, epigenetic, metabolic, and signaling pathway alterations that contribute to the complexity of this disease process. Translational implications remain limited in clinical application, largely due to rapidly developing resistance to targeted therapy as well as inadequate preclinical models. Ultimately, ongoing research and innovative clinical trials are essential to improve outcomes for patients with PDAC, through early detection via surveillance and personalized medicine approaches.

CLINICS CARE POINTS

- Pearl: Germline testing is recommended for all individuals diagnosed with exocrine pancreatic cancer, as well as their first-degree relatives, to help guide potential targeted therapies and surgical decision-making.
- Pearl: Assess MMR and MSI status in patients with Lynch syndrome-associated pancreatic cancer, as these tumors demonstrate significantly higher response rates to immune checkpoint inhibitors.
- Pearl: Prioritize smoking cessation counseling in preventative care; smoking remains the strongest modifiable risk factor, accounting for an estimated 19 to 24% of sporadic PDAC cases.
- Pitfall: Do not rely on genetic testing to assess or rule out FPC; due to the lack of a specific driving mutation, clinical risk assessment must rely instead on a thorough family history.
- Pitfall: Do not recommend routine population-based screening for average-risk individuals; the low incidence of the disease and lack of validated early biomarkers lead to a high risk of false positives, psychological distress, and unnecessary invasive procedures.

REFERENCES

1. Siegel RL, Kratzer TB, Giaquinto AN, et al. Cancer statistics, 2025. CA Cancer J Clin 2025;75(1):10–45.
2. Stoop TF, Javed AA, Oba A, et al. Pancreatic cancer. Lancet 2025;405(10485): 1182–202.
3. NCCN clinical practice guidelines in oncology (NCCN Guidelines®): pancreatic adenocarcinoma. Version 2.2025. 2025. Available at: https://www.nccn.org. Accessed July 24, 2025.
4. Ryan DP, Hong TS, Bardeesy N. Pancreatic adenocarcinoma. N Engl J Med 2014;371(11):1039–49.
5. Raphael BJ, Hruban RH, Aguirre AJ, et al. Integrated genomic characterization of pancreatic ductal adenocarcinoma. Cancer Cell 2017;32(2):185–203.e13.
6. Park W, Chawla A, O'Reilly EM. Pancreatic cancer. JAMA 2021;326(9):851.
7. Lugo A, Peveri G, Bosetti C, et al. Strong excess risk of pancreatic cancer for low frequency and duration of cigarette smoking: a comprehensive review and meta-analysis. Eur J Cancer 2018;104:117–26.
8. Maisonneuve P, Lowenfels AB. Risk factors for pancreatic cancer: a summary review of meta-analytical studies. Int J Epidemiol 2015;44(1):186–98.
9. Than MT, O'Hara M, Stanger BZ, et al. KRAS-driven tumorigenesis and KRAS-driven therapy in pancreatic adenocarcinoma. Mol Cancer Ther 2024;23(10): 1378–88.
10. de Jesus VHF, Mathias-Machado MC, de Farias JPF, et al. Targeting KRAS in pancreatic ductal adenocarcinoma: the long road to cure. Cancers 2023; 15(20). http://dx.doi.org/10.3390/cancers15205015.
11. Hayashi A, Hong J, Iacobuzio-Donahue CA. The pancreatic cancer genome revisited. Nat Rev Gastroenterol Hepatol 2021;18(7):469–81.

12. Gurreri E, Genovese G, Perelli L, et al. KRAS-dependency in pancreatic ductal adenocarcinoma: mechanisms of escaping in resistance to KRAS inhibitors and perspectives of therapy. Int J Mol Sci 2023;24(11):9313.
13. Wei D, Wang L, Zuo X, et al. A small molecule with big impact: MRTX1133 targets the KRASG12D mutation in pancreatic cancer. Clin Cancer Res 2024;30(4): 655–62.
14. Jiang J, Jiang L, Maldonato BJ, et al. Translational and therapeutic evaluation of RAS-GTP inhibition by RMC-6236 in RAS-driven cancers. Cancer Discov 2024; 14(6):994–1017.
15. Tang B, Li Y, Qi G, et al. Clinicopathological significance of CDKN2A promoter hypermethylation frequency with pancreatic cancer. Sci Rep 2015;5(1):13563.
16. Jacobs M, Murad A, Cho N, et al. CDKN2A cancer predisposition. 2025. Available at: https://www.ncbi.nlm.nih.gov/books/NBK616232/. Accessed September 30, 2025.
17. Chou A, Froio D, Nagrial AM, et al. Tailored first-line and second-line CDK4-targeting treatment combinations in mouse models of pancreatic cancer. Gut 2018;67(12):2142–55.
18. Mello SS, Flowers BM, Mazur PK, et al. Multifaceted role for p53 in pancreatic cancer suppression. Proc Natl Acad Sci 2023;120(10):e2211937120.
19. Agrawal R, Natarajan KN. Oncogenic signaling pathways in pancreatic ductal adenocarcinoma. Adv Cancer Res 2023;251–83. http://dx.doi.org/10.1016/bs.acr.2023.02.006.
20. Tuval A, Strandgren C, Heldin A, et al. Pharmacological reactivation of p53 in the era of precision anticancer medicine. Nat Rev Clin Oncol 2024;21(2):106–20.
21. Peuget S, Zhou X, Selivanova G. Translating p53-based therapies for cancer into the clinic. Nat Rev Cancer 2024;24(3):192–215.
22. Cecerska-Heryć E, Jerzyk A, Goszka M, et al. TGF-β signaling in cancer: mechanisms of progression and therapeutic targets. Int J Mol Sci 2025;26(15):7326.
23. Dardare J, Witz A, Merlin JL, et al. SMAD4 and the TGFβ pathway in patients with pancreatic ductal adenocarcinoma. Int J Mol Sci 2020;21(10):3534.
24. Murimwa GZ, Williams NE, Alzhanova D, et al. SMAD4 deficiency promotes pancreatic cancer progression and confers susceptibility to TGFβ inhibition. Cancer Res 2025;85(16):2987–96.
25. Principe DR, Timbers KE, Atia LG, et al. TGFβ signaling in the pancreatic tumor microenvironment. Cancers 2021;13(20):5086.
26. Palamaris K, Felekouras E, Sakellariou S. Epithelial to mesenchymal transition: key regulator of pancreatic ductal adenocarcinoma progression and chemoresistance. Cancers 2021;13(21):5532.
27. Christenson ES, Jaffee E, Azad NS. Current and emerging therapies for patients with advanced pancreatic ductal adenocarcinoma: a bright future. Lancet Oncol 2020;21(3):e135–45.
28. Tindall RR, Bailey-Lundberg JM, Cao Y, et al. The TGF-β superfamily as potential therapeutic targets in pancreatic cancer. Front Oncol 2024;14. http://dx.doi.org/10.3389/fonc.2024.1362247.
29. Aslanian HR, Lee JH, Canto MI. AGA clinical practice update on pancreas cancer screening in high-risk individuals: expert review. Gastroenterology 2020; 159(1):358–62.
30. NCCN clinical practice guidelines in oncology (NCCN guidelines®): genetic/familial high-risk assessment: breast, ovarian, pancreatic, and prostate. Version 1.2026. 2025. Available at: https://www.nccn.org. Accessed July 24, 2025.

31. Rainone M, Singh I, Salo-Mullen EE, et al. An emerging paradigm for germline testing in pancreatic ductal adenocarcinoma and immediate implications for clinical practice: a review. JAMA Oncol 2020;6(5):764.
32. Gardiner A, Kidd J, Elias MC, et al. Pancreatic ductal carcinoma risk associated with hereditary cancer-risk genes. JNCI J Natl Cancer Inst 2022;114(7): 996–1002.
33. Li S, Silvestri V, Leslie G, et al. Cancer risks associated with *BRCA1* and *BRCA2* pathogenic variants. J Clin Oncol 2022;40(14):1529–41.
34. Kastrinos F, Mukherjee B, Tayob N, et al. Risk of pancreatic cancer in families with Lynch syndrome. JAMA 2009;302(16):1790.
35. Kimura H, Klein AP, Hruban RH, et al. The role of inherited pathogenic CDKN2A variants in susceptibility to pancreatic cancer. Pancreas 2021;50(8):1123–30.
36. Calderwood AH, Sawhney MS, Thosani NC, et al. American Society for Gastrointestinal Endoscopy guideline on screening for pancreatic cancer in individuals with genetic susceptibility: methodology and review of evidence. Gastrointest Endosc 2022;95(5):827–54.e3.
37. Klimkowski S, Ibrahim M, Ibarra Rovira JJ, et al. Peutz–Jeghers syndrome and the role of imaging: pathophysiology, diagnosis, and associated cancers. Cancers 2021;13(20):5121.
38. Syngal S, Brand RE, Church JM, et al, American College of Gastroenterology. ACG clinical guideline: genetic testing and management of hereditary gastrointestinal cancer syndromes. Am J Gastroenterol 2015;110(2):223–62.
39. Lowenfels AB, Maisonneuve P, DiMagno EP, et al. Hereditary pancreatitis and the risk of pancreatic cancer. JNCI J Natl Cancer Inst 1997;89(6):442–6.
40. Singh VK, Yadav D, Garg PK. Diagnosis and management of chronic pancreatitis: a review. JAMA 2019;322(24):2422.
41. Rebours V, Boutron-Ruault MC, Schnee M, et al. Risk of pancreatic adenocarcinoma in patients with hereditary pancreatitis: a national exhaustive series. Am J Gastroenterol 2008;103(1):111–9.
42. Hsu FC, Roberts NJ, Childs E, et al. Risk of pancreatic cancer among individuals with pathogenic variants in the *ATM* gene. JAMA Oncol 2021;7(11):1664.
43. Sawhney MS, Calderwood AH, Thosani NC, et al. ASGE guideline on screening for pancreatic cancer in individuals with genetic susceptibility: summary and recommendations. Gastrointest Endosc 2022;95(5):817–26.
44. Chari ST, Maitra A, Matrisian LM, et al. Early detection initiative: a randomized controlled trial of algorithm-based screening in patients with new onset hyperglycemia and diabetes for early detection of pancreatic ductal adenocarcinoma. Contemp Clin Trials 2022;113:106659.
45. Frank RC, Shim B, Lo T, et al. Pancreatic cancer screening in new-onset and deteriorating diabetes: preliminary results from the PANDOME study. J Clin Endocrinol Metab 2025. http://dx.doi.org/10.1210/clinem/dgaf319.
46. Mahajan UM, Oehrle B, Goni E, et al. Validation of two plasma multimetabolite signatures for patients at risk of or with suspected pancreatic ductal adenocarcinoma (METAPAC): a prospective, multicentre, investigator-masked, enrichment design, phase 4 diagnostic study. Lancet Gastroenterol Hepatol 2025;10(7): 634–47.
47. Shah I, Silva-Santisteban A, Germansky KA, et al. Pancreatic cancer screening for At-Risk individuals (pancreas scan study): yield, harms, and outcomes from a prospective multicenter study. Am J Gastroenterol 2023;118(9):1664–70.
48. Blackford AL, Canto MI, Dbouk M, et al. Pancreatic cancer surveillance and survival of high-risk individuals. JAMA Oncol 2024;10(8):1087.

49. Dbouk M, Katona BW, Brand RE, et al. The multicenter cancer of pancreas screening study: impact on stage and survival. J Clin Oncol 2022;40(28): 3257–66.
50. Maitra A, Adsay NV, Argani P, et al. Multicomponent analysis of the pancreatic adenocarcinoma progression model using a pancreatic intraepithelial neoplasia tissue microarray. Mod Pathol 2003;16(9):902–12.
51. Shalaby A, Sadri N, Xue Y. Molecular pathology of pancreatic ductal adenocarcinoma. Cancers 2025;17(21):3549.
52. Tsuda M, Fukuda A, Kawai M, et al. The role of the SWI/SNF chromatin remodeling complex in pancreatic ductal adenocarcinoma. Cancer Sci 2021;112(2): 490–7.
53. Pandey S, Gupta VK, Lavania SP. Role of epigenetics in pancreatic ductal adenocarcinoma. Epigenomics 2023;15(2):89–110.
54. Oyon D, Lopez-Pascual A, Castello-Uribe B, et al. Targeting of the G9a, DNMT1 and UHRF1 epigenetic complex as an effective strategy against pancreatic ductal adenocarcinoma. J Exp Clin Cancer Res 2025;44(1). http://dx.doi.org/10.1186/s13046-024-03268-5.
55. Shi H, Liu X, Xing C, et al. DNMT1 -induced downregulation of CBX7 inhibits ERK phosphorylation and promotes pancreatic ductal adenocarcinoma progression. FASEB J 2025;39(10):e70571.
56. Perkhofer L, Gout J, Roger E, et al. DNA damage repair as a target in pancreatic cancer: state-of-the-art and future perspectives. Gut 2021;70(3):606–17.
57. Perkhofer L, Golan T, Cuyle PJ, et al. Targeting DNA damage repair mechanisms in pancreas cancer. Cancers 2021;13(17):4259.
58. Bensi M, Minucci A, Ribelli M, et al. DNA damage repair (DDR) germline mutations (GMs) in pancreatic ductal adenocarcinoma (PDAC): a mono-institutional retrospective study. J Clin Oncol 2022;40(16_suppl):10587.
59. Pasca Di Magliano M, Biankin AV, Heiser PW, et al. Common activation of canonical wnt signaling in pancreatic adenocarcinoma. In: Hatakeyama M, editor. PLoS One 2007;2(11):e1155.
60. Pećina-Šlaus N, Aničić S, Bukovac A, et al. Wnt signaling inhibitors and their promising role in tumor treatment. Int J Mol Sci 2023;24(7):6733.
61. Yabuuchi S, Pai SG, Campbell NR, et al. Notch signaling pathway targeted therapy suppresses tumor progression and metastatic spread in pancreatic cancer. Cancer Lett 2013;335(1):41–51.
62. Notch signaling pathway in pancreatic tumorigenesis. In: Advances in cancer research. Elsevier; 2023. p. 1–36. http://dx.doi.org/10.1016/bs.acr.2023.02.001.
63. Papadakos SP, Dedes N, Gkolemi N, et al. The EPH/ephrin system in pancreatic ductal adenocarcinoma (PDAC): from pathogenesis to treatment. Int J Mol Sci 2023;24(3):3015.
64. Furuhashi S, Morita Y, Ida S, et al. Ephrin receptor A4 expression enhances migration, invasion and neurotropism in pancreatic ductal adenocarcinoma cells. Anticancer Res 2021;41(4):1733–44.
65. Liu J, Yuan Q, Chen X, et al. Prognostic and therapeutic value of the Eph/Ephrin signaling pathway in pancreatic cancer explored based on bioinformatics. Sci Rep 2024;14(1):17650.
66. Tomuleasa C, Tigu AB, Munteanu R, et al. Therapeutic advances of targeting receptor tyrosine kinases in cancer. Signal Transduct Target Ther 2024;9(1):201.
67. Huang XL, Khan MI, Wang J, et al. Role of receptor tyrosine kinases mediated signal transduction pathways in tumor growth and angiogenesis—New insight and futuristic vision. Int J Biol Macromol 2021;180:739–52.

68. Barzi A, Weipert CM, Espenschied CR, et al. ERBB2 (HER2) amplifications and co-occurring KRAS alterations in the circulating cell-free DNA of pancreatic ductal adenocarcinoma patients and response to HER2 inhibition. Front Oncol 2024;14. http://dx.doi.org/10.3389/fonc.2024.1339302.
69. Li Z, Shao C, Liu X, et al. Oncogenic ERBB2 aberrations and KRAS mutations cooperate to promote pancreatic ductal adenocarcinoma progression. Carcinogenesis 2019. http://dx.doi.org/10.1093/carcin/bgz086.
70. Knepper TC, Kim DW, Mauer E, et al. Comparative analysis of the targetable landscape in *KRAS* -mutant and wild-type pancreatic adenocarcinoma. J Clin Oncol 2022;40(16_suppl):4155.
71. Philip PA, Azar I, Xiu J, et al. Molecular characterization of *KRAS* wild-type tumors in patients with pancreatic adenocarcinoma. Clin Cancer Res 2022;28(12): 2704–14.
72. Tong Y, Sun M, Chen L, et al. Proteogenomic insights into the biology and treatment of pancreatic ductal adenocarcinoma. J Hematol Oncol 2022;15(1):168.
73. Huang A, Burke J, Bunker RD, et al. Regulation of human 4-hydroxy-2-oxoglutarate aldolase by pyruvate and α-ketoglutarate: implications for primary hyperoxaluria type-3. Biochem J 2019;476(21):3369–83.
74. Coleman JC, Hallett SR, Grigoriadis AE, et al. LARP4A and LARP4B in cancer: the new kids on the block. Int J Biochem Cell Biol 2023;161:106441.
75. Tu J, Zhang L. LARP4B inhibits ferroptosis and accelerates the progression of pancreatic cancer by activating WNK1-induced NRF2/GCH1/BH4 pathway. Integr Biol 2025;17:zyaf019.
76. Grützmann R, Lüttges J, Sipos B, et al. ADAM9 expression in pancreatic cancer is associated with tumour type and is a prognostic factor in ductal adenocarcinoma. Br J Cancer 2004;90(5):1053–8.
77. Slapak EJ, El Mandili M, Brink MST, et al. Preclinical assessment of ADAM9-Responsive mesoporous silica nanoparticles for the treatment of pancreatic cancer. Int J Mol Sci 2023;24(13):10704.
78. Chen J, Wang X, Wang J, et al. Cyclin-dependent kinase 1 (CDK1) in cancers: from upstream regulation to downstream substrates and therapeutic inhibitors. Eur J Med Chem 2025;299:118090.

The Genetics and Screening of Gastroenteropancreatic Neuroendocrine Tumors and Adrenal Tumors

William Wong, DO, MPH[a], Sofia W. Viana, MD[b], Mecker G. Möller, MD, FACS[a,*]

KEYWORDS

• Neuroendocrine neoplasms • GEP-NET • Adrenal tumors • Genetics • Screening

KEY POINTS

- Neuroendocrine malignancies and adrenal tumors are biologically heterogenous; so, management relies on integrating clinical symptomatology, histopathology, and molecular profiling.
- Surgical decision-making in hereditary syndromes for neuroendocrine tumors (NETs) and adrenal tumors balances function preservation with extent of resection.
- Screening and surveillance are more frequent and, occasionally, reflexive to rule out NETs and adrenal tumors when it is associated with a germline mutation.
- Molecular profiling has advanced the recent utilization and development of targeted therapy especially in NETs.

INTRODUCTION

Endocrine malignancies make up about 55% of all global cancer cases if all organ sites are included.[1] Neuroendocrine neoplasms (NENs) and malignant adrenal tumors account for 2% and less than 0.001%, of all malignancies overall, respectively.[2,3] With some overlap in cellular origin between NENs and adrenal tumors, the National Comprehensive Cancer Network (NCCN) combines the 2 endocrine tumor types within 1 guideline.[4]

NENs are heterogenous in biochemical function and location. The incidence of NENs continues to increase but with current advanced therapies, survival outcomes

[a] Section of Surgical Oncology, Department of Surgery, University of Chicago Pritzker School of Medicine, Chicago, IL, USA; [b] Division of Thoracic Surgery, Department of Surgery, University of Cincinnati College of Medicine, Cincinnati, OH, USA

* Corresponding author. Section of Surgical Oncology, Director Surgical Oncology Fellowship Program and Regional Therapies (HIPEC) Program, University of Chicago Pritzker School of Medicine, 5841 S Maryland Avenue, Room G212, Chicago, IL 60637.

E-mail address: mmoller@uchicago.edu

Surg Clin N Am 106 (2026) 555–569
https://doi.org/10.1016/j.suc.2026.03.011 surgical.theclinics.com

Abbreviations	
ACC	adrenocortical carcinoma
GEP	gastroenteropancreatic
MEN	multiple endocrine neoplasia
NCCN	neuroendocrine neoplasms
NECs	neuroendocrine carcinomas
NENs	neuroendocrine neoplasms
NETs	neuroendocrine tumors
NGS	next-generation sequencing
PNET	pancreatic neuroendocrine tumor
PPGL	pheochromocytoma and paraganglioma
SSA	somatostatin analogs
VHL	Von Hippel-Landau

appear to be improving for all stages and locations of primary tumors.[5] Based on the 2022 World Health Organization (WHO) classification system, it is essential to clarify nomenclature when discussing NENs. NENs can be subcategorized into neuroendocrine tumors (NETs) or neuroendocrine carcinomas (NECs). Distinguishing the 2 as well as the grade of NETs (grade 1–3) are generally based on pathologic features including Ki-67 index, presence of necrosis, frequency of mitoses, regularity of cell shape, and nuclear/cytoplasm ratio.[6]

NENs can originate in all organs of the human body, with the most common locations being gastroenteropancreatic (GEP).[5] Workup includes determining whether the NEN is functionally active with a combination of biochemical workup and imaging modalities. While serum chromogranin A, serum serotonin levels, and 24-hour urinary 5-Hydroxyindoleacetic acid (5-HIAA) metabolite continue to be traditional biochemical tests to obtain for NENs, other tests to evaluate excess levels of other hormones are based on clinical presentation and/or location of the tumor. However, NENs are commonly associated with hereditary syndromes so it is important for clinicians to have an understanding on their genetics to guide screening, workup, personalized management, and prognostic consultation.[7] For example, in paragangliomas and pheochromocytomas, unique subtypes of NENs and commonly associated with adrenal neoplasms, initial testing includes plasma free or 24-hour urine fractionate metanephrine and normetanephrines.[8] However, especially if a hereditary syndrome is present, functional NENs may produce excessive levels of hormones in a synchronous (or even metachronous) manner, creating complex, overlapping clinical manifestations.[6]

Adrenal tumors can arise from either the adrenal cortex or medulla and encompass a wide spectrum of benign and malignant neoplasms with variable hormonal activity.[9] Evaluation of adrenal tumors includes determining functional status through a combination of targeted biochemical testing and imaging modalities. While screening for cortisol, aldosterone, and catecholamine excess remains central to the workup of adrenal neoplasms, additional hormonal assays are guided by clinical presentation and suspected tumor subtype.[9] Hereditary adrenal tumors account for a minority of all adrenal neoplasms. However, they represent a higher burden in specific clinical context including pediatric adrenocortical carcinoma (ACC), bilateral pheochromocytomas, and recurrent or multifocal adrenal disease.[10] In contrast to sporadic adrenal tumors, hereditary cases often present earlier in life and may demonstrate distinct biological behavior. Some tumors exhibit more indolent growth patterns, such as medullary tumors associated with germline mutations, whereas others display aggressive clinical behavior, particularly ACC, arise in the setting of tumor suppressor gene alterations.

This article will review relevant genetic, screening, and surveillance patterns behind 2 major categories of NENs for the general surgeon: GEP-NENs and adrenal tumors.

Gastroenteropancreatic-Neuroendocrine Neoplasias

Genetic mutations in gastroenteropancreatic-neuroendocrine neoplasias

Genomic studies on NENs remain sparse due to the rarity of the malignancy itself and majority of the genetic data are based on pancreatic neuroendocrine tumors (PNET).[7] Besides being heterogenous in terms of location and clinical symptoms, GEP-NENs are heterogenous in regards to their genetic mutations. Besides pathologic findings to distinguish NETs from NECs, their distinction can be determined genetically. NEC of the pancreas displays the inactivation of RB1 and TP53 genes, both involved in cell cycle regulation, which are commonly intact in PNETs.[11] KRAS and BRAF mutations have been detected in NENs and are suggestive of NEC.[7,11] Prognoses of NECs are significantly worse than NETs, including grade 3 NETs, altering treatment strategies.[12] Therefore, it is important for the initial pathology slides and reports suggestive of NEC be reviewed by multiple pathologists and/or major institutions with multidisciplinary teams.

Common somatic genetic alterations within PNETs include DAXX and ATRX, both of which are involved in chromatin remodeling.[13] Specifically in small bowel NETs, there is no single dominant driver mutation identified at this time. Researchers have appreciated occasional loss of chromosome 18 and sometimes extra copies of other chromosomes (4,5,7,14, and 20).[7,14] This suggests carcinogenesis via multiple mechanisms including chromatin remodeling, DNA damage, apoptosis, and axon guidance.[14]

While there are other somatic mutations reported to be involved with NENs, it is the germline mutations with associated hereditary syndromes that have helped elucidate the major cellular pathways that lead to NENs (cyclin-dependent cell cycle regulation and PI2K/mTOR pathway).[7] These major germline mutations include multiple endocrine neoplasia (MEN)1, MEN4, VHL, NF1, and TSC. **Table 1** is a summary of the hereditary syndromes associated with these germline mutations that also have high propensity for developing GEP-NETs. About 5% of all NENs are appreciated in hereditary syndromes.[15] GEP-NETs penetrance, especially PNET, in MEN1 is up to 90% in MEN1.[15] All these syndromes have autosomal dominant inheritance patterns. Small intestinal NETs are rarely associated with hereditary syndromes.[7] Attributing endocrine malignancies to specific syndromes are essential to both frequency of surveillance and aggressiveness of treatment to optimize oncologic outcomes and quality of life.

Screening and surveillance for gastroenteropancreatic-neuroendocrine tumors in patients with known germline mutations

When GEP-NET is a common cause of morbidity and mortality in hereditary syndromes, like MEN1, screening and surveillance for timely intervention seem reasonable. However, guidelines for patients with germline mutation-associated GEP-NET are sparse.

Genetic evaluation is also recommended if patients have a combination of MEN-related conditions and/or with family history with related conditions. First degree relatives of patients with confirmed diagnoses of syndromes should be genetically tested. Patients with diagnoses of gastrinomas and multifocal PNET should also be considered for genetic evaluation.[4] With isolated NETs, it is not recommended to perform germline testing.[16]

For MEN1, while annual biochemical test is recommended for hyperparathyroidism and functional pituitary adenomas, biochemical workup for functional NETs and adrenal tumor are indicated once symptoms are present.[17] Updated guidelines no longer recommend workup to rule out the presence of asymptomatic, functional NETs.[4,16]

Table 1
Hereditary syndromes associated with gastroenteropancreatic-neuroendocrine tumors

Hereditary Syndrome	Gene (Chromosome Location)	Risk of Developing Gastroenteropancreatic-Neuroendocrine Tumors (%)	Most Common Gastroenteropancreatic-Neuroendocrine Tumor	Screening Frequency for Gastroenteropancreatic-Neuroendocrine Tumors	Timing for Initial Screening Gastroenteropancreatic-Neuroendocrine Neoplasiasfor Family Members	Other Associated Diseases	Ref
MEN Type 1	MEN1 (11q13)	7%–90% (varies based on location)	Pancreas	Biochemical workup 1–3 y Imaging based on clinical and biochemical suspicion. (as often as every 2–3 y)	As early as possible (early childhood)	Multiglandular primary hyperparathyroidism, pituitary adenoma, adrenal tumors, breast cancer, benign skin tumors	15,17–19
MEN4	CDKN1B(12p13)	25%	Pancreas	See MEN1	See MEN1	Primary hyperparathyroidism, pituitary adenoma	15,19
von Hippel-Lindau	VHL (3p25)	8%–17%	Pancreas	Every 2 y	15 year old	Renal cell carcinoma, hemangioblastoma, pheochromocytoma	4,15,21,70
Neurofibromatosis Type 1	NF1 (17q11.2)	1%–3%	Duodenal- periampullary	Based on clinical suspicion		Neurofibroma, peripheral nerve sheath tumors, pheochromocytoma, cafe au lait cutaneous spots	15,22,71,72
Tuberous Sclerosis complex	TSC1(9q34)/TSC2 (16p13.3 more common)	3%–4%	Pancreas			Renal angiomyolipoma, renal cell carcinoma	73,74

Cross sectional imaging should be performed based on these biochemical results or symptoms suspicious for tumors.[17,18] Subsequent imaging should be based on previous findings. Imaging for asymptomatic individuals remains controversial and should be individualized, but some guidelines have recommended imaging as often as 2 to 3 years after diagnosis of MEN1 syndrome.[17,19] It must be noted that biochemical and radiographic screening for patients with germline mutations can be a social and financial burden to patients and their families. One study calculated that an aggressive screening schedule for patients with MEN1 will expect at least 200 blood tests and 70 surveillance scans by age 40.[20] Therefore, experts are advocating for an individualized, patient centered approach in screening and surveillance.[20] MEN4 is a relatively new germline mutation compared to MEN1/2. Thus, the management approach to MEN4 associated GEP-NET is similar to MEN1.[4,15]

For patients with Von Hippel-Landau (VHL) syndrome, MRI of the abdomen is recommended to rule out intra-abdominal tumors including renal cell carcinoma and pancreatic tumors every 2 years starting at age 15.[4,21]

Screening for NF-1 associated GEP-NET and pheochromocytoma is limited. The European Reference Network for Genetic Tumor Risk Syndromes recommended guidelines to obtain biochemical workup or radiographic imaging based on clinical suspicion.[22] There are no screening guidelines for tuberous sclerosis complex (TSC) associated GEP-NET.[23]

There is no consensus with duration of surveillance of treated sporadic GEP-NETs in addition to hereditary-associated NETs.[16] It is generally recommended to continue imaging at least annually (more often for patients with advanced disease and biochemical evidence of recurrence) for up to 10 years.[16] Such recommendations can be extrapolated to include hereditary associated NETs, although some guidelines have recommended it continue indefinitely.[20,24] There are some data that suggests slower progression of nonfunctional, small (<2 cm) MEN1-associated PNETs compared with small sporadic PNETs, which may allow less-frequent surveillance.[4,25] However, evidence to support the difference in follow-up remains low.

Considerations in management of germline mutated gastroenteropancreatic-neuroendocrine tumors compared with somatic-mutated gastroenteropancreatic-neuroendocrine tumors

The technical aspects of resections and medical treatment modalities remain the same between GEP-NET of somatic and germline mutations.[4] However, with a higher propensity of muti-centric PNETs and recurrence in patients with germline mutations (21%–37% in MEN1),[26] it is important to weigh the oncologic implications of the cancer and treatment goals with the possible morbid endocrine imbalances that may come from aggressive interventions. For example, with the multifocal nature of PNETs (or even functional gastric NETs) in germline mutations, the goal is to attempt to avoid surgical resection to avoid the morbidities that arise from pancreas resection (ie, pancreatic leak, new onset or worsening diabetes, malabsorption among others). For patients with MEN1, NCCN recommends surgical consideration if the tumor is greater than 2 cm in size, rapidly growing on surveillance imaging, or refractory to medical management.[4] Even if surgery is necessary, it is important to first localize the tumor and then consider parenchymal sparing approaches, such as enucleation, if technically feasible. Because of its morbidity and no evidence of survival benefit, pancreaticoduodenectomies are not recommended in germline-mutated NETs regardless of functionality.[24] Especially as most NETs are grade 1, well differentiated, indolent in nature, survival remains excellent with medical management alone or minor resection.[24] Therefore, preserving quality of life for these patients should be considered to be of utmost importance.

Novel medical strategies in managing gastroenteropancreatic-neuroendocrine tumors based on molecular profile. Upregulation of somatostatin receptors (SSTRs) is a well-known element of well differentiated NENs. This has led to standard use of drugs like somatostatin analogs (SSAs) to slow progression of disease in GEP-NETs.[27,28] In addition, peptide receptor radionuclide therapy has demonstrated to be effective for SSTR positive GEP-NETs, increasing progression free survival and clinically relevant overall survival compared with long acting SSA alone in advanced, well differentiated NETs.[29,30] At this time, routine next generation sequencing of GEP-NETs is not recommended.[16] However, it remains a possibility in the future with advances in targetable mutations, adding both prognostic and therapeutic value to management of these rare malignancies. For example, everolimus is a second-line agent that focuses on inhibiting known mTOR pathway, mutated in about 15% of PNETs.[31] Currently, use of this inhibitory drug is not determined by first identifying molecular biomarkers.[15,31]

Consideration for the use of belzutifan in patients with VHL-associated NET is now mentioned in the recent NCCN guidelines.[4] FDA approved in 2021, belzutifan inhibits HIF-2 alpha, which is upregulated in VHL.[32] It is considered for small, resectable NETs but there is not enough data to support belzutifan's use on large, locally advanced, or unresectable disease.[4,32]

There is growing research on using leflunomide to target or prevent MEN1 associated NET.[33] Leflunomide, approved to treat rheumatoid arthritis has been suggested to have antitumor activities as a kinase inhibitor of DHODH. DHODH has been found to be overexpressed in MEN1 mutated cell lines, which upregulate DNA and RNA synthesis.[33,34] Leflunomide has been shown to decrease incidence of PNET in mice and some early reports of progressive free benefit in patients with advanced MEN1-associated NETs.[34]

Adrenal Neoplasms

Genetic mutations of malignant adrenal neoplasms

Somatic mutations have a central role in the development of sporadic adrenal tumors and help to determine hormonal phenotype and malignant potential.[35] In adrenocortical adenomas, somatic alterations commonly affect intracellular signaling pathways involved in steroidogenesis with the activation of mutations in the cAMP–PKA signaling pathway (eg, PRKACA, GNAS, and PRKAR1A), which are strongly associated with cortisol-producing adenomas.[36] Aldosterone-producing adenomas frequently harbor mutations in ion channels and adenosine triphosphatases (ATPases) (KCNJ5, ATP1A1, ATP2B3, and CACNA1D), leading to calcium-mediated aldosterone excess.[37] ACC somatic mutations reflect aggressive tumor biology and genomic instability rather than hormone specificity.[38]

The most common alterations include tumor suppressor gene mutations (TP53, RB10),[39,40] dysregulation of the Wnt/β-catenin pathway (CTNNB1, ZNRF3),[41,42] and telomere maintenance and chromatin remodeling abnormalities.[43] In pheochromocytoma, somatic mutations may activate kinase signaling or hypoxia-related pathways, contributing to tumor growth and catecholamine secretion.[44]

Several germline mutations and subsequent hereditary cancer syndromes predispose to adrenal tumors, most notably pheochromocytoma and paraganglioma (PPGL).[44,45] Germline mutations may affect tumor suppressor genes, kinase signaling pathways, or cellular hypoxia responses.[46,47] Adrenal tumors arising in hereditary settings are more likely to be bilateral or multifocal, diagnosed at a younger age, associated with other synchronous or metachronous malignancies (**Table 2**).[48] Hereditary PPGL syndromes involve mutations in the SDHx genes (SDHB, SDHD, SDHC, SDHA, SDHAF2), with SDHB mutations conferring a higher risk of malignant and

Table 2
Hereditary syndromes associated with adrenal tumors

Hereditary Syndrome	Gene (Chromosome Location)	Risk of Developing Adrenal Tumors	Adrenal Tumor Type	Other Associated Diseases	Ref
Hereditary PPGL syndromes (SDHx syndrome)	SDHB (1p36.13), SDHD (11q23.1), SDHC (1q.23.3), SDHA (5p15.33), SDHAF2 (11q12.2)	Penetrance: 20%–40% (highest with SDHB) by age 60	Axtra-adrenal paragangliomas	Renal tumors, GIST, head and neck paragangliomas, pheochromocytomas	75,76
MAX-associated PPGL	MAX (14q23.3)	Penetrance: 100% by age 60	Pheochromocytoma	Paraganglioma	75,77
TMEM127-associated PPGL	TMEM127 (2q11.2)	Penetrance: 80% by age 60	Pheochromocytoma	Paraganglioma	75,77
Li-Fraumeni syndrome	TP53 (12p13.1)	6%–13%	ACC	Various sarcomas, choroid plexus carcinoma, breast cancer, brain tumors, leukemia, colorectal cancer, lung cancer, prostate cancer, pancreatic cancer, melanoma	78
Beckwith–Wiedemann syndrome	CDKN1C, H19, IGF2, KCNQ10T1, KCNQ1 (11p15.5)	1.10%	ACC	Wilms tumor, hepatoblastoma, neuroblastoma, rhabdomyosarcoma	79
Carney Complex (Primary pigmented nodular adrenocortical disease)	PRKAR1A (17q22–24)	25%	Cushing syndrome	Cardiac myxomas, pituitary adenomas, thyroid tumors, schwannoma, breast tumors, cutaneous mycoma	80

(*continued on next page*)

Table 2
(*continued*)

Hereditary Syndrome	Gene (Chromosome Location)	Risk of Developing Adrenal Tumors	Adrenal Tumor Type	Other Associated Diseases	Ref
von Hippel–Lindau	VHL (3p25.3)	25%–35%	Pheochromocytoma	Renal cell carcinoma, hemangioblastoma, NETs	4,15,21,70
MEN Type 2	RET (10q11.21)	50%	Pheochromocytoma	Medullary thyroid carcinoma, parathyroid adenoma/hyperplasia, neuromas	4
Neurofibromatosis Type 1	NF1 (17q11.2)	<5.7%	Pheochromocytoma	Neurofibroma, peripheral nerve sheath tumors, NETs, cafe au lait cutaneous spots	15,22,71,72

metastatic disease.[49] Other PPGL-associated germline mutations include MAX and TMEM127, alter kinase signaling pathways. MEN2 is established from a RET mutation, which disrupt hypoxia-inducible factor signaling.[50] Additional hereditary syndromes linked to adrenal tumors include VHL syndrome (VHL mutation), Li-Fraumeni syndrome (TP53 mutations), Beckwith–Wiedemann syndrome (alterations in 11p15), Carney Complex (PRKAR1A mutations), and Carney–Stratakis syndrome (germline SDHx mutations).[51–53] Tumors arising in these hereditary contexts are more likely to be bilateral or multifocal, present at a younger age, and may coexist with other synchronous or metachronous malignancies.

Screening and surveillance for adrenal tumors in patients with known germline mutations

Preventative strategies differ significantly between hereditary and sporadic adrenal tumors. In sporadic adrenal tumors, screening is generally reactive and initiated only after an adrenal mass is incidentally identified.[54] Proactive screening in the hereditary populations allows for earlier detection and optimized surgical timing.

For adrenal tumors, the NCCN recommends patients be referred to a geneticist for genetic testing if they are diagnosed with ACC, PPGL.[4] PPGL follow a systematic approach that differs from sporadic adrenal neoplasms due to its high prevalence in hereditary disease, such as MEN2, VHL, and NF1.[55] Germline-associated pheochromocytoma is commonly multifocal or bilateral. NCCN recommends annual and syndrome-directed biochemical screening for hormone excess and longitudinal surveillance.[56]

In VHL, annual physical examination and blood pressure monitoring start at age 2, with plasma-free metanephrines or 24-hour urine catecholamines beginning at age 5.[4,57] In contrast, workup of sporadic adrenal tumors is generally performed either after they are identified incidentally or there is clinical concern for PPGL.

For ACC surveillance, MRI is generally preferred for children and young adults to reduce radiation exposure, while CT may be used for surgical planning or detecting metastases. It is critical to identify and treat pheochromocytomas before any other germline-mutation–associated surgery to avoid catastrophic perioperative catecholamine crises. Bilateral or multifocal adrenal tumors are more frequently observed in hereditary mutations compared with somatic cases, emphasizing the need for longitudinal surveillance and individualized, syndrome-specific management.[58]

It must be emphasized that patients with germline mutations such as MEN2, PPGL must be ruled out and subsequently treated before definitive management of any other germline-mutation associated disease to avoid catastrophic perioperative from massive catecholamine release.[59] It is important to note that bilateral pheochromocytomas are seen more often in many notable germline mutations compared to somatic mutations.[60]

Considerations in management of germline-mutated adrenal tumors compared with somatic-mutated adrenal tumors

Management of adrenal tumors in the setting of hereditary cancer syndromes differs from that of sporadic adrenal neoplasms and requires a multidisciplinary, genetics-informed approach.[17,61] Similar to GEP-NETs, in hereditary syndromes, treatment strategies prioritize not only oncologic control of the index tumor but also preservation of adrenal function, anticipation of multifocal or bilateral disease, and long-term surveillance.[60,62] For example, in patients with VHL disease or MEN2 who develop bilateral pheochromocytomas, NCCN guidelines support consideration of cortical-sparing adrenalectomy to reduce the risk of permanent adrenal insufficiency, a strategy less commonly employed in sporadic cases where unilateral adrenalectomy is typically curative.[4,63] Similarly, patients with succinate dehydrogenase (SDHx)-associated PPGL syndromes require management strategies that account for a higher risk of multifocality, recurrence, and metastatic potential, particularly in SDHB mutation carriers, influencing surgical planning, intensity of surveillance, and use of functional imaging modalities.[64] In contrast, ACC arising in the context of tumor suppressor gene mutations, such as TP53 in Li-Fraumeni syndrome, may demonstrate aggressive behavior, often necessitating earlier intervention, more extensive resection, and closer postoperative monitoring.[53]

Novel diagnostic modalities for adrenal tumors based on molecular profile

Recent advances in the biochemical and molecular characterization of adrenal tumors have significantly improved diagnostic accuracy and opened new opportunities for personalized management. On the biochemical level, development of automated immunochemical assays, including chemiluminescence-based methods (chemiluminescent Immunoassay [CLIA] and electrochemiluminescence immunoassay [ECLIA]), has expanded access to reliable and cost-effective screening for functional adrenal masses.[65] Chromatographic and metabolomic techniques, particularly liquid chromatography–tandem mass spectrometry (LC-MS/MS), allow simultaneous assessment of multiple steroid and catecholamine metabolites, improving diagnostic precision and facilitating individualized biochemical profiling.[66,67] Advances in molecular studies have substantially improved the genetic characterization of adrenal tumors. In pheochromocytomas, early studies reported germline variants in 10% to 15% of cases, whereas next-generation sequencing (NGS) has increased detection to 35% to 40%, reflecting the discovery of additional susceptibility genes such as CSDE1, H3F3A, MET, MERTK, and IRP1.[68] In ACC, potentially targetable alterations have been described in genes including TP53, TERT, CTNNB1, CDK4, and MDM2, and blood-based NGS detects genomic alterations in over 80% of advanced cases. Overall, these genetic advances have improved tumor classification, personalized management, and genetic counseling for patients and their families.[69]

SUMMARY

Diagnosis and management of adrenal tumors and NETs require careful consideration of the endocrine function(s) involved as well as oncologic prognosis of the disease when managed operatively and nonoperatively. It requires mindful discussion with patients and a multidisciplinary team on whether resection with curative intent is worth risking the morbidity of surgery itself as well as the morbidity of removing an endocrine organ in patients who now may require exogenous hormonal replacement. Such deliberations are important in germline-associated NETs and adrenal tumors because of the multifocal nature of the disease. Identifying germline mutations guide screening and surveillance to be more frequent compared to sporadic-associated mutations. With improvements in molecular profiling, mutational patterns are more efficiently detected, allowing for more individualized treatment plans including future targeted therapies for patients.

CLINICS CARE POINTS

- Aggressive screening schedules for patients with germline mutations can be a social and financial burden. Therefore, screening and surveillance should be individualized and patient-centered.

- In patients with germline mutations with high propensity for multifocal GEP-NETs and recurrence, it is important to weigh the oncologic benefit of resection with morbid postoperative endocrine deficiencies that worsen quality of life.
- In patients known or suspected of having certain germline mutations such as MEN2, pheochromocytoma and paragangliomas must be ruled out or treated prior to definitive management of any other germline-mutation associated disease to avoid symptoms of massive catecholamine release.

DISCLOSURE

The authors have nothing to disclose.

REFERENCES

1. Liu. Endocrine cancer trends 1990–2021: global disparities and health inequalities. Endocr Relat Cancer 2024;31(11). https://doi.org/10.1530/ERC-23-0363.
2. Sultana Q, Kar J, Verma A, et al. A comprehensive review on neuroendocrine neoplasms: presentation, pathophysiology and management. J Clin Med 2023; 12(15):5138.
3. Rashed WM, Saad A, Al-Husseini M, et al. Incidence of adrenal gland tumor as a second primary malignancy: SEER-based study. Endocr Connect 2018;7(10): 1040–8.
4. National Comprehensive Cancer Network, *NCCN Clinical Practice Guidelines in oncology: neuroendocrine and adrenal tumors.* Version 3.2025, *National Comprehensive Cancer Network*, 2025. Available at: https://www.nccn.org. Accessed April 30, 2026.
5. Dasari A, Shen C, Halperin D, et al. Trends in the incidence, prevalence, and survival outcomes in patients with neuroendocrine tumors in the United States. JAMA Oncol 2017;3(10):1335–42.
6. Rindi G, Mete O, Uccella S, et al. Overview of the 2022 WHO classification of neuroendocrine neoplasms. Endocr Pathol 2022;33(1):115–54.
7. Mafficini A, Scarpa A. Genetics and epigenetics of gastroenteropancreatic neuroendocrine neoplasms. Endocr Rev 2019;40(2):506–36.
8. Mete O, Juhlin CC. Recent progress in the pathologic classification of pheochromocytomas and paragangliomas. Best Pract Res Clin Endocrinol Metab 2024; 38(6):101958.
9. Fuß CT, Megerle F, Fassnacht M. [Adrenal tumors: current standards in clinical management]. Inn Med 2024;65(7):632–41.
10. Burciulescu SML, Gheorghiu ML, Muresan A, et al. Bilateral pheochromocytomas: clinical presentation and morbidity rate related to surgery technique and genetic status. Endocr Connect 2024;13(4). https://doi.org/10.1530/EC-23-0466.
11. Yachida S, Vakiani E, White CM, et al. Small cell and large cell neuroendocrine carcinomas of the pancreas are genetically similar and distinct from well-differentiated pancreatic neuroendocrine tumors. Am J Surg Pathol 2012;36(2): 173–84.
12. Sorbye H, Hjortland GO, Vestermark LW, et al. Characteristics and treatment outcome in a prospective cohort of 639 advanced high-grade digestive neuroendocrine neoplasms (NET G3 and NEC). The NORDIC NEC 2 study. Br J Cancer 2025;133(3):316–24.

13. Heaphy CM, de Wilde RF, Jiao Y, et al. Altered telomeres in tumors with ATRX and DAXX mutations. Science 2011;333(6041):425.
14. Banck MS, Kanwar R, Kulkarni AA, et al. The genomic landscape of small intestine neuroendocrine tumors. J Clin Investig 2013;123(6):2502–8.
15. Ruggeri RM, Benevento E, De Cicco F, et al. Neuroendocrine neoplasms in the context of inherited tumor syndromes: a reappraisal focused on targeted therapies. J Endocrinol Investig 2023;46(2):213–34.
16. North American Neuroendocrine Tumor Society (NANETS). NANETS 2024 symposium guidelines compendium. 2024. Available at: https://nanets.net/net-guidelines-library.
17. Rivero JD, Gangi A, Annes JP, et al. American association of clinical endocrinology consensus statement on management of multiple endocrine neoplasia type 1. Endocr Pract 2025;31(4):403–18.
18. Romei C, Pardi E, Cetani F, et al. Genetic and clinical features of multiple endocrine neoplasia types 1 and 2. J Oncol 2012;2012(1):705036.
19. Halperin R, Tirosh A. Progress report on multiple endocrine neoplasia type 1. Fam Cancer 2025;24(1):15.
20. Newey PJ, Newell-Price J. MEN1 surveillance guidelines: time to (re)Think? J Endocr Soc 2022;6(2):bvac001.
21. Laks S, van Leeuwaarde R, Patel D, et al. Management recommendations for pancreatic manifestations of von Hippel-Lindau disease. Cancer 2022;128(3): 435–46.
22. Carton C, Evans DG, Blanco I, et al. ERN GENTURIS tumour surveillance guidelines for individuals with neurofibromatosis type 1. eClinicalMedicine 2023;56: 101818.
23. Krueger DA, Northrup H, International Tuberous Sclerosis Complex Consensus Group. Tuberous sclerosis complex surveillance and management: recommendations of the 2012 International Tuberous Sclerosis Complex Consensus Conference. Pediatr Neurol 2013;49(4):255–65.
24. Thakker RV, Newey PJ, Walls GV, et al. Clinical practice guidelines for multiple endocrine neoplasia type 1 (MEN1). J Clin Endocrinol Metab 2012;97(9): 2990–3011.
25. Pieterman CRC, de Laat JM, Twisk JWR, et al. Long-term natural course of small nonfunctional pancreatic neuroendocrine tumors in MEN1—Results from the Dutch MEN1 study group. J Clin Endocrinol Metab 2017;102(10):3795–805.
26. Ratnayake CBB, Loveday BP, Windsor JA, et al. Patient characteristics and clinical outcomes following initial surgical intervention for MEN1 associated pancreatic neuroendocrine tumours: a systematic review and exploratory meta-analysis of the literature. Pancreatology 2019;19(3):462–71.
27. Albertelli M, Nazzari E, Sciallero S, et al. Anti-tumoral effects of somatostatin analogs: a lesson from the CLARINET study. J Endocrinol Investig 2017;40(11): 1265–9.
28. Rinke A, Müller HH, Schade-Brittinger C, et al. Placebo-controlled, double-blind, prospective, randomized study on the effect of octreotide LAR in the control of tumor growth in patients with metastatic neuroendocrine midgut tumors: a report from the PROMID study group. J Clin Oncol 2009;27(28):4656–63.
29. Strosberg JR, Caplin ME, Kunz PL, et al. 177Lu-Dotatate plus long-acting octreotide versus high-dose long-acting octreotide in patients with midgut neuroendocrine tumours (NETTER-1): final overall survival and long-term safety results from an open-label, randomised, controlled, phase 3 trial. Lancet Oncol 2021;22(12): 1752–63.

30. Loree JM, Chan D, Lim J, et al. Biomarkers to inform prognosis and treatment for unresectable or metastatic GEP-NENs. JAMA Oncol 2024;10(12):1707.
31. Yao JC, Fazio N, Singh S, et al. Everolimus for the treatment of advanced, non-functional neuroendocrine tumours of the lung or gastrointestinal tract (RADIANT-4): a randomised, placebo-controlled, phase 3 study. Lancet 2016; 387(10022):968–77.
32. Pelle E, Al-Toubah T, Morse B, et al. Belzutifan in a patient with VHL-associated metastatic pancreatic neuroendocrine tumor. J Natl Compr Cancer Netw JNCCN 2022;20(12):1285–7.
33. Boharoon H, Grossman A. A new medical therapy for multiple endocrine neoplasia type 1? Eur Endocrinol 2022;18:86.
34. Ma Y, Wang X, Zhao H, et al. Molecular alterations and therapeutic targets in pancreatic neuroendocrine tumors. J Pancreatol 2023;6(3).
35. Gao X, Yamazaki Y, Ono Y, et al. Histopathological features of aldosterone-producing lesions according to their different somatic genetic mutations. Vitam Horm 2025;129:125–41.
36. Molecular and genetics perspectives on primary adrenocortical hyperfunction disorders. Available at: https://www.mdpi.com/1422-0067/25/21/11341. Accessed January 24, 2026.
37. Mohd Rizam NS, Mustangin M, Pauzi FA, et al. Prevalence of KCNJ5 mutations in aldosterone-producing adenomas among Malaysian primary aldosteronism patients: genotype-phenotype correlation. Malays J Pathol 2025;47(1):63–76.
38. Dybal E, Decaussin-Petrucci M, Descotes F, et al. From hyperplasia to carcinoma: a molecular driven adrenal disease. Eur J Endocrinol 2025;192(6):K55–9.
39. Baliakas P, Soussi T. The TP53 tumor suppressor gene: from molecular biology to clinical investigations. J Intern Med 2025;298(2):78–96.
40. Kitajima S, Li F, Takahashi C. Tumor milieu controlled by RB tumor suppressor. Int J Mol Sci 2020;21(7):2450.
41. Maharjan R, Backman S, Åkerström T, et al. Comprehensive analysis of CTNNB1 in adrenocortical carcinomas: identification of novel mutations and correlation to survival. Sci Rep 2018;8:8610.
42. Structural insights into the LGR4-RSPO2-ZNRF3 complexes regulating WNT/β--catenin signaling | nature communications. Available at: https://www.nature.com/articles/s41467-024-55431-3. Accessed January 24, 2026.
43. van der Lugt R, Jacobs JJL. Structural organization and function of telomeric chromatin. Nat Cell Biol 2026;1–14. https://doi.org/10.1038/s41556-025-01844-1.
44. Cascón A, Robledo M. Clinical and molecular markers guide the genetics of pheochromocytoma and paraganglioma. Biochim Biophys Acta BBA - Rev Cancer 2024;1879(5):189141. https://doi.org/10.1016/j.bbcan.2024.189141.
45. Lu Y, Ek WE, Whiteman D, et al. Most common 'sporadic' cancers have a significant germline genetic component. Hum Mol Genet 2014;23(22):6112–8.
46. Kamilaris CDC, Hannah-Shmouni F, Stratakis CA. Adrenocortical tumorigenesis: lessons from genetics. Best Pract Res Clin Endocrinol Metab 2020;34(3):101428.
47. Pitsava G, Stratakis CA. Genetic alterations in benign adrenal tumors. Biomedicines 2022;10(5):1041.
48. Ohmoto A, Hayashi N, Takahashi S, et al. Current prospects of hereditary adrenal tumors: towards better clinical management. Hered Cancer Clin Pract 2024; 22(1):4.
49. Lussey-Lepoutre C, Pacak K, Grossman A, et al. Overview of recent guidelines and consensus statements on initial screening and management of

phaeochromocytoma and paraganglioma in *SDHx* pathogenic variant carriers and patients. Best Pract Res Clin Endocrinol Metab 2025;39(1):101938.
50. Carmona Alexandrino H, Martins Fernandes A, Godinho R, et al. Pathogenic MAX variant in bilateral adrenal paragangliomas: the dilemma of cortical-sparing surgery. Cureus 2025;17(11):e97541.
51. Altun İ, Turan H, Dağdeviren A, et al. Case reports: exploring the varied presentations and clinical features of carney complex, A detailed report on three distinct cases. J Clin Res Pediatr Endocrinol 2026. https://doi.org/10.4274/jcrpe.galenos.2026.2025-8-10. Online ahead of print.
52. Creswell L, Pandya P, Hillman S, et al. A case of familial CDKN1C-related beckwith-wiedemann syndrome. Prenat Diagn 2026;46(3):458–62.
53. Kratz CP, Frone MN, Khincha PP, et al. Urgent need to recognize that disease-causing TP53 variants with atypical penetrance require distinct clinical recommendations. J Natl Cancer Inst 2026;24:djag015.
54. Lee JM, Kim MK, Ko SH, et al. Clinical guidelines for the management of adrenal incidentaloma. Endocrinol Metab 2017;32(2):200–18.
55. Korpershoek E, van Nederveen FH, Komminoth P, et al. Familial endocrine tumours: pheochromocytomas and extra-adrenal paragangliomas – an update. Diagn Histopathol 2017;23(8):335–45.
56. Liang Y, Yu XJ, Chen J. [The diagnosis and treatment of G3 neuroendocrine tumors according to the new NCCN guideline]. Zhonghua Yixue Zazhi 2022;102(14):982–7.
57. Jackson BS. Adrenal incidentaloma controversial size recommendations. Urol Res Pract 2023;49(2):96–9.
58. Fassnacht M, Puglisi S, Kimpel O, et al. Adrenocortical carcinoma: a practical guide for clinicians. Lancet Diabetes Endocrinol 2025;13(5):438–52.
59. Wells SA, Asa SL, Dralle H, et al. Revised American Thyroid Association Guidelines for the management of medullary thyroid carcinoma. Thyroid 2015;25(6):567–610.
60. Mathiesen JS, Effraimidis G, Rossing M, et al. Multiple endocrine neoplasia type 2: a review. Semin Cancer Biol 2022;79:163–79.
61. Yip L, Duh QY, Wachtel H, et al. American Association of Endocrine Surgeons Guidelines for adrenalectomy: executive summary. JAMA Surg 2022;157(10):870–7.
62. Kuhlen M, Virgone C, Rigaud C, et al. European clinical guidance for the management of adrenal and extra-adrenal paraganglioma in children and adolescents: a consensus by the EXPeRT group. Eur J Endocrinol 2025;193(6):G13–126.
63. Shah MH, Goldner WS, Benson AB, et al. Neuroendocrine and adrenal tumors, version 2.2021, NCCN Clinical Practice Guidelines in oncology. J Natl Compr Cancer Netw JNCCN 2021;19(7):839–68.
64. Cole Y, Howarth S, Javaid A, et al. Expanding the clinical tumor phenotype of the EPAS1-associated tumor syndrome. J Clin Endocrinol Metab 2026;dgag003. https://doi.org/10.1210/clinem/dgag003.
65. Khan M, Shah SH, Salman M, et al. Enzyme-linked immunosorbent assay versus chemiluminescent immunoassay: a general overview. Glob J Med Pharm Biomed Update 2023;18. https://doi.org/10.25259/GJMPBU_77_2022.
66. Knuchel R, Erlic Z, Gruber S, et al. Association of adrenal steroids with metabolomic profiles in patients with primary and endocrine hypertension. Front Endocrinol 2024;15:1370525.

67. Kulyyassov A, Fresnais M, Longuespée R. Targeted liquid chromatography-tandem mass spectrometry analysis of proteins: basic principles, applications, and perspectives. Proteomics 2021;21(23–24):e2100153.
68. Cioppi F, Cantini G, Ercolino T, et al. Targeted next generation sequencing molecular profiling and its clinical application in adrenocortical cancer. Eur J Endocrinol 2024;191(1):17–30.
69. Messina E, Puglisi S, Scatolini M, et al. Germline targeted next-generation sequencing in patients with adrenal incidentalomas. Endocr Abstr 2024;99-(Bioscientifica). https://doi.org/10.1530/endoabs.99.P417.
70. Tsoli M, Panagaki M, Tasouli E, et al. New developments in VHL-associated neuroendocrine neoplasms. Curr Oncol Rep 2025;27(1):59–67.
71. Hirbe AC, Gutmann DH. Neurofibromatosis type 1: a multidisciplinary approach to care. Lancet Neurol 2014;13(8):834–43.
72. Stewart DR, Korf BR, Nathanson KL, et al. Care of adults with neurofibromatosis type 1: a clinical practice resource of the American College of Medical Genetics and Genomics (ACMG). Genet Med 2018;20(7):671–82.
73. Evans LM, Geenen KR, O'Shea A, et al. Tuberous sclerosis complex-associated nonfunctional pancreatic neuroendocrine tumors: management and surgical outcomes. Am J Med Genet 2022;188(9):2666–71.
74. Li R, Miguel C, Schienda J, et al. Prevalence, characteristics, and management of pancreatic tumors among children with Tuberous sclerosis complex. J Pediatr Surg 2025;60(7):162339.
75. Else T, Greenberg S, Fishbein L. Hereditary paraganglioma-pheochromocytoma syndromes. In: Adam MP, Bick S, Mirzaa GM, et al, editors. GeneReviews®. University of Washington, Seattle; 1993. Available at: http://www.ncbi.nlm.nih.gov/books/NBK1548/. Accessed January 31, 2026.
76. Andrews KA, Ascher DB, Pires DEV, et al. Tumour risks and genotype–phenotype correlations associated with germline variants in succinate dehydrogenase subunit genes SDHB, SDHC and SDHD. J Med Genet 2018;55(6):1–11.
77. Bausch B, Schiavi F, Ni Y, et al. Clinical characterization of the pheochromocytoma and paraganglioma susceptibility genes SDHA, TMEM127, MAX, and SDHAF2 for gene-informed prevention. JAMA Oncol 2017;3(9):1204–12.
78. Schneider K, Zelley K, Nichols KE, et al. Li-Fraumeni syndrome. In: Adam MP, Bick S, Mirzaa GM, et al, editors. GeneReviews®. University of Washington, Seattle; 1993. Available at: http://www.ncbi.nlm.nih.gov/books/NBK1311/. Accessed January 31, 2026.
79. Shuman C, Kalish JM, Weksberg R. Beckwith-Wiedemann syndrome. In: Adam MP, Bick S, Mirzaa GM, et al, editors. GeneReviews®. University of Washington, Seattle; 1993. Available at: http://www.ncbi.nlm.nih.gov/books/NBK1394/. Accessed January 31, 2026.
80. Bouys L, Bertherat J. Management of endocrine disease: carney complex: clinical and genetic update 20 years after the identification of the CNC1 (PRKAR1A) gene. Eur J Endocrinol 2021;184(3):R99–109.

The Role of Genetics in Malignant Melanoma

A Comprehensive Review

Shannon M. Smith, MD[a,*], G. Paul Wright, MD, FACS[a,b]

KEYWORDS

- Cutaneous malignancy • Malignant melanoma • Familial melanoma syndrome
- Melanoma genetics • Germline mutation • Somatic mutation
- Genetic screening guidelines • Polygenic risk scoring

KEY POINTS

- Most patients, greater than 80%, diagnosed with cutaneous malignant melanoma result from somatic genetic mutations within BRAF, KRAS, or c-KIT.
- Familial melanoma syndrome represents less than 15% of patients with cutaneous melanoma and within this subset of patients, only 45% have an identifiable associated germline mutation.
- Several inheritable gene mutations are implicated in the development of melanoma dominant syndromes including cyclin-dependent kinase inhibitor 2A, cyclin-dependent kinase 4, BRCA1-associated protein-1, telomerase reverse transcriptase, protection of telomeres 1, adrenocortical dysplasia protein/TERF2IP, and ataxia-telangiectasia mutated.
- Genetic screening guidelines are currently dictated by the *rule of twos, threes, fours* based on the disease prevalence of sporadic melanoma within the region.

INTRODUCTION

Cutaneous malignancies represent one of the most frequently diagnosed cancers in the Western world.[1] Among these, malignant melanoma (MM) is the most lethal form despite being less common than basal or squamous cell carcinoma.[1] The global distribution of melanoma correlates strongly with ultraviolet (UV) radiation intensity, reinforcing UV exposure as a major etiologic driver of cutaneous malignancy in combination with acquired genetic factors.[2] The disproportionate mortality associated with melanoma has led to its prominence in contemporary oncologic and genomic research to promote early recognition, diagnosis, and treatment.

[a] Department of General Surgery, Corewell Health West/Michigan State Univeristy College of Human Medicine, Grand Rapids, MI, USA; [b] Division of Surgical Oncology, Corewell Health West/Michigan State University College of Human Medicine, Grand Rapids, MI, USA
* Corresponding author.
E-mail address: Shannon.smith4@corewellhealth.org

Surg Clin N Am 106 (2026) 571–584
https://doi.org/10.1016/j.suc.2026.03.010 surgical.theclinics.com
0039-6109/26/

Abbreviations	
ACD	adrenocortical dysplasia protein
BAP1	BRCA1-associated protein-1
c-KIT	cellular KIT
CDK4	cyclin-dependent kinase 4
CDKN2A	cyclin-dependent kinase inhibitor 2A
FANCI	Fanconi anemia complementation group I
FMS	familial melanoma syndrome
MAPK	mitogen-activated protein kinase
MM	malignant melanoma
NRAS	neuroblastoma RAS
RB	retinoblastoma
SNP	single nucleotide polymorphism
TERF2IP	telomeric repeat-binding factor 2 interacting protein
TERT	telomerase reverse transcriptase
UV	ultraviolet

Most melanoma cases arise sporadically. Approximately 7% to 15% of patients exhibit a hereditary predisposition, constituting the familial melanoma subset.[3,4] Familial melanoma syndrome (FMS) is defined as 2 first-degree relatives or 3 or more first- and second-degree relatives on the same side of a family who all develop melanoma.[5] The concept of *melanoma-dominant* and *melanoma-subordinate* syndromes provides further granularity in characterizing FMS hereditary predisposition.[6] Individuals with melanoma-dominant syndromes fulfill formal criteria for FMS and present with multiple primary melanomas with other malignancies driven by the same germline mutation being less prevalent. Conversely, melanoma-subordinate syndromes describe patients whose germline mutation predisposes to melanoma among other cancers, but in whom nonmelanoma malignancies predominate clinically.

Within the population of FMS patients, there is an even smaller subpopulation of individuals who harbor a specific, identified gene mutation (45%) as noted in **Table 1**.[3,4] The remaining 55% of individuals who exhibit FMS do not have an identified germline genetic mutation on current algorithms. This review aims to collate information on high- and medium-penetrance germline mutations involved in the development of FMS while also exploring the genetic evolution of melanoma lesions, the role that inconsistencies in global screening thresholds and the emergence of polygenetic risk stratification (PRS) will play in future genetic screening recommendations.

Major Somatic Genetic Mutations

Melanoma often arises from a clinically identifiable precursor lesion that evolved from normal melanocytes through a staged morphologic and molecular progression.[7] This transformation occurs through accumulation of somatic mutations in a well-defined fashion, analogous to the stepwise progression observed in other malignancies. Although most pre-existing melanocytic lesions (30%–50%) will remain stable or regress, a small subset undergo malignant transformation following an initial oncogenic insult.[8] UV radiation is the principle environmental driver typically inducing a driver gain of function point mutation within v-Raf murine sarcoma viral oncogene homolog B1(BRAF) to initiate oncogenic transformation.[7,9] Subsequent genetic alterations often involve additional components of the mitogen-activated protein kinase (MAPK) signaling cascade pathway including mutations affecting neuroblastoma RAS (NRAS) viral oncogene homolog.[7,8] The MAPK signaling cascade is critical for regulating cellular proliferation, differentiation, and survival.[8] As these alterations

Table 1
Germline genetic mutation overview

Gene	Function/Pathway	Penetrance/Frequency	Histopathology/Notes	Other Associated Malignancies
CDKN2A	Tumor suppressor; regulates cellular senescence	20%–40% of FMS cases, ~65-fold increase risk melanoma	Similar to sporadic melanoma	Pancreas, mesothelioma, renal cell carcinoma, astrocytoma
CDK4	Promotes G1 → S phase via RB protein phosphorylation	Rare, ~74% lifetime risk of melanoma	Similar to sporadic melanoma	Breast, pancreas, ovarian, cervical, stomach
BAP1	Deubiquitinating enzyme; regulates DNA repair, apoptosis, cell cycle	~1% of cutaneous melanoma; 3% of uveal melanoma	No histopathologic predilection noted	Uveal melanoma, basal cell carcinoma malignant mesothelioma, renal cell carcinoma
TERT	Telomerase catalytic subunit; telomere length regulation	High penetrance, ~1% of FMS cases	Associated with superficial spreading and nodular melanoma	Bladder, colon, prostate, testicular, breast, kidney, CNS tumors
POT1	Shelterin complex; telomere protection	0.6%–3.8% depending on population	Spitzoid morphology	Angiosarcoma, glioma, chronic lymphocytic leukemia, thyroid, colorectal
ACD/TERF2IP	Shelterin complex; telomere protection	High penetrance	Superficial spreading or lentigo meligna at a young age, occasional spitzoid morphology	B cell lymphomas, esophagus, breast, lung, kidney, cervical, bladder, colon, prostate
ATM	DNA damage response kinase; double-strand break repair	Low-to-moderate penetrance, 2–3 × lifetime risk of melanoma	No histopathologic predilection noted	Breast, pancreas, prostate, stomach, ovarian, colorectal
FANCI	Fanconi anemia pathway; DNA repair	Novel likely pathogenic variants identified in small cohorts	Uncertain; more studies needed	Ovarian

accumulate, melanocytic lesions progress along a continuum from benign nevi to melanoma in situ and ultimately invasive lesions.[8]

BRAF

In Western melanoma populations, BRAF mutations account for approximately 50% to 60% of all somatic genetic alterations, with more than 90% occurring at codon 600 within exon 15 as a substitution of glutamic acid for valine (V600 E).[9,10] The prevalence of this mutation demonstrates an inverse relationship with patient age, occurring more frequently in younger patient and rapidly declining in those of advance age.[9] *BRAF* encodes a serine–threonine kinase that functions as a key regulator within the MAPK signaling pathway. Mutations in *BRAF* result in constitutive MAPK pathway activation, promoting uncontrolled cellular proliferation independent of upstream RAS-mediated signaling.[9,11] Given its central role in melanoma pathogenesis, substantial effort has been directed toward developing reliable diagnostic assays, predictive biomarkers, and targeted therapies aimed at exploiting BRAF-driven oncogenesis.

Neuroblastoma RAS

Mutations in NRAS represent the second most common somatic driver genetic mutation in cutaneous melanoma, occurring in approximately 15% to 25% of cases.[12,13] NRAS encodes a small GTPase that functions upstream of the MAPK and PI3K signaling pathways, acting as a molecular switch to cellular proliferation, differentiation, and survival. Activating mutations within NRAS commonly affect codon 61 at exon 2 or 3 leading to constitutive activation of MAPK independent of extracellular growth signals, thereby promoting melanocyte proliferation and oncogenic progression.[12] Substitutions at codons 12 and 13 have also been described but are rare.[12]

NRAS mutations also promote tumor-mediated evasion from immune cell surveillance, increasing tumor pathogenicity.[13] NRAS mutations are commonly associated with nodular melanoma subtype, advanced age and chronically sun-damaged skin.[7,12,13] These tumors display an aggressive biological behavior and are difficult to target with existing pharmacologic agents.

Cellular KIT

Cellular KIT (c-*KIT*) proto-oncogene encodes a receptor tyrosine kinase which plays a central role in melanocyte development, migration, and survival through downstream pathway stimulation.[14] Mutations in c-KIT occur in approximately 3% to 8% of cutaneous melanomas. Unlike *BRAF* and *NRAS* mutations, c-KIT mutations are also commonly observed in acral lentiginous and mucosal melanoma (up to 50% of patients).[15,16] The frequency of c-KIT mutations is directly influenced by the primary tumor location.[16] The identification of c-*KIT* mutant melanoma has important therapeutic implications. Certain tumors demonstrate a strong sensitivity to tyrosine kinase inhibitors such as imatinib. However, its efficacy varies significantly depending on the mutation location within the protein. For example, tumors harboring mutations in exons 11 and 13 exhibit favorable treatment response to therapeutic agents, whereas mutations in other locations show a much more variable treatment response.[15,16]

MAJOR GERMLINE MUTATIONS

Cyclin-Dependent Kinase Inhibitor 2A

The cyclin-dependent kinase inhibitor 2A (CDKN2A) gene remains the most extensively studied and clinically relevant germline mutation in FMS.[5,17,18] Mutations in CDKN2A account for approximately 20% to 40% of FMS cases.[5] The pathogenicity of this gene lies in its regulation of cellular senescence. Under normal conditions,

UV-induced DNA damage triggers melanocytes to enter irreversible cell cycle arrest, a process mediated by tumor suppressor pathways such as TP53/P21 and $P16^{INK4a}$/retinoblastoma (RB). Mutations in CDKN2A lead to impaired $P16^{INK4a}$ expression and ultimately preventing transition into a senescent state.[5] Without senescence, melanocytes with critical DNA damage are allowed to proliferate and expand resulting in melanoma development.

Individuals harboring CDKN2A mutations exhibit melanoma-dominant phenotypes and have up to a 65-fold increased personal risk of developing melanoma.[1] Patients who progress to develop MM have a poor overall survival in stage III/IV melanoma patients.[17,19] Harboring this mutation confers an increased risk of first-degree relatives also carrying the mutation (standardized incident ratio [SIR], 7.47; 95% confidence interval [CI], 3.97–12.77) as well as the risk for other cancer types such as pancreatic cancer, mesothelioma, renal cell carcinoma, and other neurologic tumors such as astrocytoma resulting in melanoma-astrocytoma syndrome.[6,18,20–22] Histopathologically CDKN2A-associated melanomas are largely indistinguishable from sporadic forms, and there is no consistent anatomic predilection for lesion development.[18,23]

Cyclin-Dependent Kinase 4

Cyclin-dependent kinase 4 (CDK4) is a downstream product of CDKN2A. CDK4 with CDK6 facilitates cell cycle progression from G1 to S phase via phosphorylation of the RB protein.[1] Germline mutations that result in MM always occur as a substitution for arginine within the codon critical for p16 protein binding.[1,18] Without p16 binding, constitutive kinase activation and uncontrolled cellular proliferation occurs. Although rare, CDK4 mutations confer a lifetime melanoma risk of approximately 74%.[1] Similar to CDKN2A-mutant tumors, CDK4-associated melanomas exhibit no distinct histologic or anatomic features.[23]

BRCA1-Associated Protein-1

Germline mutation in BRCA1-associated protein-1 (BAP1) represents a high penetrance mutation responsible for 1% of all MM.[1] Functionally, BAP1 is a deubiquitinating enzyme that regulates DNA repair, cell cycle progression, and apoptosis.[1] On UV-induced DNA damage, BAP1 activation promotes cell cycle arrest through serine/threonine kinase-mediated pathways.[18] Loss-of-function mutation within the BAP1 gene disrupt this checkpoint control predisposing cells to malignant transformation as there is no enzyme to trigger cell cycle arrest. Its impact in uveal melanoma is higher, cited at 3%, and when there is a concurrent uveal and cutaneous melanoma patients, one study cited 29% of families had germline mutations.[18] Mutations in BAP1 are also linked with the development of other cancers such as basal cell carcinoma, malignant mesothelioma and renal cell carcinoma.[24,25]

Telomerase Reverse Transcriptase

Germline mutations in telomerase reverse transcriptase (TERT) are uncommon but of high penetrance contributing to approximately 1% of FMS cases.[1,18] This gene encodes a protein involved in the shelterin protein complex, a complex of 8 proteins involved in telomere length regulation.[1,18,26] Shorting of cellular telomeres is a trigger for the cell to enter a senescent state, preventing further replication. Mutations in this protein allow for telomere lengthening and thus unchecked cellular growth. TERT mutations typically occur in the promoter region and other proteins involved include in this complex and result in high penetrance germline mutations including adrenocortical dysplasia protein (ACD), TERF21P, and protection of telomeres 1 (POT1).[18] This mutation is directly associated with superficial spreading and nodular subtypes of melanoma.[1]

Protection of Telomeres 1

The POT1 gene is another critical component of the shelterin complex, functioning in telomere length regulation and genomic stability.[18,27,28] POT1 variants have been associated with a significantly increased risk of melanoma, though reported frequencies vary among populations. In a US familial cohort, individuals with pathogenic POT1 variants demonstrated a markedly elevated melanoma risk (Odds Ratio [OR]] 7.03; 95% CI, 4.7–10.5; *P*<.001) and a higher incidence of multiple primary tumors.[29] Conversely, the MelaNostrum database reported variant frequencies of 3.8%, a separate study of CDKN2A/CDK4 wild-type Spanish families revealed and incidence of 1.75% and finally a Swedish cohort of 168 FMS cases identified POT1 pathogenic variants in only 0.6% of families, underscoring population variability.[27,28,30] Consistent with these findings, UK clinical practice guidelines recognize POT1 as a rare but relevant high-risk germline mutation.[31] These guidelines encourage POT1 germline genetic testing in individuals; however, if discovered, no additional clinical monitoring is required beyond yearly skin exams.[31] Histologically, POT1-associated melanomas frequently exhibit Spitzoid morphology.[23,27]

Adrenocortical Dysplasia Protein/Telomeric Repeat-Binding Factor 2 Interacting Protein

ACD and telomeric repeat-binding factor 2 interacting protein (TERF2IP) both play a role in comprising the shelterin complex in addition to POT1.[21,32,33] Their main role is in telomere maintenance, and they represent high-penetrance germline mutations.[21,32,34] Melanoma resultants due to these mutations typically present at a young age with superficial spreading or lentigo meligna subtypes.[32] Spitzoid morphology may also be seen.[35]

Ataxia-Telangiectasia Mutated

The ataxia-telangiectasia mutated (ATM) gene encodes a serine/threonine kinase that mediates DNA double-strand break repair and cellular response to oxidative and ionizing radiation or UV radiation. Biallelic ATM mutations cause the autosomal recessive disorder ataxia-telangiectasia or Louis-Barr syndrome, while heterozygous loss-of-function variants confer susceptibility to several cancers, including breast carcinoma and melanoma.[36–38] A large case–control evaluation performed between 2 centers demonstrate a higher frequency of deleterious or uncertain ATM variants among FMS cases compared with sporadic cases (*P*=.027).[36] Additional evidence indicates a low-to-moderate melanoma risk associated with ATM mutations (OR 1.46; 95% CI, 1.18–1.81).[27,28] Although rare, carriers exhibit a 2- to 3-fold increased lifetime melanoma risk compared to the general population.[39]

Fanconi Anemia Complementation Group I

Emerging data have implicated Fanconi anemia complementation group I (FANCI) variants in melanoma predisposition. In a small Hungarian cohort (n = 17) with FMS, novel FANCI variants were identified, one of which was classified as likely pathogenic.[40] However, most reported variants represent low- to moderate-penetrance alleles without confirmed clinical relevance. Further large-scale studies are required to clarify the role of FANCI and related Fanconi pathway genes in melanoma susceptibility.[40,41]

Melanoma Subordinate Syndromes

Melanoma subordinate syndromes arise in the context of other well-established inherited gene mutations such as those associated with breast cancer or ovarian cancer. Although melanoma may be seen in these instances, it does not predominate likely secondary to variable gene expressivity and incomplete penetrance.[6] Examples of melanoma subordinate syndromes include Cowden Syndrome, xeroderma pigmentosum, and Li Fraumeni syndrome.[6] Each of these well-studied syndromes are governed by their own genetic screening recommendations, surveillance guidelines, and gene panels. Recognition of melanoma's role within these syndromes remains clinically important and requires appropriate patient counsel.

Genetic Screening Recommendations

With respect to somatic genetic mutations, current National Comprehensive Cancer Network (NCCN) guidelines recommend germline testing primarily in stage III/IV disease, high-risk stage II disease based on pathologic features, or stage I or II melanoma only when results may inform clinical trial participation.[42] The goal of genetic testing is to identify mutations for which targeted medical therapy can be administered.

Germline genetic screening in familial melanoma facilitates early detection and intervention, improving melanoma-specific survival to near that of the general population.[43,44] Advances in genetic testing for both germline and somatic mutations have increased affordability, accessibility, and accuracy, prompting updates to clinical screening strategies. Early screening guidelines, established in 2009, focused only on CDKN2A testing.[6] Currently, these guidelines have evolved and are now indicated in patients who meet the "rule of twos or threes".[42]

The *rule of twos and threes* aids in estimating the pretest probability of detecting clinically actionable germline mutations and to guide the decision to pursue genetic testing.[6] The *rule of threes* is used in higher-prevalence melanoma regions such as the United States and is defined as 3 or more primary melanomas in the patient or first-/second-degree relatives. Inclusion of certain nonmelanoma cancers known to be caused by similar germline mutations is permitted. Cancers considered for inclusion include breast, colon, pancreatic, and prostate cancers.[4,6,45,46] Similarly, the *rule of twos* is used in lower-prevalence regions, requiring 2 primary melanomas or one primary melanoma plus a first-/second-degree relative with a relevant malignancy. Regions that constitute lower prevalence include European countries like Italy, Spain and France.[6] In lower- to medium-prevalence regions, some studies are emerging to suggest that the *rule of threes* may be an acceptable guideline for genetic testing; however, strict abidance by the *rule of twos* should be used if the individual diagnosed with melanoma is younger than age 40.[45] The *rule of fours* is used in Australia given the high prevalence of sporadic disease.[6,19] Although the concept is similar, global consensus on whether including melanoma in situ lesions as a *hit* remains lacking.

In addition to using the guidelines stated above, providers must also account for their clinical acumen for ultimate decision making. This is guided by a thorough history including detailed oncologic family history followed by physical exam. The decision to pursue genetic testing requires shared decision-making with patients and families. Overscreening can increase health care costs, laboratory utilization, procedural risks, and patient burden, without improving outcomes. A survey of clinicians recently performed believe that over screening for melanoma has become a public health concern.[47] However, underscreening can confer elevated risks for additional malignancies within the patient as well as their first- and second-degree relatives, such as pancreatic cancer, which carry significant prognostic implications. Therefore, when pursing genetic testing of family members, it is recommended to begin by screening the youngest affected individual within a family.[6] By screening an affected individual at a young age, the hope is to maximize identifying an actionable mutation while minimizing the risks of over screening additional family members as noted above.

Polygenic Risk Scoring

The genetic interplay within melanoma cells is complex. PRS has a role in stratifying patients who could be at genetically high risk for melanoma development but without a clearly identified germline mutation, representing ~55% of the FMS population.[48–50] PRS scoring combines many single nucleotide polymorphisms (SNPs) that have previously been previously identified and validated as holding melanoma risk in genome-wide association studies and combines them into an assessment tool.[48,51] Based on a genetic assessment, a score is then generated, and patients are placed into low- intermediate- or high-quartiles.

PRS helps to supplement current melanoma risk assessments as it provides a more comprehensive picture of an individual's genetic interplay.[52] PRS scoring allows clinicians to better identify and stratify patients into a high-risk category who may have otherwise been overlooked.[50,52] Consideration of a patient's genetic ancestry is important when consider SNPs to analyze when calculating PRS as it may influence the type and frequency of melanoma subtype a patient develops.[52] Validation studies of the multiple PRS risk prediction models are ongoing but have shown promising results.[53,54]

DISCUSSION

In summary, most melanotic lesions arise in a staged morphologic progression as accumulation of driver genetic mutations are acquired. There are 3 major identified somatic mutations: BRAF, NRAS, and c-KIT. The first major genetic mutation most often occurs in BRAF and results in autologous activation of the MAPK pathway. As the precursor lesion progresses, it next acquires activating mutations within NRAS. NRAS mutations promote independent cell cycle proliferation in addition to tumor-mediated immune cell evasion increased its pathogenicity. The third most encountered somatic mutation is c-KIT; however, these mutations have a predilection for mucosal melanoma as opposed to cutaneous. All melanoma tissue in unresected stage III and IV disease or stage II-III disease under consideration for adjuvant therapy undergoes BRAF testing to facilitate targeted medical therapy.[42] However, NCCN guidelines caution providers that current gene expression profiling (GEP) data are not robust enough to provide clinically actionable prognostic information.[42] Validation studies are ongoing.

There are 7 well-established germline mutations identified as principal drivers of MM development; however, these account for only approximately 45% of FMS cases, leaving more than half of hereditary susceptibility unexplained. Efforts to identify additional high-penetrance loci have been hindered by the rarity, heterogeneity, and inconsistent presence of variants even within affected first degree relatives.[40] Many large-scale genomic analyses documented in the literature have revealed numerous rare mutations of uncertain pathogenicity, underscoring the complexity of the genetic landscape underlying melanoma predisposition. PRS offers a promising avenue for quantifying cumulative genetic risk by integrating the additive effects of multiple SNP variants that are not currently tested for on widely established genetic tests. Implementation of PRS may enhance clinicians' ability to identify individuals at elevated risk for developing multiple primary melanomas or those who might harbor undetected susceptibility within the 55% of familial cases unexplained by current genetic testing. Ultimately, the integration of polygenic models with established screening frameworks represents a critical next step toward a comprehensive, precision-based approach to melanoma risk assessment and prevention.

When looking at genetic testing from a patient-centered approach, studies examining patient attitudes toward genetic testing before conception indicate that motivations are predominantly centered on control over personal and familial oncologic risk management.[55] Concerns exist regarding potential additional living costs (eg, mortgage and insurance), as well as availability of life insurance coverage.[55] Ultimately, family planning appeared to be unaffected because patients have a relatively poor understanding of germline genomic inheritance and wish to continue meeting their family planning goals.[55] Examination of psychological distress among high-risk MM patients do not significantly differ from the general population.[56] As expected, patients who are at known increased risk for MM desire the additional appropriate screening.[56]

Despite all ongoing work in the genetics space, NCCN guidelines currently state that GEP does not provide clinically actionable prognostic information and it is unclear whether they are a reliable tool for clinically actionable decisions.[42] This evidence is supported by recent meta-analysis. However, FMS patients were excluded from analysis in this study.[57] To date, there are no meta-analysis that have been performed investigating GEP effectiveness in FMS patients. Lastly, armed with evidence that screening in FMS facilitates early detection, intervention, and improves melanoma-specific survival to near that of the general population, further work should continue in this space.[43,44]

LIMITATIONS AND FUTURE DIRECTIONS

Several limitations affect the interpretation and application of genetic testing within the cutaneous melanoma population. Currently, gene expression profile panels for somatic genetic mutations are not adequately validated within literature, limiting their ability to be used for clinical prognostication.[42] In addition, there are multiple gene expression panels available ranging in evaluation from anywhere between 11 to 31 genes and there is no standardization among their utilization. Most studies in the current literature evaluating the efficacy of these profiles are retrospective in nature and more robust evaluations are ongoing in the form of large meta-analyses and prospective randomized trials.[58–60]

In terms of germline genetics, only 45% of FMS patients have a detectable high-penetrance mutation leaving over half the population without a clear germline mutation association.[6] This is likely as a result from low- or medium-penetrance genes in combination with epigenetic, environmental and geographic factors. Identifying true driver, high-penetrance mutations remains challenging. In review of the literature, there are many studies published regarding rare or new variants with uncertain clinical relevance, and larger studies are required to validate their pathogenicity.[61]

In addition to the extreme difficulty identifying high penetrance gene mutations among a sea of many unique, but nongeneralizable mutations, the FMS population is small. Within the FMS population, patients with the same genetic mutations are even smaller. Most studies focus on highly selected, high-risk populations, limiting power analysis. Data on specific gene mutations at population-level cohorts remain sparse. The development of consortium and gene databanks is growing; ongoing work is required to help identify genes that are likely to be driver mutations for further development is required. Large-scale genomic databases and collaborative networks are essential for identifying novel driver mutations and clarifying the penetrance of rare variants.

Lastly, global variability in genetic screening criteria for melanoma exists. Differences in melanoma classification for screening thresholds complicate cross-study comparisons. For example, some countries include melanoma in situ as a qualifying lesion, whereas others do not.[6] Future directions could include standardizing these definitions.

Emerging strategies in melanoma genomics aim to enhance risk stratification and personalize oncologic surveillance. Many gene expression profile panels are currently undergoing validation with hopes that soon they can be used to provide clinically actionable prognostic information. Incorporating the use of polygenic risk scores (PRS) to assist in risk, stratifying patients into low or high-risk categories for further assist in advancing precision medicine within the melanoma population.[62] Using PRS, patients and their first-degree relatives with pathogenic or likely pathogenic variants in high-risk genes (eg, CDKN2A) who currently fall outside the *rule of twos and threes* could benefit from more inclusive testing strategies.[46]

CLINICS CARE POINTS

- 45% of FMS patients have a detectable high-penetrance mutation leaving over half the population without a clear germline mutation association.
- NCCN guidelines recommend germline testing primarily in stage III/IV disease, high-risk stage II disease based on pathologic features, or stage I or II melanoma only when results may inform clinical trial participation.
- Current screening guidelines have evolved and are now indicated in patients who meet the "rule of twos or threes".
- Gene expression profile panels for somatic genetic mutations are not adequately validated within literature, limiting their ability to be used for clinical prognostication.

DISCLOSURE

The authors of this article have no financial disclosures to report.

REFERENCES

1. Truderung OA, Sagi JC, Semsei AF, et al. Melanoma susceptibility: an update on genetic and epigenetic findings. Int J Mol Epidemiol Genet 2021;12(5):71–89. PMID: 34853632; PMCID: PMC8611230.
2. Bruno W, Dalmasso B, Barile M, et al. Predictors of germline status for hereditary melanoma: 5 years of multi-gene panel testing within the Italian Melanoma Intergroup. ESMO Open 2022;7(4):100525.
3. Toussi A, Mans N, Welborn J, et al. Germline mutations predisposing to melanoma. J Cutan Pathol 2020;47(7):606–16. Epub 2020 May 11. PMID: 32249949; PMCID: PMC8232041.
4. Funchain P, Ni Y, Heald B, et al. Germline cancer susceptibility in individuals with melanoma. J Am Acad Dermatol 2024;91(2):265–72.
5. Subramanian P, Sayegh S, Laphanuwat P, et al. Multiple outcomes of the germline $p16^{INK4a}$ mutation affecting senescence and immunity in human skin. Aging Cell 2025;24(2):e14373. https://doi.org/10.1111/acel.14373. Epub 2024 Oct 17. Erratum in: Aging Cell. 2025 Aug;24(8):e70157. doi: 10.1111/acel.70157. PMID: 39420514; PMCID: PMC11822638.

6. Leachman SA, Lucero OM, Sampson JE, et al. Identification, genetic testing, and management of hereditary melanoma. Cancer Metastasis Rev 2017;36(1):77–90. PMID: 28283772; PMCID: PMC5385190.
7. Shain AH, Yeh I, Kovalyshyn I, et al. The genetic evolution of melanoma from precursor lesions. N Engl J Med 2015;373(20):1926–36. PMID: 26559571.
8. Elder DE, Bastian BC, Cree IA, et al. The 2018 World Health Organization classification of cutaneous, mucosal, and uveal melanoma: detailed analysis of 9 distinct subtypes defined by their evolutionary pathway. Arch Pathol Lab Med 2020;144(4):500–22. Epub 2020 Feb 14. PMID: 32057276.
9. Wang W, Lian B, Xu C, et al. Expert consensus on the diagnosis and treatment of solid tumors with BRAF mutations. Innovation 2024;5(6):100661. https://doi.org/10.1016/j.xinn.2024.100661. PMID: 39529955; PMCID: PMC11551471.
10. Schirosi L, Strippoli S, Gaudio F, et al. Is immunohistochemistry of BRAF V600E useful as a screening tool and during progression disease of melanoma patients? BMC Cancer 2016;16(1):905. PMID: 27863476; PMCID: PMC5116153.
11. Johnson DB, Menzies AM, Zimmer L, et al. Acquired BRAF inhibitor resistance: a multicenter meta-analysis of the spectrum and frequencies, clinical behaviour, and phenotypic associations of resistance mechanisms. Eur J Cancer 2015;51-(18):2792–9. Epub 2015 Nov 19. PMID: 26608120; PMCID: PMC4666799.
12. Chatziioannou E, Lallas K, Sinnberg T, et al. Insights into RAS-driven melanoma and its therapeutic implications. Cancer Treat Rev 2026;143:103090. https://doi.org/10.1016/j.ctrv.2026.103090. Epub 2026 Jan 15. PMID: 41576808.
13. Anastacio Da Costa Carvalho L, Tovbis Shifrin N, Phadke MS, et al. RAS(ON) multiselective inhibition drives antitumor immunity in preclinical models of NRAS-mutant melanoma. Cancer Immunol Res 2026;14(1):90–106. PMID: 41186497; PMCID: PMC12666865.
14. Kaveti A, Sullivan RJ, Tsao H. KIT-mutant melanoma: understanding the pathway to personalized therapy. Cancers (Basel) 2025;17(22):3644. PMID: 41301010; PMCID: PMC12650433.
15. Kawczak P, Bączek T. Pathway-specific therapeutic modulation of melanoma: Small-molecule inhibition of BRAF-MEK and KIT signaling in contemporary precision oncology with a special focus on vemurafenib, trametinib, and imatinib. J Clin Med 2025;14(22):7906. PMID: 41302945; PMCID: PMC12653686.
16. Sergi MC, Filoni E, Triggiano G, et al. Mucosal melanoma: epidemiology, clinical features, and treatment. Curr Oncol Rep 2023;25(11):1247–58. Epub 2023 Sep 29. PMID: 37773078; PMCID: PMC10640506.
17. Aoude LG, Bonazzi VF, Brosda S, et al. Pathogenic germline variants are associated with poor survival in stage III/IV melanoma patients. Sci Rep 2020;10(1): 17687. https://doi.org/10.1038/s41598-020-74956-3. PMID: 33077847; PMCID: PMC7572377.
18. Zocchi L, Lontano A, Merli M, et al. Familial melanoma and susceptibility genes: a review of the most common clinical and dermoscopic phenotypic aspect, associated malignancies and practical tips for management. J Clin Med 2021;10(16): 3760. PMID: 34442055; PMCID: PMC8397216.
19. Helgadottir H, Höiom V, Tuominen R, et al. Germline CDKN2A mutation status and survival in familial melanoma cases. J Natl Cancer Inst 2016;108(11). 545-452.
20. Chen X, Meyer MA, Kemppainen JL, et al. Risk of syndrome-associated cancers among first-degree relatives of patients with pancreatic ductal adenocarcinoma with pathogenic or likely pathogenic germline variants. JAMA Oncol 2023;9(7): 955–61. PMID: 37200008; PMCID: PMC10196930.

21. Zheng C, Sarin KY. Unveiling the genetic landscape of hereditary melanoma: from susceptibility to surveillance. Cancer Treat Res Commun 2024;40:100837. https://doi.org/10.1016/j.ctarc.2024.100837. Epub 2024 Aug 6. PMID: 39137473.
22. Sargen MR, Kim J, Potjer TP, et al. Estimated prevalence, tumor spectrum, and neurofibromatosis type 1-like phenotype of CDKN2A-Related melanoma-astrocytoma syndrome. JAMA Dermatol 2023;159(10):1112–8. PMID: 37585199; PMCID: PMC10433137.
23. Sargen MR, Calista D, Elder DE, et al. Histologic features of melanoma associated with germline mutations of CDKN2A, CDK4, and POT1 in melanoma-prone families from the United States, Italy, and Spain. J Am Acad Dermatol 2020;83(3):860–9. Epub 2020 Apr 10. PMID: 32283231; PMCID: PMC7505133.
24. Ochoa-Mellado IG, Padua-Bracho A, Cabrera-Galeana P, et al. Skin signals: exploring the intersection of cancer predisposition syndromes and dermatological manifestations. Int J Mol Sci 2025;26(13):6140. PMID: 40649916; PMCID: PMC12250388.
25. Elsayed AM, Kittaneh M, Cebulla CM, et al. An overview of BAP1 biological functions and current therapeutics. Biochim Biophys Acta Rev Cancer 2025;1880(2): 189267. https://doi.org/10.1016/j.bbcan.2025.189267. Epub 2025 Jan 21. Erratum in: Biochim Biophys Acta Rev Cancer. 2025 Jul;1880(3):189301.
26. Harland M, Petljak M, Robles-Espinoza CD, et al. Germline TERT promoter mutations are rare in familial melanoma. Fam Cancer 2016;15(1):139–44. PMID: 26433962; PMCID: PMC4698275.
27. Papadakis K, Portelli F, Schultz K, et al. POT1 genetic testing in melanoma-prone families in Sweden: germline variant prevalence and tumor spectrum in identified carriers. Acta Oncol 2025;64:1102–8.
28. Potrony M, Puig-Butille JA, Ribera-Sola M, et al. POT1 germline mutations but not TERT promoter mutations are implicated in melanoma susceptibility in a large cohort of Spanish melanoma families. Br J Dermatol 2019;181(1):105–13. Epub 2019 Feb 27. PMID: 30451293; PMCID: PMC6526091.
29. Herrera-Mullar J, Fulk K, Brannan T, et al. Characterization of POT1 tumor predisposition syndrome: tumor prevalence in a clinically diverse hereditary cancer cohort. Genet Med 2023;25(11):100937. https://doi.org/10.1016/j.gim.2023.100937. Epub 2023 Jul 17. PMID: 37466057.
30. Pellegrini C, Cardelli L, Ghiorzo P, et al. High- and intermediate-risk susceptibility variants in melanoma families from the mediterranean area: a multicentre cohort from the MelaNostrum consortium. J Eur Acad Dermatol Venereol 2023;37(12): 2498–508. Epub 2023 Sep 5. PMID: 37611275; PMCID: PMC10842987.
31. Tsoulaki O, Evans DG, Sinha K, et al. UK clinical practice guidelines for the management of patients with constitutional *POT1* pathogenic variants. J Med Genet 2025;62(9):559–65. PMID: 40350252; PMCID: PMC12418547.
32. Fiasconaro CA, Carbone A, Giordano S, et al. Germline Non-CDKN2A variants in melanoma and associated hereditary cancer syndromes. Diseases 2025;13(6): 180. PMID: 40558591; PMCID: PMC12191738.
33. Rice C, Shastrula PK, Kossenkov AV, et al. Structural and functional analysis of the human POT1-TPP1 telomeric complex. Nat Commun 2017;8:14928. https://doi.org/10.1038/ncomms14928. PMID: 28393830; PMCID: PMC5394233.
34. Pastorino L, Andreotti V, Dalmasso B, et al. Insights into genetic susceptibility to melanoma by gene panel testing: potential pathogenic variants in ACD, *ATM, BAP1,* and *POT1*. Cancers (Basel) 2020;12(4):1007. PMID: 32325837; PMCID: PMC7226507.

35. Goldstein AM, Qin R, Chu EY, et al. Association of germline variants in telomere maintenance genes (*POT1, TERF2IP, ACD,*and *TERT*) with spitzoid morphology in familial melanoma: a multi-center case series. JAAD Int 2023;11:43–51. PMID: 36876055; PMCID: PMC9978843.
36. Dalmasso B, Pastorino L, Nathan V, et al. Germline ATM variants predispose to melanoma: a joint analysis across the GenoMEL and MelaNostrum consortia. Genet Med 2021;23(11):2087–95. Epub 2021 Jul 14. PMID: 34262154; PMCID: PMC8553617.
37. Hall MJ, Bernhisel R, Hughes E, et al. Germline pathogenic variants in the ataxia telangiectasia mutated (*ATM*) gene are associated with high and moderate risks for multiple cancers. Cancer Prev Res 2021;14(4):433–40. Epub 2021 Jan 28. PMID: 33509806; PMCID: PMC8026745.
38. Goldstein AM, Xiao Y, Sampson J, et al. Rare germline variants in known melanoma susceptibility genes in familial melanoma. Hum Mol Genet 2017;26(24): 4886–95. PMID: 29036293; PMCID: PMC5886297.
39. LaDuca H, Polley EC, Yussuf A, et al. Clinical guide to hereditary cancer panel testing: evaluation of gene-specific cancer associations and sensitivity of genetic testing criteria in a cohort of 165,000 high-risk patients. Genet Med 2020;22(2): 407–15. Epub 2019 Aug 13. PMID: 31406321; PMCID: PMC7000322.
40. Bokor BA, Abdolreza A, Kaptás F, et al. Novel *FANCI* and *RAD54B* variants and the observed clinical outcomes in a Hungarian melanoma cohort. Int J Mol Sci 2024;26(1):23. PMID: 39795882; PMCID: PMC11719457.
41. Fierheller CT, Alenezi WM, Serruya C, et al. Molecular genetic characteristics of *FANCI*, a proposed new ovarian cancer predisposing gene. Genes 2023;14(2): 277. PMID: 36833203; PMCID: PMC9956348.
42. National Comprehensive Cancer Network. NCCN clinical practice guidelines in oncology: melanoma: cutaneous (version 2.2025). 2025. Available at: https://www.nccn.org.
43. Sargen MR, Pfeiffer RM, Elder DE, et al. The impact of longitudinal surveillance on tumor thickness for melanoma-prone families with and without pathogenic germline variants of *CDKN2A* and *CDK4*. Cancer Epidemiol Biomarkers Prev 2021; 30(4):676–81. PMID: 33811164; PMCID: PMC8049096.
44. Pissa M, Lapins J, Sköldmark C, et al. Melanoma-specific survival before and after inclusion in a familial melanoma dermatologic surveillance program in CDKN2A mutation carriers and non-carriers. J Eur Acad Dermatol Venereol 2023;37(2):284–92. Epub 2022 Oct 1. PMID: 36156317; PMCID: PMC10091727.
45. Delaunay J, Martin L, Bressac-de Paillerets B, et al. Improvement of genetic testing for cutaneous melanoma in countries with low to moderate incidence: the rule of 2 vs the rule of 3. JAMA Dermatol 2017;153(11):1122–9. PMID: 28903138; PMCID: PMC5710425.
46. Villa-Gonzalez JM, Carrera Revilla S, Lombardero Gutiérrez L, et al. Retrospective study of germline variants in patients with hereditary melanoma study criteria in a real clinical practice setting. Clin Exp Dermatol 2024;49(12):1532–6. PMID: 38833603.
47. Kerr KF, Eguchi MM, Piepkorn MW, et al. Dermatopathologist perceptions of overdiagnosis of melanocytic skin lesions and association with diagnostic behaviors. JAMA Dermatol 2022;158(6):675–9. PMID: 35442415; PMCID: PMC9021983.
48. Potjer TP, van der Grinten TWJ, Lakeman IMM, et al. Association between a 46-SNP polygenic risk score and melanoma risk in Dutch patients with familial melanoma. J Med Genet 2021;58(11):760–6. Epub 2020 Sep 29. PMID: 32994281; PMCID: PMC8551976.

49. Pellegrini S, Potjer TP, Del Bianco P, et al. Polygenic risk score improves melanoma risk assessment in a patient cohort from the Veneto region of Italy. Biology 2024;13(11):954.
50. Cust AE, Drummond M, Kanetsky PA, et al. Assessing the incremental contribution of common genomic variants to melanoma risk prediction in two population-based studies. J Invest Dermatol 2018;138(12):2617–24.
51. Landi MT, Bishop DT, MacGregor S, et al. Genome-wide association meta-analyses combining multiple risk phenotypes provide insights into the genetic architecture of cutaneous melanoma susceptibility. Nat Genet 2020;52(5):494–504. Epub 2020 Apr 27. PMID: 32341527; PMCID: PMC7255059.
52. Tovar-Parra D, Gutiérrez-Castañeda LD. Polygenic risk score analysis of 37 SNPs associated with melanoma risk in Colombian population. Int J Mol Sci 2025;26-(10):4674. PMID: 40429816; PMCID: PMC12112468.
53. Steinberg J, Iles MM, Lee JY, et al. Independent evaluation of melanoma polygenic risk scores in UK and Australian prospective cohorts. Br J Dermatol 2022;186(5):823–34. Epub 2022 Mar 31. PMID: 34921685; PMCID: PMC9545863.
54. Bakshi A, Yan M, Riaz M, et al. Genomic risk score for melanoma in a prospective study of older individuals. J Natl Cancer Inst 2021;113(10):1379–85. PMID: 33837773; PMCID: PMC8921762.
55. Onnekink AM, Klatte DCF, van Hooft JE, et al. Attitudes toward genetic testing, family planning and preimplantation genetic testing in families with a germline CDKN2A pathogenic variant. Fam Cancer 2024;23(3):255–65. Epub 2024 Jun 1. PMID: 38822936; PMCID: PMC11255069.
56. Onnekink AM, Klatte DCF, van Hooft JE, et al. Psychological distress and quality of life in families with a germline CDKN2A pathogenic variant. Mol Genet Genom Med 2025;13(2):e70045. https://doi.org/10.1002/mgg3.70045. PMID: 39936490; PMCID: PMC11815477.
57. Johansson M, Brodersen J, Gøtzsche PC, et al. Screening for reducing morbidity and mortality in malignant melanoma. Cochrane Database Syst Rev 2019;6(6): CD012352. https://doi.org/10.1002/14651858.CD012352.pub2. PMID: 31157404; PMCID: PMC6545529.
58. Greenhaw BN, Covington KR, Kurley SJ, et al. Molecular risk prediction in cutaneous melanoma: a meta-analysis of the 31-gene expression profile prognostic test in 1,479 patients. J Am Acad Dermatol 2020;83(3):745–53. Epub 2020 Mar 27. PMID: 32229276.
59. Hsueh EC, DeBloom JR, Lee JH, et al. Long-term outcomes in a multicenter, prospective cohort evaluating the prognostic 31-Gene expression profile for cutaneous melanoma. JCO Precis Oncol 2021;5. https://doi.org/10.1200/PO.20.00119. PO.20.00119.
60. Bartlett EK, O'Donoghue C, Boland G, et al. Society of surgical oncology gene expression profiling consensus statement work group. Society of surgical oncology consensus statement: assessing the evidence for and utility of gene expression profiling of primary cutaneous melanoma. Ann Surg Oncol 2025;32(3):1429–42. Epub 2024 Oct 29. PMID: 39470890; PMCID: PMC11811439.
61. Iversen GT, Loeng M, Holth AL, et al. Germline variants in CDKN2A wild-type melanoma prone families. Mol Oncol 2025;19(5):1493–507. Epub 2025 Mar 12. PMID: 40072281; PMCID: PMC12077288.
62. Ingold N, Seviiri M, Ong JS, et al. Exploring the germline genetics of in situ and invasive cutaneous melanoma: a genome-wide association study meta-analysis. JAMA Dermatol 2024;160(9):964–71. PMID: 39141363; PMCID: PMC11325244.

Role of Genetics in Gynecologic Malignancies

Corbyn M. Nchako, MD[a], Kara C. Long, MD, MSc[a],
Ying L. Liu, MD, MPH[b], Yukio Sonoda, MD[a,*]

KEYWORDS

• *BRCA* • Risk-reducing • Mismatch repair • Molecular subtype • Tubo-ovarian
• Endometrial carcinoma

KEY POINTS

- Universal germline and tumor testing, including *BRCA1/2* and mismatch repair/microsatellite instability analyses, are essential in gynecologic cancers to guide targeted therapy, identify hereditary syndromes, and inform family risk.
- Molecular classification should complement histopathology to refine prognosis and direct adjuvant treatment, de-escalation strategies, and clinical trial eligibility.
- Targeted and immune therapies must be biomarker-driven, with poly (ADP-ribose) polymerase inhibitors, immune checkpoint inhibitors, and HER2-directed agents selected based on tumor molecular profiles.
- Risk-reducing surgery should be individualized using gene-specific cancer risks, patient age, and reproductive goals, with counseling on menopausal and quality-of-life implications.
- Genetic counseling is integral to care, enabling appropriate test interpretation, cascade testing, fertility planning, and long-term survivorship management.

INTRODUCTION

Advances in cancer genomics have fundamentally reshaped the understanding, classification, and clinical management of gynecologic malignancies. Historically defined by histopathology and anatomic site, these cancers are now increasingly recognized as diseases driven by distinct molecular alterations that influence risk, tumor biology, prognosis, and therapeutic responsiveness. Across tubo-ovarian, endometrial, cervical, and rare gynecologic tumors, germline predisposition and somatic evolution together establish the genetic landscape that underpins modern

[a] Department of Surgery, Gynecology Service, Memorial Sloan Kettering Cancer Center, New York, NY, USA; [b] Department of Medicine, Gynecologic Medical Oncology Service and Clinical Genetics Service, Memorial Sloan Kettering Cancer Center, New York, NY, USA
* Corresponding author.
E-mail address: sonoday@mskcc.org

Surg Clin N Am 106 (2026) 585–602
https://doi.org/10.1016/j.suc.2026.03.004 **surgical.theclinics.com**

Abbreviations	
BSO	bilateral salpingo-oophorectomy
GCT	germ cell tumor
GCT	granulosa cell tumor
HBOC	hereditary breast and ovarian cancer
HGSOC	high-grade serous ovarian carcinoma
HPV	human papillomavirus
LGSC	low-grade serous carcinoma
MMR	mismatch repair
MMRd	mismatch repair deficient
MSI	microsatellite instability
NCCN	National Comprehensive Cancer Network
OS	overall survival
PARP	poly (ADP-ribose) polymerase
PFS	progression-free survival
PJS	Peutz-Jeghers syndrome
RRSO	risk-reducing salpingo-oophorectomy
SCSTs	sex-cord stromal tumors
SEE-FIM	Sectioning and Extensively Examining the Fimbriated end
TCGA	The Cancer Genome Atlas

clinical decision-making. As genomic testing becomes more accessible and deeply integrated into routine oncologic care, the role of genetics in gynecologic cancer has expanded from a specialized consideration to a central component of prevention, diagnosis, and treatment.

The genetic basis of gynecologic cancers encompasses a broad spectrum of alterations in tumor suppressor genes, oncogenes, and DNA repair pathways that contribute to tumor initiation and progression. Germline pathogenic variants (ie, mutations) in genes such as *BRCA1*, *BRCA2*, and DNA mismatch repair (MMR) genes define hereditary cancer syndromes including hereditary breast and ovarian cancer (HBOC) and Lynch syndrome—conditions that collectively account for up to 20% of gynecologic malignancies.[1] Somatic mutations, though not inherited, provide equally critical insights into tumor behavior and therapeutic vulnerabilities, particularly through identification of homologous recombination deficiency (HRD), *TP53* abnormalities, PI3K-pathway alterations, and MMR deficiency.

These genetic insights have catalyzed major shifts in risk assessment and prevention. Identification of hereditary syndromes guides individualized surveillance, cascade testing of at-risk relatives, and risk-reducing surgical procedures such as salpingo-oophorectomy, salpingectomy, or hysterectomy. In parallel, molecular classification systems—exemplified by The Cancer Genome Atlas (TCGA) framework for endometrial carcinoma—have refined prognostic stratification and informed treatment de-escalation or intensification strategies. Similar advances in tubo-ovarian, cervical, and rare tumor subtypes highlight the increasing necessity of molecularly guided management.

Crucially, the therapeutic landscape has also evolved with the advent of targeted and immune-based therapies that exploit specific genetic vulnerabilities. Poly (ADP-ribose) polymerase (PARP) inhibitors for homologous recombination-deficient tubo-ovarian cancers, HER2-targeted therapies in uterine serous carcinoma, and immune checkpoint inhibitors for microsatellite instability (MSI)-high or PD-L1-expressing tumors exemplify precision oncology in practice. As recurrent disease increasingly prompts repeat molecular profiling, genetic information continues to guide clinical decisions throughout the patient's disease course.

Collectively, the integration of genetic and molecular data has transformed gynecologic oncology, enabling more precise prevention strategies, refined tumor classification, and personalized therapeutic approaches. This article explores these developments, outlining the genetic foundations, hereditary syndromes, molecular classifications, and clinical implications that define contemporary care in gynecologic malignancies.

GENETIC BASIS OF GYNECOLOGIC CANCERS

Key Genetic Pathways and Mutations

Cancer arises from the accumulation of genetic and epigenetic alterations that disrupt normal cellular regulation. Among the most important contributors to tumorigenesis are changes in tumor suppressor genes, oncogenes, and DNA MMR pathways. These alterations influence cellular growth, genomic stability, and response to therapy, making them central to contemporary oncology practice.

Tumor suppressor genes act as guardians of genomic integrity, promoting cell-cycle arrest, apoptosis, or DNA repair in response to cellular stress. Loss-of-function mutations in these genes remove critical constraints on cell proliferation. *BRCA1* and *BRCA2* are classic examples involved in homologous recombination repair of double-stranded DNA breaks. Germline or somatic inactivation of *BRCA1* or *BRCA2* results in HRD, leading to genomic instability and an increased risk of breast, tubo-ovarian, prostate, and pancreatic cancers.[2] These defects create actionable therapeutic vulnerabilities, particularly to PARP inhibitors, which exploit synthetic lethality. *TP53*, often called the "guardian of the genome," is the most frequently mutated tumor suppressor across human cancers.[3] In normal cells, TP53 responds to genotoxic stress by inducing cell-cycle arrest, senescence, or apoptosis. Mutations—typically missense alterations—impair this function and may also produce dominant-negative or gain-of-function effects that enhance tumor aggressiveness. *TP53*-mutated tumors often exhibit resistance to conventional therapy and harbor high genomic instability, factors that influence prognosis and treatment selection.

Oncogenes, in contrast, drive malignant transformation when *activated* by mutation, amplification, or overexpression. *KRAS*, a key GTPase regulating cell proliferation and survival pathways, is among the most commonly mutated oncogenes, particularly in colorectal, pancreatic, and lung cancers.[4] *KRAS* mutations promote constitutive activation of downstream *MAPK/ERK* signaling, fostering uncontrolled growth and resistance to targeted therapies. Although historically considered "undruggable," recent advances have produced allele-specific inhibitors for *KRAS* and related variants, reshaping therapeutic strategies in lung and colorectal cancers. *HER2* (ERBB2) is another clinically significant and recently emerged target oncogene, initially known for its role in a subset of breast and gastric cancers. HER2 amplification leads to overactive receptor tyrosine kinase signaling that enhances cellular proliferation and survival.[5] HER2-driven cancers tend to be aggressive but are highly responsive to targeted therapy. It has recently become a target in gynecologic malignancies as well. The development of monoclonal antibodies, antibody–drug conjugates, and small-molecule inhibitors has transformed outcomes in HER2-positive disease.

MMR genes, including *MLH1*, *MSH2*, *MSH6*, and *PMS2*, maintain genomic fidelity by correcting base–base mismatches and insertion–deletion loops during DNA replication. Deficiency in MMR function leads to MSI, a hypermutator phenotype resulting in widespread frameshift mutations.[6] MSI-high tumors occur in colorectal, endometrial, gastric, and other cancers and have distinct biological behavior. Importantly, MSI-high or MMR-deficient tumors are highly immunogenic due to their elevated mutational burden, making them exceptionally responsive to immune checkpoint inhibitors.[7] MSI testing is now standard in multiple malignancies for prognostication and therapeutic decision-making.

Germline and Somatic Mutations

To fully understand the risk-stratification and treatment approaches of the various genetically driven gynecologic tumors, the types of mutational variants must be discussed. Germline and somatic mutations play distinct but complementary roles in the development, progression, and clinical movement of these malignancies. Germline mutations are inherited pathogenetic variants present in *all* cells of the body and are transmitted across generations, thus conferring a lifelong predisposition to cancer. They form the molecular basis of several hereditary cancer syndromes. In tubo-ovarian, endometrial, and less commonly, cervical cancers, germline mutations frequently involve DNA repair pathways such as homologous recombination and mismatch repair. In contrast, somatic mutations arise spontaneously within tumor tissue and inform the biology of the tumor but do not imply any inherited risk. They reflect the acquired spontaneous events that drive carcinogenesis. Though not heritable, these mutations provide an important layer of biological and sometime actionable information that may even overlap with germline findings. For example, tumors with somatic *BRCA* mutations behave similarly to their germline *BRCA*-associated counterparts[8] and also demonstrate similar sensitivity to PARP inhibitors—a class of drugs commonly used for *BRCA*-derived breast or gynecologic cancer.[9] Tumors with somatic MMR deficiency also exhibit MSI and are responsive to immune checkpoint blockade drugs.[10]

Identifying a germline mutation has implications for the patient's relatives, enabling cascade testing and risk-reducing interventions for family members. Somatic mutations do not affect familial risk. When a pathogenic variant is found in tumor testing; confirmatory germline testing is necessary to determine heritability and guide counseling. National bodies, such as the National Comprehensive Cancer Network (NCCN) and Society of Gynecologic Oncology, recommend patients meeting criteria for germline testing undergo dedicated germline analysis, even if tumor profiling is negative or inconclusive.[11,12]

HEREDITARY SYNDROMES AND RISK ASSESSMENT

Hereditary cancer syndromes account for approximately 10% to 20% of gynecologic malignancies (proportion varying by cancer type) and have substantial implications for prevention, early detection, and individualized treatment. Among these, HBOC and Lynch syndrome are the most common, while less frequent conditions—such as Peutz-Jeghers and Cowden syndromes—also confer elevated gynecologic cancer risks. Understanding their associated genetics, clinical manifestations, and recommended management enables clinicians to implement appropriate surveillance strategies and risk-reducing interventions.

Hereditary Breast and Ovarian Cancer

HBOC results predominantly from germline pathogenic variants in the autosomal dominant genes, *BRCA1* and *BRCA2*. These tumor suppressor genes are central to homologous recombination repair of double-stranded DNA breaks. Pathogenic variants impair DNA repair capacity, leading to genomic instability and significantly increased lifetime risk of breast, ovarian, fallopian tube, and peritoneal cancers. For women, the cumulative risk of tubo-ovarian cancer is approximately 39% to 46% for *BRCA1* carriers and 12% to 20% for *BRCA2* carriers[13]; breast cancer risk likewise rises to over 45% to 75% for *both* genes, with *BRCA1* carriers more likely to develop triple-negative disease.[14] In patients with pathogenic *BRCA* mutations who develop tubo-ovarian cancer, the overwhelming majority are of a serous histology. These patients typically present with advanced and high-grade disease, and 10% to 15% of the cases of high-grade serous carcinomas are linked to hereditary causes.[1] More data are needed to establish the relationship, if any, between non-serous epithelial subtypes (eg, endometrioid, clear cell, mucinous) and HBOC, but some studies have suggested *BRCA1* mutation may result in an increased risk of high-grade histology endometrial carcinoma.[15] Aside from *BRCA1/2*, there are a host of other pathogenic genetic mutations that confer an increased risk of tubo-ovarian and/or breast cancer that should be mentioned (**Table 1**).

Risk management and surveillance combine both imaging and risk-reducing strategies. Breast surveillance for *BRCA1/2* mutation carriers includes annual breast MRI with contrast beginning at the age of 25 years and annual mammography from age 30, alternating at 6-month intervals.[2] Clinical breast examinations every 6 to 12 months complement imaging. Tubo-ovarian cancer screening, such as with transvaginal ultrasound and serum CA-125—which has been studied in numerous trials—has not been shown to be beneficial with no improvement in mortality.[16–19]

Lynch Syndrome (HNPCC)

Lynch syndrome is the most common hereditary cause of endometrial cancer and arises from autosomal dominant germline mutations in DNA MMR genes—*MLH1*, *MSH2*, *MSH6*, and *PMS2*—or *EPCAM* deletions leading to *MSH2* silencing. Loss of MMR function results in an MSI-high tumor phenotype. Approximately 3% of endometrial cancer cases can be attributed to Lynch syndrome.[20] Compared with the general population's lifetime risk of endometrial cancer of 2% to 3%, women with Lynch syndrome have a 20% to 60% lifetime risk, often occurring before age 50 years, although this varies by gene.[21] The tumor tends to be located more in the lower uterine segment (vs uterine corpus), sometimes leading to misdiagnosis as cervical adenocarcinoma.

An increased risk of tubo-ovarian cancer is also associated with Lynch syndrome (**Table 2**). Risks range from 8% to 20% for those with *MLH1* mutations, 12% to 38% for *MSH2* mutations, and 1% to 11% for those with *MSH6* mutations, versus 1.3% for the general population, and is controversial for *PMS2* (approximately 3% risk). Tubo-ovarian cancer in these patients tend to occur the fourth decade of life versus the sixth decade in the general population and are thought to be driven by endometriosis with an enrichment in endometrioid and clear cell histologies. When diagnosed, the tubo-ovarian cancer is also more likely to be at an earlier stage (FIGO stage I or II), and invasive epithelial ovarian carcinoma is more likely to be well (Grade 1) or moderately (Grade 2) differentiated.

Risk management and surveillance include annual or biennial endometrial sampling starting between ages 30 and 35 years and consideration of transvaginal ultrasound in postmenopausal women,[11] although evidence supporting screening efficacy is limited. Patients should be counseled about early recognition of abnormal uterine bleeding. Like in HBOC, screening for Lynch-related tubo-ovarian cancer with transvaginal ultrasound or CA-125 has not been shown to be effective. Whether endometrial or tubo-ovarian screening, continue until total abdominal hysterectomy with bilateral salpingo-oophorectomy is performed. Colorectal cancer surveillance is mandatory, starting at 20 to 25 years of age (or 2–5 years prior to earliest diagnosis in first-degree relative, whichever is earlier),[2] due to substantially elevated risk with some variation by gene, with delayed initiation potentially in *MSH6* and *PMS2* Lynch syndrome.

Table 1
Genetic mutations associated with hereditary breast and ovarian cancer

Gene	Breast Cancer Risk	Tubo-Ovarian Cancer Risk	Other Associated Cancers
ATM	Mildly Increased	Mildly Increased	Pancreas, Prostate, Colorectal
BARD1	Increased	No increased risk	Unknown
BRCA1	Highly Increased	Highly Increased	Pancreas, Prostate
BRCA2	Highly Increased	Highly Increased	Pancreas, Prostate, Melanoma
BRIP1	Insufficient Evidence	Moderately Increased	Unknown
CDH1	Moderately Increased	No increased risk	Gastric
CHEK2	Moderately Increased	No increased risk	Prostate
Lynch Syndrome MMR genes: *MSH2, MLH1, MSH6, PMS2,* and *EPCAM*	Insufficient Evidence	Moderately Increased	Colorectal, Endometrium, Gastric, Hepatobiliary, Urothelial, Small Bowel, Pancreas
NF1	Moderately Increased	No increased risk	Peripheral nerve sheath tumors, GIST
PALB2	Mildly Increased	Mildly Increased	Pancreas, Prostate
PTEN	Increased	No increased risk	Cowden Syndrome, Thyroid, Colorectal, Endometrial, Renal
RAD51C	Moderately Increased	Moderately Increased	Unknown
RAD51D	Moderately Increased	Moderately Increased	Unknown
STK11	Increased	Increased risk of sex cord stromal tumors	Peutz-Jeghers Syndrome, Pancreatic
TP53	Highly Increased	No increased risk	Li-Fraumeni Syndrome, Pancreas, Prostate

Table 2
Lynch syndrome related cancers

Colorectal	Small Bowel	Hepatobiliary	Gastric
Endometrium	Ovary	Urothelial[a]	Brain[b]
Pancreas	Sebaceous gland tumors		

[a] Renal pelvis, ureter, bladder.
[b] Typically glioblastoma.

Peutz-Jeghers, Cowden, and Li-Fraumeni Syndromes

Peutz-Jeghers syndrome (PJS) results from autosomal dominant *STK11* mutations and is characterized by mucocutaneous pigmentation and gastrointestinal hamartomatous polyps.[1] Women with PJS have an elevated risk of sex-cord stromal tumors (SCST)—particularly ovarian sex cord tumors with annular tubules—and a modestly increased risk of cervical adenoma malignum, a highly differentiated form of mucinous adenocarcinoma. Gynecologic surveillance strategies include annual pelvic examinations and consideration of transvaginal ultrasound and CA-125 monitoring, though evidence is limited. Risk-reducing surgery is not routinely recommended but may be individualized based on polyp burden, tumor markers, or family history.

Cowden syndrome, caused by autosomal dominant *PTEN* mutations, predisposes individuals to endometrial carcinoma with a lifetime risk estimated at 20% to 30%.[1] Because onset can be early and endometrial cancer often arises from PTEN-driven hyperplasia, annual or biennial endometrial biopsy beginning at age 30 to 35 years is recommended.[2] Hysterectomy may be considered for women with completed childbearing and significant additional cancer risks, especially if endometrial hyperplasia develops.

Li-Fraumeni syndrome, associated with autosomal dominant *TP53* mutations, confers a broad cancer spectrum including early-onset breast cancer, soft tissue sarcomas, osteosarcomas, central nervous system tumors, and adrenocortical carcinomas.[1] Because ionizing radiation carries additional risk for these patients, surveillance emphasizes MRI-based imaging. *TP53* testing is recommended for patients with pathogenic *TP53* variants identified on tumor testing, especially if the diagnosis occurs before age 30 years.[22] Risk-reducing surgical procedures are considered on a case-by-case basis, particularly prophylactic mastectomy, but no routine gynecologic prophylactic surgery is recommended given unclear associations with tubo-ovarian cancer.

Among all 33 syndromes, pre-test and post-test genetic counseling is essential, with multigene panel testing being increasingly utilized to capture genetic heterogeneity and better guide management. From this, tailored surveillance and risk-reducing strategies can be created for the patient and family members.

Genetic Counseling and Testing

Genetic counseling should integrate personal and family history, tumor characteristics, and patient values to assess hereditary cancer risk and guide informed decision-making regarding genetic testing. Universal germline testing for epithelial ovarian cancer and consideration of germline testing with universal tumor testing for MMR deficiency in endometrial cancer have become standard practice. These approaches facilitate identification of patients who may benefit from targeted therapies, such as PARP inhibitors or immune checkpoint inhibitors, while also informing surgical decision-making and long-term surveillance.

Beyond implications for the individual patient, genetic counseling and testing extend their impact to families through cascade testing, allowing at-risk relatives to pursue risk-reducing interventions and appropriate screening. As multigene panel testing becomes more widely adopted and tumor–germline integration continues to evolve, the role of genetic counseling is expanding with criteria for referral including, but not limited to[12]:

- Early-onset cancers (age <50 years)
- Multiple primary cancers
- Epithelial ovarian, tubal, or primary peritoneal cancer

- Strong family history of breast, tubo-ovarian, or endometrial cancers
- High-risk ethnic backgrounds (eg, Ashkenazi Jewish)
- Known familial pathogenic variants
- Tumor features suggesting hereditary disease (eg, MSI-high or MMR-deficient endometrial cancer, triple-negative breast cancer before age 60 years, serous tubo-ovarian cancer at any age).

Interpreting genetic test results requires distinguishing pathogenic and likely pathogenic variants—which warrant surveillance and risk-reduction—from variants of uncertain significance, which should not guide clinical decisions. Cascade testing of at-risk relatives is essential for familial risk mitigation.[23] Genetic counseling ensures patients understand inheritance patterns, surveillance recommendations, and the implications of surgical prevention strategies.

MOLECULAR CLASSIFICATIONS OF GYNECOLOGIC CANCERS

Across almost all types of gynecologic tumors, molecular profiling has transformed the landscape of understanding and management. Traditional histopathologic classification remains fundamental, but integrating genomic, transcriptomic, and proteomic features allows for more precise prognostication and individualized therapy. Specific molecular signatures increasingly guide therapeutic decision-making and clinical trial stratification.

Endometrial

In 2013, a landmark study by TCGA introduced a molecular classification system for endometrial carcinoma that has started to reshape the landscape of risk-assessment and clinical relevance.[24] The framework defined 4 major molecular subtypes (**Fig. 1**):

1. *POLE-ultramutated:* Characterized by exonuclease domain mutations in *POLE*, these tumors exhibit extremely high mutational burden and robust immune infiltration. Despite often high-grade histology, they carry an excellent prognosis. Multiple prospective trials (PORTEC-4a,[25] NRG-GY032) are investigating safe de-escalation protocols, even in high-risk cases, given the very low recurrence risk.
2. *Mismatch repair deficient (MMRd)/MSI-high:* Resulting from somatic or germline MMR gene loss, this group shows elevated mutational burden, lymphocytic infiltration, and intermediate prognosis. MSI-high status predicts sensitivity to immune checkpoint inhibitors and informs Lynch syndrome evaluation.
3. *Copy-number high (p53-abnormal):* Includes most serous carcinomas and a minority of high-grade endometrioid tumors. Defined by *TP53* mutations and extensive chromosomal instability, this group has the *worst* prognosis. HER2 amplification in serous carcinomas is therapeutically actionable.
4. *Copy-number low (no specific molecular profile [NSMP]):* Typically, endometrioid, low-grade tumors with mutations in *PTEN*, *PIK3CA*, *KRAS*, and *CTNNB1*. Prognosis is generally favorable, though *CTNNB1* exon 3 mutations identify a subgroup at higher risk of recurrence.[26]

Overall, this classification has begun to drive adjuvant therapy decision-making in endometrial cancer and is reflected in the latest NCCN guidelines.

Ovarian

High-grade serous ovarian carcinoma (HGSOC), likely arising from the fimbriated end of the fallopian tube, is the most common and lethal ovarian cancer subtype

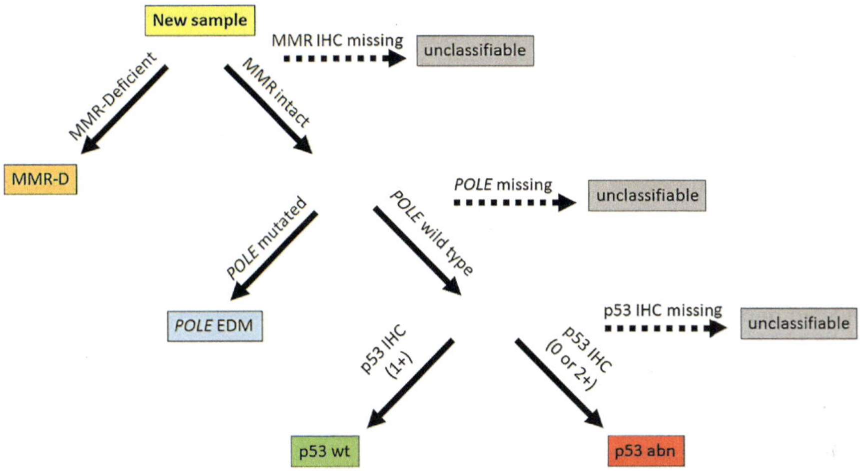

Fig. 1. Endometrial carcinoma ProMisE algorithm. IHC, immunohistochemistry; IHC score 0, complete loss; IHC score 1+, normal expression IHC score 2+, accumulation; MMR-d, mismatch-repair-deficient (15%–27%); NSMP, no specific molecular profile (50%); POLEmut, Polymerase Epsilon exonuclease domain mutated (8%–10%); p53abn, p53 mutated/copy-number-high (15%); wt, wild type. (Talhouk, A. et al., (2017), Confirmation of ProMisE: A simple, genomics-based clinical classifier for endometrial cancer. Cancer, 123: 802-813. https://doi.org/10.1002/cncr.30496.)

and is defined by distinctive molecular features. Nearly all HGSOCs harbor *TP53* mutations and exhibit widespread genomic instability. Approximately 50% demonstrate HRD, driven by germline or somatic *BRCA1/2* mutations or alterations in other HR-associated genes.[27] HRD-positive status predicts response to platinum-based chemotherapy and PARP inhibitors; positivity is associated with increased sensitivity, as well as longer progression-free survival (PFS) and improved overall survival (OS) compared with HRD-negative tumors. Gene expression–based classification further delineates mesenchymal, immunoreactive, proliferative, and differentiated subtypes, which correlate with prognosis and potential immunotherapeutic responsiveness.

Low-grade serous carcinoma (LGSC), in contrast, is characterized by MAPK pathway mutations, particularly *KRAS*, *BRAF*, and *NRAS*.[28] These molecular features support emerging use of MEK inhibitors and distinguish LGSC from HGSOC both biologically and therapeutically.[29] Endometrioid and clear-cell ovarian carcinomas often arise from endometriosis and are enriched for *ARID1A* loss, *PTEN* mutations, and *PIK3CA* mutations.[30,31] Clear-cell tumors demonstrate HNF-1β overexpression,[32] metabolic reprogramming, and frequent MMR deficiency, providing rationale for immunotherapy in select cases. Mucinous ovarian carcinomas display *KRAS* mutations and HER2 amplification in a subset, opening consideration for HER2-directed therapy.[33]

Cervical Cancer

Cervical cancer is predominantly driven by persistent infection with high-risk human papillomavirus (HPV). The molecular hallmarks stem from viral oncoproteins E6 and E7, which inactivate p53 and Rb, respectively, leading to unchecked proliferation and chromosomal instability.[3,34] HPV-associated cancers (primarily squamous cell carcinoma and usual-type adenocarcinoma) are genomically and immunologically distinct from their HPV-independent counterparts. These HPV-associated cervical carcinomas have enhanced AKT/mTOR signaling through viral mechanisms, while pathway alterations in HPV-independent carcinoma are frequently due to the significantly increased number of somatic mutations. HPV-independent cervical adenocarcinomas, including gastric-type carcinomas, display *TP53* and *STK11* mutations and carry a worse prognosis.[35] Their distinct molecular profile underscores the need for separate treatment algorithms.

Other Gynecologic Tumors

Ovarian germ cell tumors

Germ cell tumor (GCTs) are molecularly and clinically distinct from epithelial ovarian cancers. Dysgerminomas exhibit KIT overexpression and *KIT* or *RAS* mutations in a subset. They demonstrate exceptional chemosensitivity, which underlies their favorable outcomes. Yolk sac tumors express AFP-related gene signatures and frequently activate PI3K/AKT/mTOR signaling.[36] Embryonal carcinoma and mixed GCTs reflect pluripotency pathways, including NANOG and OCT3/4 expression.

Sex-cord stromal tumors

Granulosa cell tumors (GCTs), particularly adult-type, are characterized by the pathognomonic *FOXL2 C134W* mutation,[37] which alters transcriptional regulation of granulosa cell differentiation. This mutation aids diagnosis and may influence hormonal signaling-based therapeutics. Juvenile GCTs lack *FOXL2* mutations and instead show alterations in *GNAS* and *AKT1* pathways.[38] Sertoli-Leydig cell tumors harbor *DICER1* mutations in approximately 50%, linking them to hereditary DICER1 syndrome and influencing recommendations for genetic testing and long-term surveillance.[39]

Other rare SCSTs, such as small cell carcinoma of the ovary hypercalcemic type, are defined by *SMARCA4 (BRG1)* loss and are considered within the spectrum of SWI/SNF-deficient cancers. These tumors behave aggressively but may respond to targeted therapies exploiting epigenetic vulnerabilities.

IMPLICATIONS FOR TREATMENT AND MANAGEMENT STRATEGIES

Targeted Therapies

The clearest example of genomically informed therapy in gynecologic oncology is the use of PARP inhibitors in tubo-ovarian cancer. High-grade serous tubo-ovarian carcinomas exhibit high rates of HRD, driven by germline or somatic *BRCA1/2* mutations or alterations in other DNA repair genes (*RAD51C/D*, *BRIP1*, *PALB2*). HRD renders tumor cells more vulnerable to PARP-mediated synthetic lethality (**Fig. 2**). Agents such as olaparib, niraparib, and rucaparib significantly prolong PFS in both frontline maintenance and recurrent disease settings, with the greatest benefit in *BRCA*-mutated tumors but meaningful activity in HRD-positive, *BRCA*-wild-type disease as well.[40]

HER2 amplification is present in a subset of uterine serous carcinomas. Trastuzumab combined with chemotherapy has demonstrated improved outcomes in HER2-positive uterine serous carcinoma, establishing HER2 testing as standard.[41] Emerging agents, including antibody-drug conjugates such as trastuzumab deruxtecan, have been shown to be efficacious as biomarker-directed therapy options in patients with HER2-positive (immunohistochemistry 3+ or 2+) recurrent endometrial carcinoma.[42]

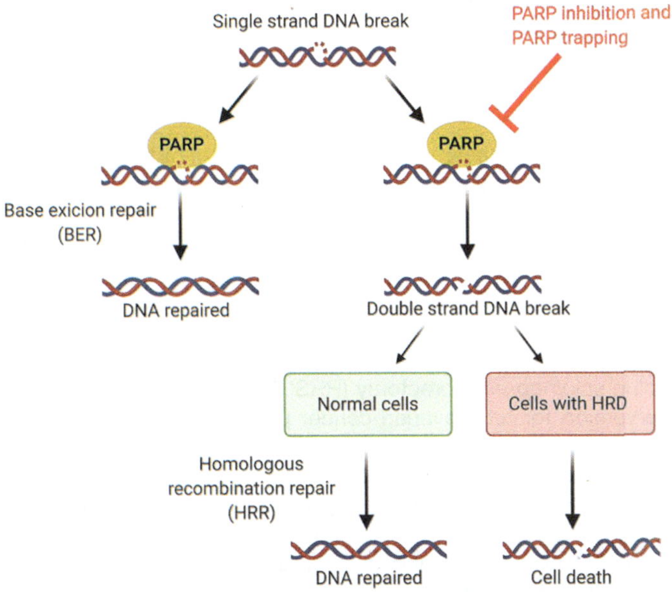

Fig. 2. PARP inhibitor mechanism of action. (*From* 'Pharmacokinetics and Pharmacodynamics of PARP Inhibitors in Oncology' by Bruin MAC, Sonke GS, Beijnen JH, et al. Pharmacokinetics and Pharmacodynamics of PARP Inhibitors in Oncology. Clin Pharmacokinet 2022;61(12):1649–1675. https://doi.org/10.1007/s40262-022-01167-6; with permission.)

MMRd and MSI-high tumors exhibit high neoantigen loads and strong immune responsiveness. In endometrial carcinoma, PD-1 inhibitors such as pembrolizumab and dostarlimab have produced durable responses in recurrent MMRd tumors and are now key components of second-line and combination frontline therapy.[43,44] Even in MMR-proficient disease, combination regimens (eg, pembrolizumab + lenvatinib[45]) provide benefit, highlighting the expanding role of immunotherapy. Cervical cancers driven by HPV often express PD-L1 and exhibit immunogenic signatures. Immune checkpoint inhibitors (pembrolizumab, cemiplimab),[46,47] with or without standard chemotherapy, are now standard in recurrent or metastatic cervical cancer. *PIK3CA* and *KRAS* mutations have also been targeted with inhibitors used in HPV-independent tumors.

Genetic Testing in Recurrent Disease

Routine germline *BRCA1/2* testing is recommended for all patients with epithelial ovarian, fallopian tube, or primary peritoneal cancer, regardless of family history. Universal tumor testing for HRD and somatic *BRCA* alterations further refines the selection of PARP inhibitors and identifies individuals who require germline confirmatory testing.

In endometrial carcinoma, universal MMR immunohistochemistry or MSI testing is standard to identify Lynch syndrome and to determine eligibility for immunotherapy. Additionally, germline genetic testing is also being considered in all endometrial cancer given presence of germline mutations in non-Lynch genes including *BRCA1/2*. In recurrent cervical cancer, genetic testing is less standardized but may identify HER2 amplification, PI3K pathway alterations, or actionable biomarkers for clinical trials. As targeted options expand—especially after failure of first-line therapy—re-testing tumors at recurrence is increasingly common. Tumor evolution may reveal new actionable alterations, such as *ESR1* mutations, secondary *BRCA* reversion, or emerging gene amplifications.

Risk-Reducing Strategies and Surgical Procedures

The management of individuals with hereditary susceptibility to gynecologic malignancies necessitates a multifaceted approach integrating surgical, pharmacologic, and reproductive strategies. Genetic predisposition—most commonly involving *BRCA1, BRCA2*, and DNA MMR genes associated with Lynch syndrome—significantly alters both the timing and nature of preventive interventions. As a result, risk-reducing strategies must be personalized, evidence-based, and attentive to the long-term quality-of-life implications for patients who often face decisions at younger ages than the general population.

Risk-reducing salpingo-oophorectomy (RRSO) remains the most evidence-based, effective intervention for tubo-ovarian cancer prevention in patients with *BRCA1/2* germline pathogenic variants. For *BRCA1* carriers, RRSO is recommended between ages 35 to 40 years, and for *BRCA2* carriers between 40 and 45 years of age,[2] or earlier based on family history or completion of childbearing (**Box 1**). RRSO in this patient population decreases tubo-ovarian cancer risk by over 80% to 90%[48] and reduces premenopausal breast cancer risk by approximately 40% to 50% through the removal of estrogen production.

Risk-reducing salpingectomy with later or *delayed* oophorectomy is an emerging risk-reduction strategy in premenopausal patients who are not ready for oophorectomy and its associated fertility and endocrine implications. The advantage of this two-stage approach, especially in women with pathogenic *BRCA* variants, has been demonstrated from a quality-of-life standpoint in studies such as the WISP and TUBA trials.[49,50] The oncologic efficacy of such an approach is still under investigation with multiple prospective observational studies ongoing (ie, SOROCk, TUBA-WISP-II, and PROTECTOR), with maturity of data expected within the next 5 to 10 years.

After the specimens have been removed, pathologic evaluation using the "Sectioning and Extensively Examining the Fimbriated end" (SEE-FIM) pathologic dissection protocol enhances detection of occult serous tubal intraepithelial carcinoma, a precursor lesion in high-grade serous carcinoma. Hormone replacement therapy is recommended for premenopausal individuals without a breast cancer history.

Risk-reducing hysterectomy with bilateral salpingo-oophorectomy (BSO) is a validated strategy in patients with Lynch syndrome. Prophylactic surgery markedly

Box 1
Risk-reducing BSO considerations

- *BRCA1*: 35 to 40 year old, or completion of childbearing
- *BRCA2*: 40 to 45 year old, or completion of childbearing
- Thoroughly inspect peritoneal cavity and perform cytologic washings
- Ensure removal of all ovarian and fallopian tube tissue:
  - Isolate and ligate the infundibulopelvic (IP) ligament ~2cm *proximal* to any identifiable ovarian tissue
  - The fallopian tube should be divided at its cornual insertion site
  - Isolate and divide the utero-ovarian ligament as close to the uterus as possible
  - Serially section pathology specimens with microscopic examination (SEE-FIM protocol)

reduces endometrial cancer and tubo-ovarian cancer risk.[51] It is generally recommended once childbearing is complete, or between ages 40 and 50 years, with timing individualized by gene: *MLH1* and *MSH2* carriers warrant earlier intervention around age 40 years due to higher risk, while *MSH6* and *PMS2* carriers may defer to later ages based on a more moderate risk profile.[52] In terms of delayed oophorectomy, similar strategies can be applied with gene-specific timing: in *MSH6* carriers, hysterectomy with salpingectomy can be considered starting at age 40 years, with delayed bilateral oophorectomy at 45-50 years of age. In *MLH1* and/or *MSH2* carriers who face earlier age risk, delayed oophorectomy is generally not considered.

Patients who carry pathogenic variants of *RAD51C* or *RAD51D* face up to a 20% lifetime risk of tubo-ovarian cancer and a median age at diagnosis of 60 years. Those who are *BRIP1* carriers have a 5% to 15% lifetime risk of tubo-ovarian cancer with a median age at diagnosis of 65 years. While these variants are more "moderate-risk" for tubo-ovarian cancer, societies such as the American College of Medical Genetics recommend that when tubo-ovarian cancer risk exceeds 3% to 5%,[53] risk-reducing BSO should be considered around ages 45 to 50 years.[2] In these patient populations, risk-reducing BSO could be delayed until age 50 years, due to the comparable age of onset to the general population.

Despite their proven efficacy, risk-reducing procedures carry significant considerations. Premenopausal oophorectomy induces abrupt surgical menopause, with associated vasomotor, sexual, bone, and cardiovascular effects.[54–56] Surgical risks and the psychological impact of early menopause underscore the need for careful shared decision-making. All discussions of surgical risk reduction should include counseling on menopausal management strategies. Hormone replacement therapy is recommended in premenopausal patients without personal breast cancer history and can help to mitigate the adverse effects of premature menopause.[2] In patients receiving hormone replacement therapy, estrogen can be administered via various routes (eg, transdermal, oral, intravaginal) with slight variations in absorption and side effect profile. In those who still have a uterus, progesterone must also be administered to temper any abnormal endometrial proliferation.

Pharmacologic and hormonal interventions provide additional avenues for risk reduction. Oral contraceptive use has consistently demonstrated an approximately 50% reduction in tubo-ovarian cancer risk in both average-risk and high-risk women, including *BRCA1/2* carriers.[57,58] In Lynch syndrome, progestin-based therapies—either through systemic regimens or intrauterine devices—may mitigate endometrial neoplasia risk by counteracting unopposed estrogen exposure, like that in the general population.[59] Lifestyle modifications, including weight management, physical activity, and smoking cessation, also contribute to lowering endometrial cancer risk, even in genetically susceptible individuals.

Given the implications of early surgical intervention, fertility preservation and reproductive counseling are essential components of care. Oocyte and embryo cryopreservation should be discussed with patients facing recommended surgical procedures that threaten reproductive potential. Furthermore, pre-implantation genetic testing for monogenic conditions provides an opportunity to *prevent* transmission of pathogenic variants to future offspring and thus has become an integral counseling point for many high-risk families.

Overall, risk-reduction strategies for hereditary gynecologic cancer syndromes require a comprehensive, anticipatory, and multidisciplinary approach. Genetic information not only guides the timing and extent of surgical management but also influences reproductive decision-making, hormonal interventions, and long-term health considerations. As genetic testing becomes increasingly widespread, the integration of personalized risk-reduction strategies will remain foundational to contemporary gynecologic oncology practice.

SUMMARY

The integration of genetic and molecular insights into gynecologic oncology has fundamentally reshaped prevention, diagnosis, and treatment paradigms. Across tubo-ovarian, endometrial, cervical, and rare gynecologic malignancies, an improved understanding of germline predisposition and somatic evolution has led to more refined risk stratification and increasingly precise clinical interventions. Genetic testing now informs hereditary cancer risk assessment, guides cascade testing for families, and supports evidence-based implementation of risk-reducing strategies such as prophylactic surgery. At the tumor level, molecular classification systems—exemplified by the TCGA framework in endometrial cancer—have moved beyond traditional histopathology to define biologically distinct subgroups with differing prognoses and therapeutic susceptibilities.

The future of gynecologic oncology lies in deeper and more universal integration of genetic testing into routine clinical practice. Expanded access to germline and somatic sequencing, harmonized testing guidelines, and improved interpretation frameworks will be essential to ensure equitable application of these advances. Continued discovery of novel biomarkers, refinements in molecular classification, and development of increasingly targeted therapies promise to further individualize patient care. Ultimately, the advancing genomic landscape offers a path toward earlier detection, more effective prevention, and more durable therapeutic response—driving meaningful improvements in outcomes for patients with gynecologic cancers.

CLINICS CARE POINTS

- A substantial proportion of patients with germline pathogenic variants (particularly BRCA1/BRCA2) lack a strong family history; reflex testing in epithelial ovarian cancer and universal tumor testing in endometrial cancer reduce missed diagnoses.
- Identifying a germline mutation should trigger systematic efforts to test at-risk relatives.
- Homologous recombination deficiency (HRD) status—not just BRCA—should guide PARP inhibitor use. Patients without BRCA mutations may still derive benefit if HRD positive.
- p53-abnormal endometrial cancers behave aggressively regardless of histologic subtype.
- Fertility and reproductive planning should be addressed early. These should occur prior to risk-reducing surgery.
- Planned premenopausal oophorectomy should prompt a preoperative discussion of menopause management.
- Decisions on the use of immunotherapy should be biomarker driven, not only dependent on tumor histology.
- Tumor evolution (eg, reversion mutations restoring BRCA function or new actionable amplifications) may alter sensitivity to prior therapies and open new treatment options.

DISCLOSURES

Y. Sonoda: None. C.M. Nchako: None. K.C. Long: None. Y.L. Liu: research funding from AstraZeneca, GSK, Artios Pharma, and Repare Therapeutics as well as advisory board participation for Myriad Genetics, Gilead, and Abbvie unlreated to this work.

REFERENCES

1. Hereditary cancer syndromes and risk assessment: ACOG COMMITTEE OPINION, number 793. Obstet Gynecol 2019;134(6):e143–9. https://doi.org/10.1097/AOG.0000000000003562.
2. National Comprehensive Cancer Network: NCCN Clinical Practice Guidelines in Oncology: Genetic/Familial High-Risk Assessment: Breast, Ovarian, Pancreatic, and Prostate. Version 2.2026.
3. Baliakas P, Soussi T. The TP53 tumor suppressor gene: from molecular biology to clinical investigations. J Intern Med 2025;298(2):78–96.
4. Huang L, Guo Z, Wang F, et al. KRAS mutation: from undruggable to druggable in cancer. Sig Transduct Target Ther 2021;6:386.
5. Cheng X. A comprehensive review of HER2 in cancer biology and therapeutics. Genes 2024;15(7):903.
6. Sijmons RH, Hofstra RMW. Review: clinical aspects of hereditary DNA mismatch repair gene mutations. DNA Repair (Amst) 2016;38:155–62.
7. Johannet P, Rousseau B, Aghajanian C, et al. Therapeutic targeting of mismatch repair-deficient cancers. Nat Rev Clin Oncol 2025;22(10):734–59.
8. Winter C, Nilsson MP, Olsson E, et al. Targeted sequencing of BRCA1 and BRCA2 across a large unselected breast cancer cohort suggests that one-third of mutations are somatic. Ann Oncol 2016;27(8):1532–8.
9. Mohyuddin GR, Aziz M, Britt A, et al. Similar response rates and survival with PARP inhibitors for patients with solid tumors harboring somatic versus germline BRCA mutations: a meta-analysis and systematic review. BMC Cancer 2020;20(1):507.
10. Le DT, Durham JN, Smith KN, et al. Mismatch repair deficiency predicts response of solid tumors to PD-1 blockade. Science 2017;357(6349):409–13.
11. National Comprehensive Cancer Network. NCCN clinical practice guidelines in oncology: genetic/familial high-risk assessment: colorectal, endometrial, gastric. Version 1. J Natl Compr Canc Netw 2025;14(8):1010–30.
12. Lancaster JM, Powell CB, Chen LM, et al, SGO Clinical Practice Committee. Society of gynecologic oncology statement on risk assessment for inherited gynecologic cancer predispositions. Gynecol Oncol 2015;136(1):3–7 [Epub 2014 Sep 17. Erratum in: Gynecol Oncol. 2015 Sep;138(3):765. PMID: 25238946].
13. Kuchenbaecker KB, Hopper JL, Barnes DR, et al. Risks of breast, ovarian, and contralateral breast cancer for BRCA1 and BRCA2 mutation carriers. JAMA 2017;317(23):2402–16.
14. Antoniou A, Pharoah PD, Narod S, et al. Average risks of breast and ovarian cancer associated with BRCA1 or BRCA2 mutations detected in case series unselected for family history: a combined analysis of 22 studies. Am J Hum Genet 2003;72(5):1117–30.
15. Kotsopoulos J, Lubinski J, Huzarski T, et al. Incidence of endometrial cancer in BRCA mutation carriers. Gynecol Oncol 2024;189:148–55.
16. Rosenthal AN. Ovarian cancer screening in the high-risk population–the UK familial ovarian cancer screening study (UKFOCSS). Int J Gynecol Cancer 2012;22(Suppl 1):S27–8.
17. Gohagan JK, Prorok PC, Hayes RB, et al, Prostate, Lung, Colorectal and Ovarian Cancer Screening Trial Project Team. Prostate, lung, colorectal and ovarian cancer screening trial project team. The prostate, lung, colorectal and ovarian (PLCO) cancer screening trial of the national cancer Institute: history, organization, and status. Control Clin Trials 2000;21(6 Suppl):251S–72S.

18. Hermsen BB, Olivier RI, Verheijen RH, et al. No efficacy of annual gynaecological screening in BRCA1/2 mutation carriers; an observational follow-up study. Br J Cancer 2007;96(9):1335–42.
19. Nañez A, Stram DA, Garcia C, et al. Ovarian cancer surveillance in the clinical follow up of women with known BRCA1 or BRCA2 pathogenic variants in a large health care system. Gynecol Oncol 2021;163(1):134–41.
20. Gruber SB, Thompson WD. A population-based study of endometrial cancer and familial risk in younger women. Cancer and steroid hormone study group. Cancer Epidemiol Biomarkers Prev 1996;5(6):411–7.
21. Underkofler KA, Ring KL. Updates in gynecologic care for individuals with Lynch syndrome. Front Oncol 2023;13:1127683.
22. Frebourg T, Bajalica Lagercrantz S, Oliveira C, et al. Guidelines for the Li-Fraumeni and heritable *TP53*-related cancer syndromes. Eur J Hum Genet 2020;28:1379–86.
23. Committee on Gynecologic Practice. ACOG committee opinion no. 727: cascade testing: testing women for known hereditary genetic mutations associated with cancer. Obstet Gynecol 2018;131(1):e31–4. https://doi.org/10.1097/AOG.0000000000002457.
24. Levine D, Kandoth C, Schultz N, et al. The cancer genome atlas research network. Integrated genomic characterization of endometrial carcinoma. Nature 2013;497:67–73.
25. van den Heerik ASVM, Horeweg N, Nout RA, et al. PORTEC-4a: international randomized trial of molecular profile-based adjuvant treatment for women with high-intermediate risk endometrial cancer. Int J Gynecol Cancer 2020;30(12):2002–7.
26. Kurnit KC, Kim GN, Fellman BM, et al. CTNNB1 (beta-catenin) mutation identifies low grade, early stage endometrial cancer patients at increased risk of recurrence. Mod Pathol 2017;30(7):1032–41.
27. Patch AM, Christie E, Etemadmoghadam D, et al. Whole–genome characterization of chemoresistant ovarian cancer. Nature 2015;521:489–94.
28. Manning-Geist B, Gordhandas S, Liu YL, et al. MAPK pathway genetic alterations are associated with prolonged overall survival in low-grade serous ovarian carcinoma. Clin Cancer Res 2022;28(20):4456–65.
29. Gershenson DM, Miller A, Brady WE, et al. Trametinib versus standard of care in patients with recurrent low-grade serous ovarian cancer (GOG 281/LOGS): an international, randomised, open-label, multicentre, phase 2/3 trial. Lancet 2022;399(10324):541–53.
30. Iida Y, Okamoto A, Hollis RL, et al. Clear cell carcinoma of the ovary: a clinical and molecular perspective. Int J Gynecol Cancer 2021;31(4):605–16.
31. Samartzis EP, Noske A, Dedes KJ, et al. ARID1A mutations and PI3K/AKT pathway alterations in endometriosis and endometriosis-associated ovarian carcinomas. Int J Mol Sci 2013;14(9):18824–49.
32. DeLair D, Han G, Irving JA, et al. HNF-1β in ovarian carcinomas with serous and clear cell change. Int J Gynecol Pathol 2013;32(6):541–6.
33. Blanc-Durand F, Leary A. Controversies in the management of mucinous ovarian tumors. Int J Gynecol Cancer 2025;35(3):101679.
34. Rasi Bonab F, Baghbanzadeh A, Ghaseminia M, et al. Molecular pathways in the development of HPV-induced cervical cancer. EXCLI J 2021;20:320–37.
35. Lei J, Ploner A, Lagheden C, et al. High-risk human papillomavirus status and prognosis in invasive cervical cancer: a nationwide cohort study. PLoS Med 2018;15(10):e1002666.

36. Van Nieuwenhuysen E, Busschaert P, Neven P, et al. The genetic landscape of 87 ovarian germ cell tumors. Gynecol Oncol 2018;151(1):61–8.
37. Jamieson S, Butzow R, Andersson N, et al. The FOXL2 C134W mutation is characteristic of adult granulosa cell tumors of the ovary. Mod Pathol 2010;23(11): 1477–85.
38. Vougiouklakis T, Zhu K, Vasudevaraja V, et al. Integrated analysis of ovarian juvenile granulosa cell tumors reveals distinct epigenetic signatures and recurrent TERT rearrangements. Clin Cancer Res 2022;28(8):1724–33.
39. Karnezis AN, Wang Y, Keul J, et al. DICER1 and FOXL2 mutation status correlates with clinicopathologic features in ovarian sertoli-leydig cell tumors. Am J Surg Pathol 2019;43(5):628–38.
40. Tew WP, Lacchetti C, Ellis A, et al. PARP inhibitors in the management of ovarian cancer: ASCO guideline. J Clin Oncol 2020;38(30):3468–93.
41. Fader AN, Roque DM, Siegel E, et al. Randomized phase II trial of carboplatin-paclitaxel versus carboplatin-paclitaxel-trastuzumab in uterine serous carcinomas that overexpress human epidermal growth factor receptor 2/neu. J Clin Oncol 2018;36(20):2044–51.
42. Meric-Bernstam F, Makker V, Oaknin A, et al. Efficacy and safety of trastuzumab deruxtecan in patients with HER2-Expressing solid tumors: primary results from the DESTINY-PanTumor02 phase II trial. J Clin Oncol 2024;42(1):47–58.
43. Eskander RN, Sill MW, Beffa L, et al. Pembrolizumab plus chemotherapy in advanced endometrial cancer. N Engl J Med 2023;388(23):2159–70.
44. Mirza MR, Chase DM, Slomovitz BM, et al. Dostarlimab for primary advanced or recurrent endometrial cancer. N Engl J Med 2023;388(23):2145–58.
45. Makker V, Colombo N, Casado Herráez A, et al. Lenvatinib plus pembrolizumab in previously treated advanced endometrial cancer: updated efficacy and safety from the randomized phase III study 309/KEYNOTE-775. J Clin Oncol 2023;41-(16):2904–10.
46. Colombo N, Dubot C, Lorusso D, et al. Pembrolizumab for persistent, recurrent, or metastatic cervical cancer. N Engl J Med 2021;385(20):1856–67.
47. Tewari KS, Monk BJ, Vergote I, et al. Survival with cemiplimab in recurrent cervical cancer. N Engl J Med 2022;386(6):544–55.
48. Eleje GU, Eke AC, Ezebialu IU, et al. Risk-reducing bilateral salpingo oophorectomy in women with BRCA1 or BRCA2 mutations. Cochrane Database Syst Rev 2018;8(8):CD012464.
49. Steenbeek MP, Harmsen MG, Hoogerbrugge N, et al. Association of salpingectomy with delayed oophorectomy versus salpingo-oophorectomy with quality of life in *BRCA1/2* pathogenic variant carriers: a nonrandomized controlled trial. JAMA Oncol 2021;7(8):1203–12.
50. Lu KH, Nebgen DR, Norquist B, et al. WISP: a prospective, multi-center trial of salpingectomy with delayed oophorectomy versus risk reducing salpingo-oophorectomy in women at increased risk for hereditary ovarian cancer. Gynecol Oncol 2019;154:22.
51. Lindor NM, Petersen GM, Hadley DW, et al. Recommendations for the care of individuals with an inherited predisposition to Lynch syndrome: a systematic review. JAMA 2006;296(12):1507–17.
52. Dominguez-Valentin M, Crosbie EJ, Engel C, et al. Risk-reducing hysterectomy and bilateral salpingo-oophorectomy in female heterozygotes of pathogenic mismatch repair variants: a Prospective Lynch Syndrome Database report. Genet Med 2021;23(4):705–12.

53. Ngeow J, Chiang J, Astiazaran-Symonds E, et al. Management of individuals with heterozygous germline pathogenic variants in RAD51C, RAD51D, and BRIP1: a clinical practice resource of the American College of Medical Genetics and Genomics (ACMG). Genet Med 2025;27(11):101557.
54. Kingsberg SA, Larkin LC, Liu JH. Clinical effects of early or surgical menopause. Obstet Gynecol 2020;135(4):853–68.
55. Hickey M, Trainer AH, Krejany EO, et al. What happens after menopause? (WHAM): a prospective controlled study of vasomotor symptoms and menopause-related quality of life 24 months after premenopausal risk-reducing salpingo-oophorectomy (RRSO). Gynecol Oncol 2024;191:201–11.
56. El Khoudary SR, Aggarwal B, Beckie TM, et al. Menopause transition and cardiovascular disease risk: implications for timing of early prevention: a scientific statement from the American heart association. Circulation 2020;142(25):e506–32.
57. Michels KA, Pfeiffer RM, Brinton LA, et al. Modification of the associations between duration of oral contraceptive use and ovarian, endometrial, breast, and colorectal cancers. JAMA Oncol 2018;4(4):516–21.
58. Chen LM, Blank SV, Burton E, et al. Reproductive and hormonal considerations in women at increased risk for hereditary gynecologic cancers: society of gynecologic oncology and American Society for reproductive medicine evidence-based review. Gynecol Oncol 2019;155(3):508–14.
59. Dashti SG, Chau R, Ouakrim DA, et al. Female hormonal factors and the risk of endometrial cancer in Lynch syndrome. JAMA 2015;314(1):61–71.

Genetics and Screening in Prostate Cancer

Joseph G.R. Partuzo, BS[a], Belén Mora-Garijo, MD[b], Jonathan Hwang, MD[a,*]

KEYWORDS

• Prostate cancer • Germline genetic testing • Somatic mutations
• Polygenic risk scores • Health disparities • Precision oncology

KEY POINTS

- Prostate cancer is one of the most heritable malignancies, with germline mutations in DNA repair pathways significantly influencing disease risk, aggressiveness, and age at onset.
- Germline and somatic genetic testing play a critical role in identifying patients who may benefit from targeted therapies, including poly (ADP-ribose) polymerase inhibitors and immune checkpoint inhibitors.
- Current guidelines recommend genetic testing based on disease stage, histology, ancestry, and family history, though growing evidence supports broader or universal testing approaches.
- Emerging technologies such as Polygenic Risk Scores, genomic classifiers, digital histopathology, and circulating tumor DNA offer new opportunities to refine risk stratification and personalize care.

INTRODUCTION

In 2022, an estimated 3 million men were living with prostate cancer in the United States. Notably, localized prostate cancer has a relatively good prognosis with an overall 5 year relative survival rate of 97.9%. However, this 5 year relative survival sharply declines to 37.9% in those with distant metastasis.[1] The discrepancy in survival between localized and metastatic disease highlights the need for evidence based screening guidelines that include recommendations on genetic testing to minimize the number of people diagnosed with advanced disease, thus limiting prostate cancer related deaths.

Prostate cancer's high prevalence results in a large mortality burden on the US health care system. The predicted number of deaths from prostate cancer in 2025

[a] Department of Urology, Georgetown University School of Medicine, Washington, DC, USA; [b] Department of Urology, Medstar Georgetown University Hospital, Washington Hospital Center, Washington, DC, USA
* Corresponding author. 106 Irving Street, NWPOB South, Room 315, Washington, DC 20010.
E-mail address: Jonathan.J.Hwang@medstar.net

Surg Clin N Am 106 (2026) 603–617
https://doi.org/10.1016/j.suc.2026.03.008 **surgical.theclinics.com**

Abbreviations	
ADT	androgen deprivation therapy
AI	artificial intelligence
ARPIs	androgen receptor pathway inhibitors
ctDNA	circulating tumor DNA
GCs	genomic classifiers
GGT	germline genetic testing
MMAI	multimodal artificial intelligence
NCCN	National Comprehensive Cancer Network
PARPi	poly (ADP-ribose) polymerase inhibitors
PGI	Polygenic Index
PRS	Polygenic Risk Score
RNA	ribonucleic acid
SNPs	single nucleotide polymorphisms

is over 35,000 men, making it the second highest cause of cancer related deaths behind cancer of the lung and bronchus. However, non-Hispanic Black men carry a disproportionate burden of prostate cancer related deaths with an incidence of 36.9 cases per 100,000 persons compared with their non-Hispanic White counterparts with an incidence of 18.4 cases per 100,000 persons.[1] This increased burden in minority populations is also reflected in the fact that non-Hispanic Black men and Hispanic men are being diagnosed with increasingly higher rates of advanced disease. An 18-year analysis of over 300,000 prostate cancer cases showed that distant stage disease is being diagnosed at increasing rates, with Hispanic and non-Hispanic black males experiencing the largest rise at 8.0% and 7.4% per year, respectively.[2]

Independent of race, prostate cancer has shown to be one of the most heritable types of cancers. One study of over 26,000 patients from the Swedish-Family Cancer Database found that if a patient's father had prostate cancer, he had a 2.1 times greater risk of developing the disease. Notably, this risk increased to 17.7 if the patient had 3 brothers diagnosed with prostate cancer.[3] Expanding upon this, the Nordic Twin Studies used a cohort of over 4000 prostate cancer cases to calculate heritability. They estimated it to be 57%, which is higher than colon, breast, and ovarian cancer. Analyses of the same cohort found a decreased time between diagnosis of prostate cancer in monozygotic twins (3.7 years) compared with dizygotic twins (6.1 years), further supporting the role that genetics plays in prostate cancer.[4–6]

It is important to distinguish between heritable prostate cancer and simply having a familial predisposition to it. Prostate cancer that is inherited aligns with the Hopkins Criteria in which one of the following is true: (1) prostate cancer in 3 or more first degree relatives, (2) prostate cancer in 3 consecutive generations, or (3) 2 family members diagnosed prior to 55 years of age.[7] In addition to this criteria, hereditary prostate cancer is often seen in patients with a family history of hereditary breast/ovarian cancer and Lynch syndrome,[8] which are associated with specific genetic mutations. As such, genetic testing plays a particularly important role for those with this type of family history.

Prostate cancer's disproportionate impact on minority populations and strong hereditary association makes genetic testing an important consideration when screening patients. The question is not if genetic testing is important, but who should be tested, when they should be tested, and how it should guide patient care. This article reviews both germline and somatic mutations, who should be genetically screened, what tests are currently being used, and future considerations for genetic testing in prostate cancer.

GERMLINE GENETIC MUTATIONS

Germline Mutations and Their Clinical Relevance

In heritable prostate cancer, the germline genetic mutations passed from parent to offspring have been observed to negatively impact the DNA repair process through 2 key mechanisms: Homologous Recombination and Mismatch Repair. Generally, Homologous Recombination is a cell's ability to repair double stranded breaks within its DNA and Mismatch Repair is a cell's ability to repair insertions, deletions, and mismatched base pairs within the strand of DNA.[8] Mutations in these pathways have been associated with an increased risk for prostate cancer, a more aggressive disease course, and an earlier onset of the disease.

The germline mutations that impact the homologous recombination repair process are BRCA1, BRCA2, ATM, CHEK2, PALB2, and HOXB13.[9] While both pathogenic variants of BRCA1/2 mutations increase a person's risk of prostate cancer, BRCA2 mutations confer a markedly increased risk compared with BRCA1. The relative risk of developing prostate cancer associated with a BRCA2 mutation ranges from 4.7 to 8.6, while the relative risk associated with a BRCA1 mutation is roughly 3.8.[10–12] Notably, the risk of being diagnosed with prostate cancer prior to 65 years of age is significantly higher in those with a BRCA2 mutation. On average, those with a BRCA2 mutation are diagnosed 3 years earlier than noncarriers.[13] Importantly, BRCA1/2 carriers are associated with more aggressive forms of prostate cancer. Compared with non-carriers, those with BRCA1/2 mutations are more frequently associated with Gleason greater than or equal to 8, T3/T4 stage, nodal involvement, and metastases at diagnosis.[14]

Of the germline mutations associated with prostate cancer, pathogenic BRCA1/2 variants are the most common and confer the greatest risk. However, ATM, PALB2, HOXB13, and CHEK2 also play significant roles. Loss of the ATM gene has shown to increase the risk of developing prostate cancer (OR 4.4) and predisposes an individual to being diagnosed with prostate cancer at an earlier age.[15] While PALB2 mutations confer only a modest risk for developing prostate cancer, their presence significantly increases the risk of developing Gleason 8 to 10 disease (OR 8.05).[16] HOXB13 mutations predispose a patient to developing prostate cancer but are not associated with higher grades of disease.[17] Lastly, CHEK2 mutations increase the likelihood of developing prostate cancer, but only specific mutations (eg, c.1100delC) have shown to be associated with poor patient outcomes.[18]

Aside from the risks that these germline mutations confer, their presence also has therapeutic and diagnostic implications. Therapeutically, the presence of BRCA1/2 often qualifies patients with metastatic castration-resistant prostate cancer (mCRPC) for treatment with poly (ADP-ribose) polymerase inhibitors (PARPi). The PROfound trial showed an improved overall survival in these patients treated with Olaparib, resulting in the American Society of Clinical Oncology recommending PARPis to patients who had previously been on androgen receptor pathway inhibitors (ARPIs).[19] From a diagnostic standpoint, PSA has been shown to be more predictive of prostate cancer in carriers of BRCA1/2 compared with non-carriers (OR 1.27).[20] Similarly, PARPis have shown efficacy in mCRPC patients with PALB2 mutations. An FDA pooled analysis demonstrated a clinically, but not statistically significant benefit for mCRPC patients with a PALB2 mutation receiving PARPis in terms of radiographic progression-free survival (HR 0.52) and overall survival (HR 0.78).[21] Notably, this effect of PARPis is not seen in those with ATM or CHEK2 mutations.[22]

Compared with homologous recombination, germline mutations in the mismatch repair pathway are relatively rare. One study of 1016 men with prostate cancer found only 7 had an MMR deficiency.[23] Despite this, these mutations confer a significant risk for developing prostate cancer and are associated with a more clinically and pathologically aggressive disease. Specifically, germline mutations in this pathway have shown to be associated with higher Gleason scores, intraductal histology, and an increased risk for metastatic disease.[24]

An important consideration in cases of MMR deficient prostate cancer is Lynch Syndrome, which is due to a mutation in 4 of the genes that control the mismatch repair process: MLH1, MSH2, MSH6, and PMS2.[25] Notably, this syndrome has shown to double a person's risk of developing prostate cancer,[26] but is only seen in 0.6% of advanced prostate cancer cases.[27] Because of the associated risk, the National Comprehensive Cancer Network (NCCN) recommends a referral to genetic counseling to assess for Lynch Syndrome if an MMR deficiency is found on tumor analysis.[28]

Notably, clinical trials have shown a good response to PD-1 inhibitors in MMR deficient patients with advanced prostate cancer. One study of 27 men with MMR deficient metastatic prostate cancer showed that 53% of the patients had a greater than or equal to 50% reduction in their PSA and that 64% had clinical/radiographic progression free survival at 6 months in response to a PD-1 Inhibitor.[29] Another study showed that the time to this greater than or equal to 50% reduction in PSA in response to Pembrolizumab was 12 weeks.[24] The therapeutic benefits of PD-1 inhibitors seen in the KEYNOTE trials resulted in the FDA giving full approval for the use of Pembrolizumab in cases of solid tumors with MMR deficiency and microsatellite instability, such as those with metastatic prostate cancer.[30–32]

Who Should Undergo Germline Genetic Testing

Per the 2026 NCCN guidelines (**Box 1**), genetic testing is indicated based on multiple factors. Most notably, it is recommended in cases of advanced prostate cancer, certain types of histology, and relevant personal/family history. If the criteria are met, the guidelines recommend testing for specific genes that have historically been associated with a more aggressive disease course.

Regarding disease specific criteria, genetic testing is currently indicated if a patient is diagnosed with Stage IVB, Stage IVA, or High/Very High-Risk prostate cancer. Stage IVA is prostate cancer that has shown regional lymph node involvement,

Box 1
Prostate cancer genetic testing recommendations

Localized prostate cancer
1. Germline testing (primary targets: BRCA2, ATM, CHEK2, HOXB13, MMR)–Strongly consider if:
   a. High risk/very high risk
   b. Strong family history
   c. Ashkenazi Jewish ancestry
2. Tissue Genomic Biomarkers (Decipher, Prolaris, GPS Oncotype Dx)
   a. Not routine for all patients
   b. Use selectively if results alter Shared Decision-Making (SDM).

Advanced prostate cancer
1. Germline Testing:
   a. Strongly recommended for all metastatic patients regardless of family history
   b. Primary targets include BRCA1/2, ATM, CHEK2, PALB2, MMR genes
2. Somatic (Tumor) Testing:
   a. Mandated to guide targeted therapy
   b. Identify eligibility for PARP inhibitors (BRCA/HRR) and immunotherapy (MSI-H/dMMR)

particularly in the pelvis. Stage IVB is prostate cancer that has shown distant metastasis, namely to the bones, liver, and lung. High Risk prostate cancer are those patients with clinical T3-T4 disease, Grade Group 4 or 5, and a PSA greater than 20 ng/mL. Very High Risk prostate cancer has the same criteria as High Risk with the caveat that the patient has a PSA greater than 40 ng/mL.[33]

Genetic testing can also be considered in patients with certain types of histology seen on biopsy. The 2 most notable types are cribriform and intraductal. These histologic variants have shown to be associated with higher rates of Gleason 4 and 5 tumors.[34] They have also been shown to more commonly contain mutations in the mismatch repair process, specifically in the MSH2 and MSH6 genes.[35] As mentioned earlier, mutations in these specific genes are also highly prevalent in Lynch Syndrome, making genetic testing in these patients more prudent.

The NCCN guidelines also recommend genetic testing in patients with a specific ancestry, family history, or diagnosis of prostate cancer less than or equal to 55 years of age. Notably, the guidelines indicate testing patients of Ashkenazi Jewish descent. Despite this population having similar rates of prostate cancer to those of European ancestry, they are more likely to harbor BRCA2 mutations.[36,37] Regarding family history, genetic testing is indicated if a patient has greater than or equal to 1 close blood relative with any of the following: breast cancer at age less than or equal to 50 years of age, male breast cancer, ovarian cancer, pancreatic cancer, or metastatic, node positive, or Very High/High risk prostate cancer. Additionally, patients should undergo genetic testing if they have greater than or equal to 3 close blood relatives with any grade of prostate cancer and/or breast cancer on the same side of the family.[33]

While guidelines currently do not address universal germline genetic testing (GGT) in patients with prostate cancer, there is growing evidence supporting the practice of universal GGT. One multisite study showed that of patients with prostate cancer and a germline pathogenic variant, roughly 30% did not meet criteria for genetic testing according to their primary cancer and 45% did not meet criteria for genetic testing according to their family history.[38] Similarly, the PROCLAIM trial found no significant difference when comparing the prevalence of pathogenic variants in patients that met criteria for genetic testing and those that did not meet criteria.[39] Notably, this disparity is further exaggerated in non-White populations where it has been shown that only 7% of GGT is performed in Black patients compared with 73% of White patients.[40] Studies that advocate for universal GGT note that it would provide potentially useful therapeutic information for patients, improve equity and access to GGT, and prevent missing patients with actionable germline mutations.[41]

Genetic Tests for Germline Mutations

Traditional genetic testing looks for the monogenic, high penetrant variants (eg, BRCA1/2, ATM, CHEK2, PALB2, and HOXB14) that have shown to be associated with an increased risk for prostate cancer. However, more studies are discovering smaller single nucleotide polymorphisms (SNPs) that influence an individual's risk for developing this disease. To date, there are over 200 known genetic variants associated with prostate cancer.[42] Individually, these SNPs do not drastically impact a person's risk. However, their effects are amplified when combined. A developing clinical tool that looks at the cumulative effects of individual genetic variants is a Polygenic Index (PGI) or Polygenic Risk Score (PRS).

Genome wide association studies have identified individual genetic variants and determined their effect size on developing prostate cancer. PGIs and PRSs calculate a patient's personal risk by adding the effect size of each genetic variant a person harbors. Currently, there are over 80 PRSs with the smallest including 4 SNPs and the largest including over 6 million.[43] Collectively, these risk assessment tools have shown modest results. A meta-analysis of 16 studies combined various PRS and found an AUC of 0.63 in regards to identifying prostate cancer in White men, which was similar in accuracy to PSA and family history. Notably, this study found that when you combined a PRS with other clinical variables the AUC rose to 0.74, indicating greater accuracy in identifying significant disease.[44]

Of the existing PRSs, there are 5 particularly reputable models that have each been validated in large, multi-ethnic populations: PRS269, PHS290, PHS2, CanRisk-Prostate, and FinRSPC. The developers of PRS269 compared 107,247 prostate cancer cases to 127,006 controls to develop a risk stratification model that incorporated 269 SNPs. The authors found that patients in the top decile of risk for developing prostate cancer had an odds ratio of 5.06, 3.74, 4.47, and 4.15 in patients of European, African, East Asian, and Hispanic descent, respectively.[42] PHS290 is a tool that was developed by looking at 590,750 veterans from the Million Veteran Program to predict the risk of developing lethal prostate cancer. When comparing those in the top 20% of risk to those in the bottom 20%, the hazard ratio for developing lethal prostate cancer was 4.42.[45] PHS2 includes 46 SNPs in its model and not only looked at risk of prostate cancer, but stratified cases by looking at risk for aggressive forms of the disease (Gleason $\geq$ 7, PSA $\geq$ 10, T3-T4 staging, metastasis). When comparing the top quintile to the bottom quintile, they found a hazard ratio of 5.88 for developing an aggressive form of prostate cancer.[46] The CanRisk-Prostate model uniquely incorporates known pathogenic variants (BRCA1/2 and HOXB13), low-risk SNPs, and personal family history of cancer into their risk calculator. Using this calculator, 86.3% of the prostate cancers developed within 10 years were within men that were in the top 50% of risk.[47] FinRSPC looked at a Finnish Population of 2783 prostate cancer patients and 2400 controls to develop a model that includes 55 SNPs in the analysis. In addition to looking at prostate cancer risk, this model uniquely found that 8.3% of patients in the bottom quartile had PSA values greater than or equal to 4 compared with 18.7% in the top quartile.[48]

PRSs have shown benefit in stratifying risk for developing prostate cancer, guiding therapeutic and diagnostic interventions, and identifying novel prostate cancer markers. While many of these PRS models have been validated and have shown clinical significance, guidelines currently do not contain recommendations pertaining to their use. Despite this, evidence has pointed to using these tools in conjunction with a patient's histologic features, personal medical history, and family cancer history to guide management more comprehensively. As these tools improve and more SNPs are revealed in genome wide association studies, the implications and impact of their daily use will become more evident.

SOMATIC MUTATIONS

Somatic Mutations and Their Clinical Relevance

Somatic mutations are genetic alterations that exist within tumor cells. Unlike germline mutations, these are not inherited but change over time due to genetic instability and/or selective pressure from therapy. Testing for somatic mutations is performed to guide therapy because specific mutations are susceptible to different treatment modalities.[49]

The 2026 NCCN guidelines recommend tumor molecular and biomarker analysis for patients with metastatic disease. They recommend testing for BRCA1/2, ATM, PALP2, FANCA, RAD51D, CHEK2, and CDK12. The guidelines also specify testing for genes associated with MSI-H and Mismatch Repair in patients with mCRPC. It is also strongly recommended to biopsy metastatic lesions, which may include a lymph node biopsy. If a metastatic biopsy cannot be performed, the recommendation is to test for somatic mutations using plasma circulating tumor DNA (ctDNA) during biochemical and/or radiographic progression. The guidelines also specify that re-evaluation may be needed at the time of cancer progression because the molecular profile of the tumor may change as a result of treatment.[28]

The most common somatic mutations seen in prostate cancer are ETS family gene fusions, alterations to the androgen receptor (AR) pathway, TP53, PTEN, and DNA damage repair genes (HRR and MMR).[27] ETS family gene fusions are the most common somatic mutation in prostate cancer and are known early drivers of disease progression.[50] While the prognostic implications of ETS family gene fusions are up for debate, they may be more responsive to androgen deprivation therapy (ADT) because they often fuse with TMPRSS2, an androgen receptor gene.[51] Mutations to the AR pathway are seen in up to 84% of mCRPC and confer a poor prognosis because these tumors are resistant to ADT and AR Pathway Inhibitors (eg, Enzalutamide, Apalutamide, Darolutamide, and Abiraterone).[52] TP53 mutations are seen in 36% of patients with metastatic prostate cancer, confer a 76% increased risk of death and 62% increased risk of disease progression, and are associated with persistence after radical prostatectomy.[27,53,54] Notably, TP53 mutations often result in resistance to standard therapies, necessitating enrollment in clinical trials or the use of novel therapies.[55] PTEN deficiencies are seen in up to 50% of mCRPC cases due to mutations in the P13K-AKT–mTOR pathway conferring resistance to ADT.[56] As such, patients with a PTEN mutation have a more aggressive disease course and worse prognosis, with one study showing a 61% increased risk of death.[57] Similar to germline mutations, genetic aberrations in the homologous recombination and mismatch repair pathways are associated with higher Gleason grades and risk for metastasis.[19] Somatic mutations in the homologous recombination and mismatch repair pathways have also shown susceptibility to PARP-1 inhibitors and PD-1 inhibitors, respectively.[30–32]

Seeing that somatic mutations are harbored by the tumor itself, testing for these mutations is centered on tissue sampling. The 3 types of testing that will be addressed in this section are tumor-derived genomic classifiers (GCs), digital histopathology-based tests, and plasma ctDNA. GCs offer prognostic and therapeutic information by analyzing the ribonucleic acid (RNA) expression profile of tumors. Digital histopathology-based tests are digitally uploaded pathology slides that use artificial intelligence (AI)-based technology to analyze for predictive biomarkers. Lastly, plasma ctDNA provides a noninvasive method of detecting actionable somatic mutations.

TUMOR-DERIVED GENOMIC CLASSIFIERS

Several prostate cancer tissue-based molecular assays have been developed to improve risk stratification and aid in clinical decision making. In general, these tools are only recommended when they have the potential to change management, and only those with high-quality, long-term clinical trial data with prospective validation should be utilized.[28] Tests range in price from $3900 to $5150.[58] Examples of patients for whom tissue-based genomic markers may help clarify risk include patients with high-volume, low-risk, or favorable intermediate-risk prostate cancer who are interested in active surveillance or men with high-risk features for treatment intensification.

Pathologists should primarily select areas of highest cellularity and specific adverse pathology growth patterns for molecular testing. For RNA-based tests, a single 1 mm core punched from the tumor is generally sufficient to obtain a test outcome, but more tissue is needed for DNA-based tests.[58]

Decipher 22 Gene Classifier

Decipher is the most extensively validated tissue-based genomic assay, analyzing 22 genes from prostate biopsy and prostatectomy specimens to predict metastatic risk and guide treatment decision. The Decipher risk score ranges from 0 to 1, with higher scores indicating more aggressive tumor biology. The assay has level 1 evidence from multiple post-hoc analyses of randomized phase III trials across different risk groups and clinical scenarios.[59]

For patients with localized intermediate-risk, high-risk, or very high-risk prostate cancer, Decipher has been shown to help inform decisions on duration of ADT. Patients with high Decipher scores (>0.6) and NCCN high- or very high-risk disease derive a greater absolute benefit from long-term ADT compared with those with low Decipher scores (<0.45). Similarly, among patients with intermediate-risk disease treated with radiation therapy alone, those with high Decipher scores have a significantly higher risk of distant metastasis at 10 years compared with those with low scores (16% vs 4%, respectively), suggesting that Decipher testing can help identify which intermediate-risk patients are most likely to benefit from the addition of ADT.[60]

In the post-biopsy and post-prostatectomy settings, Decipher independently predicts distant metastasis, prostate cancer-specific mortality, and overall survival. Among patients undergoing adjuvant radiation after prostatectomy, those with high Decipher scores demonstrate a greater benefit from the addition of systemic ADT compared with those with low scores.

Future directions lay in multiple ongoing biomarker-directed randomized trials (eg, NGR GU-009 [PREDICT-RT], GU-010), which will provide prospective evidence on whether Decipher-guided treatment intensification improves oncologic outcomes.[28]

Genomic Prostate Score

The Genomic Prostate Score (GPS), previously known as Oncotype Dx, is a 17-gene expression assay that combines mRNA gene expression results with clinical risk factors to predict the likelihood of Grade Group 3 or greater disease or extracapsular extension at radical prostatectomy. The test generates a score ranging from 0 to 100 that stratifies patients into risk categories for adverse pathology. The evidence base for GPS is primarily from retrospective studies, with more limited prospective validation compared with Decipher.[58]

In the Canary PASS active surveillance cohort (432 patients), adding GPS to clinical variables (PSA density and diagnostic grade group) did not significantly improve adverse pathology stratification (HR 1.17, 95% CI 1.00–1.43, P = .066), and there was no association with subsequent biopsy upgrade.[28] Importantly, a randomized trial raised concerns about GPS use in active surveillance candidates. Among 200 patients with NCCN very low to favorable-intermediate risk disease, GPS testing decreased the relative odds of choosing active surveillance by approximately 50%, with patients with lower health literacy being 7 fold less likely to choose active surveillance after receiving GPS results.[61]

Prolaris

Prolaris tissue-based assay uses biopsy and prostatectomy tissue to evaluate disease aggressiveness based on the expression of 31 genes (originally 46 genes) involved in cell cycle progression. Results predict the likelihood of clinical progression after treatment and prostate cancer mortality within 10 years with watchful waiting. Similarly to

GPS, the evidence for Prolaris lacks prospective data and consists primarily of retrospective institutional and tumor registry studies.[58]

For intermediate-risk prostate cancer, Prolaris has demonstrated value in appropriately identifying active surveillance candidates. A retrospective study of 3204 NCCN intermediate-risk patients showed that those recommended to active surveillance by Prolaris had a very low risk of metastasis (0.37% [95% CI 0.09%–1.47%]) within 5 years. Another study of 3208 patients found that active surveillance selection was approximately 2 times higher in patients recommended to AS by Prolaris, with 1.5 times higher 3 year AS durability.

Multiple studies have documented Prolaris's influence on clinical management. In a prospective registry study of 305 patients, 65% of cases showed a change in treatment recommendations after receiving Prolaris results, with a 37.2% reduction in interventional therapy recommendations and a 49.5% reduction in surgical interventions.[62]

Digital Histopathology-based Tests (ArteraAI)

The advent of AI has allowed for improved clinical tools that can factor in multiple variables to provide more comprehensive diagnostic, prognostic, and predictive information. In prostate cancer, a developing technology are tests centered on digital histopathology. Digital histopathology-based tests use AI-based algorithms, most often neural networks, to analyze digitally uploaded biopsy slides. These tests then factor in patient demographics, clinical staging, and biochemical information to stratify patients based on risk for metastasis, mortality, and biochemical failure, while also providing predictive information on the potential benefit of certain treatment modalities. In prostate cancer, the most studied and externally validated digital histopathology test is the ArteraAI Prostate.

ArteraAI Prostate incorporates digital biopsy images plus clinical information (baseline PSA, T stage, NCCN risk group, age, Gleason score) to provide prognostic and predictive information. Six phase III clinical trials were performed that looked at the prognostic value of this test. A meta-analysis of 1088 high risk patients in these trials showed that ArterAI Prostate was able to provide accurate and statistically significant information on 3 important prognostic values: Distant Metastasis (HR 1.9), Prostate Cancer Specific Mortality (HR 2.06), and Death with Distant Metastasis (HR 2.12).[63] Regarding predictive information, the ArteraAI Prostate model has been validated to differentiate which patients will benefit from certain treatment regimens. A study of 1192 patients compared the efficacy of long-term ADT versus short-term ADT in men with an AI predictive biomarker. The 15 year risk difference for distant metastasis in men with the biomarker was 14% when comparing long-term ADT (28 months) versus short-term ADT (4 months). Notably, there was no difference in the risk for distant metastasis in men that tested negative for the biomarker. In this study, 33% of the patients were negative for the biomarker, meaning that a substantial number of patients could have been saved from 24 extra months of ADT with the use of ArteraAI Prostate.[64]

In alignment with the research results on ArteraAI Prostate, the NCCN updated their guidelines to include recommendations on both the prognostic and therapeutic uses surrounding multimodal artificial intelligence (MMAI). Regarding prognostication, the current guideline reports that ArteraAI is superior to the standard pathologic and clinical models in terms of predicting distant metastasis and prostate cancer related mortality. Despite this, it is specifically noted that cut off thresholds have not been established to guide therapy, but instead can be used for more informed decision making. In terms of guiding therapy, the current guideline only addresses patients

Table 1
Available germline and somatic genetic testing

Mutation Type	Company	Panel Name	Included Genes	Tissue Sampling	Website
Germline Mutations	Myriad Genetics	myRisk Hereditary Cancer	ATM, BRCA1/2, CHEK2, EPCAM, HOXB13, MLH1, MSH2, MSH6, PALB2, TP53	Blood Draw, Saliva	https://myriad.com/genetic-tests/myrisk-hereditary-cancer-test/
	Invitae	Hereditary Prostate Cancer Panel	EPCAM, HOXB13, MLH1, MSH2, MSH6, PALB2, PMS2, TP53	Blood Draw; Saliva; Buccal Swab; gDNA	https://www.invitae.com/providers/test-catalog/test-01362
	Ambry Genetics	CancerNext	40 Genes (eg, ATM, BRCA1/2, CHEK2, EPCAM, HOXB13, MLH1, MSH2, MSH6, PALB2, PTEN, TP53)	Blood Draw; Saliva; Buccal Swab	https://www.ambrygen.com/providers/genetic-testing/1/oncology/cancerext
Somatic Mutations	Foundation Medicine	FoundationOne CDx	324 genes (eg, ATM, BRCA1/2, BARD1, BRIP1, CDK12, CHEK1, CHEK2, FANCL, PALB2, RAD51C, RAD51D, RAD54L, MSI)	Tumor Tissue	https://www.foundationmedicine.com/portfolio
		FoundationOne Liquid CDx	324 genes (eg, ATM, BRCA1/2, etc)	Blood Draw	https://www.foundationmedicine.com/portfolio
	Guardant Complete	Guardant360 Tissue	ATM, BRCA1/2, CDK12, CHEK1, CHEK2, FANCA, FANCL, MLH1, MRE11, NBN, PALB2, PTEN, RAD51B, RAD51C, RAD51D, RAD54L, RB1, TP53, MSI, TMB	Tumor Tissue	https://www.guardantcomplete.com/hcp
		Guardant360 CDx	ATM, BRCA1/2, CDK12, MLH1, PTEN, RB1, TP53, MSI, TMB	Blood Draw	https://www.guardant360.com

with intermediate risk prostate cancer planning to receive radiation therapy. If these patients are biomarker positive, a short-term ADT regimen is recommended, especially if they are in the unfavorable intermediate risk category. Conversely, if they are biomarker negative radiation therapy alone is sufficient.[28]

Plasma Circulating Tumor DNA

Plasma ctDNA are small fragments of DNA that have been released by tumor cells through the processes of apoptosis, necrosis, and secretion. Importantly, they contain the same somatic mutations that the tumor itself harbors essentially making it a "liquid biopsy" when measured. Currently, ctDNA is used for prognosis and disease response, but it is also used to look for actionable genetic variants. There is growing evidence for the early detection of prostate cancer using ctDNA, but this has shown to be limited with localized disease.[65]

Regarding prognosis, higher percentages of ctDNA found within plasma cell free DNA have independently shown to be associated with disease burden, progression free survival, and overall survival. One study found that patients with ctDNA% greater than 30 had a 5 times greater risk of PSA progression on first line therapy and a 5.6 times greater risk of death when compared with patients with a ctDNA% less than 2.[66] Similarly, shorter progression free survival and overall survival have been seen in mCRPC patients with persistently high levels of ctDNA following treatment with an ARPI. A multicenter observational study showed that going from detectable to undetectable ctDNA after treatment with an ARPI yielded a positive predictive value of 88% and negative predictive value of 92% when predicting which mCRPC patients would have a progression free survival greater than 6 months.[67]

ctDNA has also shown to effectively guide therapy due to its ability to detect actionable genetic mutations. The current NCCN guidelines recommend using ctDNA to test for somatic mutations in patients with metastatic prostate cancer, specifically when tissue biopsies are unsafe or not feasible. The intent of this is to look for somatic mutations in the homologous recombination, mismatch repair, and androgen receptor pathways. As outlined in the *Germline Mutations and Their Clinical Relevance* and the *Somatic Mutations and Their Clinical Relevance* sections above, certain mutations in these pathways have shown susceptibility to treatment with PARPis, PD-1 inhibitors, and ARPis (**Table 1**).

SUMMARY

Prostate cancer remains a highly prevalent disease that carries with it a disproportionate burden on the health care system, particularly in the non-Hispanic Black population. As a clinically heterogeneous disease, both germline and somatic genetic factors play a central role in shaping risk, guiding management, and informing prognosis. The increased understanding of these mutations has resulted in genetic testing serving an essential role for not only identifying individuals at increased risk, but also for selecting targeted therapies specific to individual mutations. Emerging tools such as PRS, digital histopathology platforms, tumor-derived GCs, and plasma ctDNA offer promising avenues for refining diagnosis, stratifying risk, and individualizing treatment. As these technologies advance and become increasingly integrated into clinical practice, a more personalized and precise approach to prostate cancer care is becoming possible, which has the potential to reduce mortality, limit overtreatment, and better identify those that may benefit most from targeted therapy.

DISCLOSURES

The authors have nothing to disclose.

REFERENCES

1. Cancer of the prostate - cancer stat facts. SEER. Available at: https://seer.cancer.gov/statfacts/html/prost.html. Accessed September 21, 2025.
2. Van Blarigan EL, McKinley MA, Washington SL 3rd, et al. Trends in prostate cancer incidence and mortality rates. JAMA Netw Open 2025;8(1):e2456825. https://doi.org/10.1001/jamanetworkopen.2024.56825. Published 2025 Jan 2.
3. Hemminki K. Familial risk and familial survival in prostate cancer. World J Urol 2012;30(2):143–8.
4. Lichtenstein P, Holm NV, Verkasalo PK, et al. Environmental and heritable factors in the causation of cancer–analyses of cohorts of twins from Sweden, Denmark, and Finland. N Engl J Med 2000;343(2):78–85.
5. Hjelmborg JB, Scheike T, Holst K, et al. The heritability of prostate cancer in the Nordic Twin Study of Cancer. Cancer Epidemiol Biomarkers Prev 2014;23(11): 2303–10.
6. Mucci LA, Hjelmborg JB, Harris JR, et al. Familial risk and heritability of cancer among twins in nordic countries. JAMA 2016;315(1):68–76.
7. Ostrander EA, Stanford JL. Genetics of prostate cancer: too many loci, too few genes. Am J Hum Genet 2000;67(6):1367–75.
8. Grypari IM, Tzelepi V, Gyftopoulos K. DNA damage repair pathways in prostate cancer: a narrative review of molecular mechanisms, emerging biomarkers and therapeutic targets in precision oncology. Int J Mol Sci 2023;24(14):11418. https://doi.org/10.3390/ijms241411418. Published 2023 Jul 13.
9. Khan HM, Cheng HH. Germline genetics of prostate cancer. Prostate 2022;82-(Suppl 1):S3–12.
10. Nyberg T, Frost D, Barrowdale D, et al. Prostate cancer risks for Male BRCA1 and BRCA2 mutation carriers: a prospective cohort study. Eur Urol 2020;77(1):24–35.
11. Nyberg T, Tischkowitz M, Antoniou AC. BRCA1 and BRCA2 pathogenic variants and prostate cancer risk: systematic review and meta-analysis. Br J Cancer 2022;126(7):1067–81.
12. Cheng HH, Shevach JW, Castro E, et al. BRCA1, BRCA2, and associated cancer risks and management for Male patients: a review. JAMA Oncol 2024;10(9): 1272–81.
13. Page EC, Bancroft EK, Brook MN, et al. Interim results from the IMPACT study: evidence for prostate-specific antigen screening in BRCA2 mutation carriers. Eur Urol 2019;76(6):831–42.
14. Castro E, Goh C, Olmos D, et al. Germline BRCA mutations are associated with higher risk of nodal involvement, distant metastasis, and poor survival outcomes in prostate cancer. J Clin Oncol 2013;31(14):1748–57.
15. Karlsson Q, Brook MN, Dadaev T, et al. Rare germline variants in ATM predispose to prostate cancer: a PRACTICAL consortium study. Eur Urol Oncol 2021;4(4): 570–9.
16. Wokołorczyk D, Kluźniak W, Stempa K, et al. PALB2 mutations and prostate cancer risk and survival. Br J Cancer 2021;125(4):569–75.
17. Crawford TB, Nelson T, Karunamuni R, et al. Association of HOXB13 G84E with prostate cancer among 592,158 men. J Natl Compr Cancer Netw 2025;23(10): e257055. https://doi.org/10.6004/jnccn.2025.7055. Published 2025 Sep 15.

18. Wu Y, Yu H, Zheng SL, et al. A comprehensive evaluation of CHEK2 germline mutations in men with prostate cancer. Prostate 2018;78(8):607–15.
19. Garje R, Riaz IB, Naqvi SAA, et al. Systemic therapy in patients with metastatic castration-resistant prostate cancer: ASCO guideline update. J Clin Oncol 2025;43(20):2311–34.
20. Mikropoulos C, Selkirk CGH, Saya S, et al. Prostate-specific antigen velocity in a prospective prostate cancer screening study of men with genetic predisposition. Br J Cancer 2018;118(2):266–76.
21. Fallah J, Xu J, Weinstock C, et al. Efficacy of Poly(ADP-ribose) polymerase inhibitors by individual genes in homologous recombination repair gene-mutated metastatic castration-resistant prostate cancer: a US food and drug administration pooled analysis. J Clin Oncol 2024;42(14):1687–98.
22. Naqvi SAA, Riaz IB, Bibi A, et al. Heterogeneity of the treatment effect with PARP inhibitors in metastatic castration-resistant prostate cancer: a living interactive systematic review and meta-analysis. Eur Urol 2025;87(6):626–40.
23. McNevin CS, Keogh A, Mohammed Nur M, et al. Prevalence of mismatch repair deficiency in primary prostate cancer in a large prospective cohort. Clin Cancer Res 2025;31(9):1746–53.
24. Antonarakis ES, Shaukat F, Isaacsson Velho P, et al. Clinical features and therapeutic outcomes in men with advanced prostate cancer and DNA mismatch repair gene mutations. Eur Urol 2019;75(3):378–82.
25. Bhattacharya P, Leslie SW, McHugh TW. Lynch syndrome (Hereditary Nonpolyposis Colorectal Cancer) [updated 2024 Jun 8]. In: StatPearls [Internet]. Treasure Island (FL). StatPearls Publishing; 2025. Bookshelf ID: NBK431096. Available at: https://www.ncbi.nlm.nih.gov/books/NBK431096/. Accessed November 25, 2025.
26. Raymond VM, Mukherjee B, Wang F, et al. Elevated risk of prostate cancer among men with Lynch syndrome. J Clin Oncol 2013;31(14):1713–8.
27. Sartor O, de Bono JS. Metastatic prostate cancer. N Engl J Med 2018;378(7): 645–57.
28. National Comprehensive Cancer Network (NCCN). Prostate cancer, version 1.2026. NCCN clinical practice guidelines in oncology. Available at: https://www.nccn.org/guidelines/guidelines-detail?category=2&id=1545. Accessed September 21, 2025.
29. Graham LS, Montgomery B, Cheng HH, et al. Mismatch repair deficiency in metastatic prostate cancer: response to PD-1 blockade and standard therapies. PLoS One 2020;15(5):e0233260. https://doi.org/10.1371/journal.pone.0233260. Published 2020 May 26.
30. Le DT, Kim TW, Van Cutsem E, et al. Phase II open-label study of pembrolizumab in treatment-refractory, microsatellite instability-High/Mismatch repair-deficient metastatic colorectal cancer: KEYNOTE-164. J Clin Oncol 2020; 38(1):11–9.
31. Marabelle A, Le DT, Ascierto PA, et al. Efficacy of pembrolizumab in patients with noncolorectal high microsatellite instability/mismatch repair-deficient cancer: results from the phase II KEYNOTE-158 study. J Clin Oncol 2020;38(1):1–10.
32. Geoerger B, Kang HJ, Yalon-Oren M, et al. Pembrolizumab in paediatric patients with advanced melanoma or a PD-L1-positive, advanced, relapsed, or refractory solid tumour or lymphoma (KEYNOTE-051): interim analysis of an open-label, single-arm, phase 1-2 trial. Lancet Oncol 2020;21(1):121–33.
33. National Comprehensive Cancer Network (NCCN). Genetic/Familial High-Risk Assessment: Breast, Ovarian, Pancreatic, and Prostate, version 2.2026. NCCN

Clinical Practice Guidelines in Oncology. Available at: https://www.nccn.org/professionals/physician_gls/pdf/genetics_bopp.pdf (Accessed November 25, 2025).
34. Hesterberg AB, Gordetsky JB, Hurley PJ. Cribriform prostate cancer: clinical pathologic and molecular considerations. Urology 2021;155:47–54.
35. Wyvekens N, Tsai HK, Sholl LM, et al. Histopathological and genetic features of mismatch repair-deficient high-grade prostate cancer. Histopathology 2022; 80(7):1050–60.
36. Vijai J, Kirchhoff T, Gallagher D, et al. Genetic architecture of prostate cancer in the Ashkenazi Jewish population. Br J Cancer 2011;105(6):864–9.
37. Struewing JP, Hartge P, Wacholder S, et al. The risk of cancer associated with specific mutations of BRCA1 and BRCA2 among Ashkenazi jews. N Engl J Med 1997;336(20):1401–8.
38. Choudry MM, Durant AM, Edmonds VS, et al. Germline pathogenic variants identified in patients with genitourinary malignancies undergoing universal testing: a multisite single-institution prospective study. J Urol 2024;212(4):590–9.
39. Shore N, Gazi M, Pieczonka C, et al. Efficacy of National Comprehensive Cancer Network Guidelines in identifying pathogenic germline variants among unselected patients with prostate cancer: the PROCLAIM trial. Eur Urol Oncol 2023; 6(5):477–83.
40. Briggs LG, Steele GL, Qian ZJ, et al. Racial differences in germline genetic testing for prostate cancer: a systematic review. JCO Oncol Pract 2023;19(5): e784–93.
41. Shore N, Nielsen SM, Esplin ED, et al. Implementation of universal germline genetic testing into standard of care for patients with prostate cancer: the time is now. JCO Oncol Pract 2025;21(6):747–53.
42. Conti DV, Darst BF, Moss LC, et al. Trans-ancestry genome-wide association meta-analysis of prostate cancer identifies new susceptibility loci and informs genetic risk prediction. Nat Genet 2021;53(1):65–75.
43. Viti A, Quarta L, Zaurito P, et al. The role of genomic scores in the management of prostate cancer patients: a comprehensive narrative review. Cancers (Basel) 2025;17(14):2334. Published 2025 Jul 14.
44. Siltari A, Lönnerbro R, Pang K, et al. How well do polygenic risk scores identify men at high risk for prostate cancer? Systematic review and meta-analysis. Clin Genitourin Cancer 2023;21(2):316.e1–11.
45. Pagadala MS, Lynch J, Karunamuni R, et al. Polygenic risk of any, metastatic, and fatal prostate cancer in the Million Veteran Program. J Natl Cancer Inst 2023; 115(2):190–9.
46. Huynh-Le MP, Fan CC, Karunamuni R, et al. Polygenic hazard score is associated with prostate cancer in multi-ethnic populations. Nat Commun 2021;12(1):1236. Published 2021 Feb 23.
47. Nyberg T, Brook MN, Ficorella L, et al. CanRisk-Prostate: a comprehensive, externally validated risk model for the prediction of future prostate cancer. J Clin Oncol 2023;41(5):1092–104.
48. Sipeky C, Talala KM, Tammela TLJ, et al. Prostate cancer risk prediction using a polygenic risk score. Sci Rep 2020;10(1):17075. https://doi.org/10.1038/s41598-020-74172-z. Published 2020 Oct 13.
49. Cheng HH, Sokolova AO, Schaeffer EM, et al. Germline and somatic mutations in prostate cancer for the clinician. J Natl Compr Cancer Netw 2019;17(5):515–21.
50. Sandhu S, Moore CM, Chiong E, et al. Prostate cancer. Lancet 2021;398(10305): 1075–90. https://doi.org/10.1016/S0140-6736(21)00950-8.

51. Ramanand SG, Mani RS. Genetic, environmental, and nuclear factors governing genomic rearrangements. Adv Exp Med Biol 2019;1210:57–66.
52. Virtanen T, Kwan EM, Parekh K, et al. Repertoire and clinical hierarchy of AR locus alterations in castration-resistant prostate cancer. Ann Oncol 2025;27. https://doi.org/10.1016/j.annonc.2025.10.1236. Published online October.
53. Maddah MM, Hedayatizadeh-Omran A, Moosazadeh M, et al. Evaluation of the prognostic role of TP53 gene mutations in prostate cancer outcome: a systematic review and meta-analysis. Clin Genitourin Cancer 2024;22(6):102226. https://doi.org/10.1016/j.clgc.2024.102226.
54. Nientiedt C, Budczies J, Endris V, et al. Mutations in TP53 or DNA damage repair genes define poor prognostic subgroups in primary prostate cancer. Urol Oncol 2022;40(1):8.e11–8.
55. De Laere B, Oeyen S, Mayrhofer M, et al. TP53 outperforms other androgen receptor biomarkers to predict abiraterone or enzalutamide outcome in metastatic castration-resistant prostate cancer. Clin Cancer Res 2019;25(6):1766–73.
56. Jamaspishvili T, Berman DM, Ross AE, et al. Clinical implications of PTEN loss in prostate cancer. Nat Rev Urol 2018;15(4):222–34.
57. Gupta S, To TM, Graf R, et al. Real-World overall survival and treatment patterns by PTEN status in metastatic castration-resistant prostate cancer. JCO Precis Oncol 2024;8:e2300562. https://doi.org/10.1200/PO.23.00562.
58. Eggener SE, Rumble RB, Armstrong AJ, et al. Molecular biomarkers in localized prostate cancer: ASCO guideline. J Clin Oncol 2020;38(13):1474–94.
59. Jairath Neil K, Dal Pra A, Vince R Jr, et al. A systematic review of the evidence for the decipher genomic classifier in prostate cancer. Eur Urol 2021;79(3):374–83.
60. Spratt DE, Liu VYT, Michalski J, et al. Genomic classifier performance in intermediate-risk prostate cancer: results from NRG Ooncology/RTOG 0126 randomized phase 3 trial. Int J Radiat Oncol Biol Phys 2023;117(2):370–7. Erratum in: Int J Radiat Oncol Biol Phys. 2024;120(5):1461.
61. Murphy AB, Abern MR, Liu L, et al. Impact of a genomic test on treatment decision in a predominantly African American population with favorable-risk prostate cancer: a randomized trial. J Clin Oncol 2021;39(15):1660–70.
62. Crawford ED, Scholz MC, Kar AJ, et al. Cell cycle progression score and treatment decisions in prostate cancer: results from an ongoing registry. Curr Med Res Opin 2014;30(6):1025–31.
63. Spratt DE, Liu VYT, Jia AY, et al. Meta-analysis of individual patient-level data for a multimodal artificial intelligence biomarker in high-risk prostate cancer: results from six NRG/RTOG phase 3 randomized trials. Eur Urol 2024;86(4):369–71.
64. Armstrong AJ, Liu VYT, Selvaraju RR, et al. Development and validation of an artificial intelligence digital pathology biomarker to predict benefit of long-term hormonal therapy and radiotherapy in men with high-risk prostate cancer across multiple phase III trials. J Clin Oncol 2025;43(32):3494–504.
65. Kopytov SA, Sagitova GR, Guschin DY, et al. Circulating tumor DNA in prostate cancer: a dual perspective on early detection and advanced disease management. Cancers (Basel) 2025;17(15):2589. Published 2025 Aug 6.
66. Fonseca NM, Maurice-Dror C, Herberts C, et al. Prediction of plasma ctDNA fraction and prognostic implications of liquid biopsy in advanced prostate cancer. Nat Commun 2024;15(1):1828. Published 2024 Feb 28.
67. Tolmeijer SH, Boerrigter E, Sumiyoshi T, et al. Early On-treatment changes in circulating tumor DNA fraction and response to enzalutamide or abiraterone in metastatic castration-resistant prostate cancer. Clin Cancer Res 2023;29(15):2835–44.

Role of Genetics in Sarcoma for the Practicing General Surgeon

Matthew Steensma, MD

KEYWORDS

• Sarcoma • Genetics • Hereditary sarcoma syndromes

KEY POINTS

- Most sarcomas occur sporadically.
- Germline mutations cause a small minority of sarcomas.
- Multidisciplinary care of patients with sarcoma is paramount.
- Aside from inherited syndromes, prior irradiation for other cancers can increase the risk of developing secondary sarcoma.
- Management of all hereditary sarcoma syndromes requires lifelong surveillance and multidisciplinary care to minimize death from cancer.

INTRODUCTION

Soft tissue sarcomas (STS) comprise a heterogeneous group of rare mesenchymal tumors exhibiting diverse primary site locations and clinical behavior.[1] With over 100 distinct histologic subtypes, accurate diagnosis and subtype-specific management are crucial for optimal patient outcomes.[2] The rarity and heterogeneity of these tumors frequently complicate diagnosis and treatment, often leading to delayed intervention and suboptimal therapeutic strategies.[3] The multidisciplinary management of soft tissue sarcomas in specialized sarcoma centers is highly recommended, as highlighted by consensus conference recommendations.[4] The most common soft tissue sarcoma subtypes are liposarcomas, leiomyosarcomas, pleomorphic sarcomas, and synovial sarcomas, which predominantly manifest in the extremities and trunk.[5] These mesenchymal neoplasms arise from various connective tissues including fat, muscle, nerves, and blood vessels, with retroperitoneal or intra-abdominal involvement occurring in a significant minority of cases.[6–8] A comprehensive understanding of these varied presentations, alongside the molecular and genetic underpinnings of each subtype, is essential for guiding targeted therapeutic interventions.[9]

Orthopedic Oncology, Corewell Health Regional Cancer Program, 145 Michigan Street, Grand Rapids, MI 49315, USA
E-mail address: matthew.steensma@corewellhealth.org

Surg Clin N Am 106 (2026) 619–631
https://doi.org/10.1016/j.suc.2026.04.002 **surgical.theclinics.com**

Abbreviations	
NF1	neurofibromatosis type 1
STS	soft tissue sarcomas

GENETICS

Most sarcomas occur sporadically but approximately 10% to 20% are associated with inherited genetic predisposition syndromes. Key genetic syndromes increasing sarcoma risk include Li-Fraumeni syndrome, neurofibromatosis type 1, and retinoblastoma. While rare, genetic testing can identify these inherited risks to guide surveillance when appropriate.

Inherited (Germline) Mutations:

Li-Fraumeni Syndrome: a mutation in the TP53 gene, often causing soft tissue sarcomas and other cancer.

Neurofibromatosis Type 1 (NF1): Linked to malignant peripheral nerve sheath tumors.

Retinoblastoma: Inherited eye cancer linked to higher sarcoma risk.

Other Syndromes: Gardner syndrome, Werner syndrome and familial adenomatous polyposis.

Genetic changes in tumors (somatic mutations):

Most sarcomas develop due to acquired gene mutations after birth, often involving complex genomic changes or specific chromosomal translocations that create fusion genes, such as the SS18-SSX fusion in synovial sarcoma. This will be discussed later in this article.

RISK FACTORS

Aside from inherited syndromes, prior radiation therapy for other cancers can increase the likelihood of developing a secondary sarcoma.

DIAGNOSIS

The diagnostic landscape for soft tissue sarcomas has progressively shifted from reliance on histopathological morphology alone to an integrative approach incorporating molecular analyses, which are increasingly crucial for accurate classification and treatment planning.[10] Despite the complexities, advances in diagnostic imaging, pathologic classification, and molecular profiling have significantly refined the diagnostic approach, facilitating more precise staging and treatment planning.[11] For instance, the European Society of Musculoskeletal Radiology has established guidelines to standardize imaging techniques, which are critical for early and accurate diagnosis given the considerable variability in clinical practice across regions.[12] The integration of pathologic, immunohistochemical, and molecular features is increasingly emphasized to guide histology-specific therapeutic approaches, especially given the more than 70 recognized histologic subtypes.[13,14]

While histopathological findings remain the gold standard, an integrated diagnostic approach incorporating morphology, immunohistochemistry, and advanced molecular techniques is increasingly essential for achieving diagnostic precision and refining classification, particularly given the inherent intertumoral and intratumoral heterogeneity of soft tissue sarcomas.[15–17] This detailed diagnostic workup is paramount, as misdiagnosis or inadequate initial excisions outside specialized sarcoma centers can lead to increased morbidity and mortality.[4] The challenges associated with incorrect or late diagnosis, coupled with a lack of clinical expertise, underscore the critical need for advanced diagnostic methodologies in STS.[3,18]

The initial diagnostic process for soft tissue sarcomas chiefly involves imaging and pathologic analysis.[19] Biopsy-based tumor characterization, which remains the standard of care, presents limitations such as tumor heterogeneity and procedural risks.[20] These limitations frequently result in diagnostic inconsistencies and suboptimal patient management, particularly in settings outside specialized sarcoma centers, where a lack of adherence to established diagnostic protocols often occurs.[19] The diagnostic accuracy of biopsy in soft tissue sarcoma is further complicated by interobserver variability among pathologists, leading to discrepancies in histologic grading and subtyping.[15] To mitigate these issues, expert pathology review, often augmented by molecular diagnostics, significantly enhances diagnostic precision and informs clinical management decisions.[21] This highlights the indispensable role of a multidisciplinary team approach in improving the accuracy of both diagnosis and treatment of bone and soft tissue sarcomas.[22]

The integration of radiomics, artificial intelligence, and molecular signatures further promises to bridge imaging-molecular divides, establishing a roadmap for clinically translatable, multimodal diagnostic systems in musculoskeletal oncology.[23] Case in point, extended molecular profiling, using massive parallel sequencing or next-generation sequencing technologies, has substantially advanced the diagnostic and therapeutic landscape for bone and soft tissue sarcomas, enabling a more granular understanding of their complex genetic alterations.[24] The ongoing evolution of molecular diagnostics, including integrated histomolecular approaches and specific molecular panels, is increasingly critical for tumor classification and therapeutic planning in soft tissue and bone tumors.[17]

The 5th edition of the World Health Organization (WHO) classification of soft tissue and bone sarcomas, updated in 2020, underscores the significant role of genetic mutations in diagnosis and classification, especially for sarcomas with complex karyotypes that are challenging to identify with conventional methods.[25,26] This genomic profiling, although often not directly targetable, provides critical insights for refining diagnosis, patient stratification, and treatment strategies, despite the variability in testing access and data interpretation.[24] However, next-generation sequencing offers significant advancements; its limitations in detecting complex structural variations and copy number alterations are addressed by emerging technologies such as optical genome mapping, which provides high-resolution genome-wide analysis for improved diagnostic and prognostic assessment in sarcoma.[27] Despite these advanced diagnostic tools, diagnostic errors in sarcoma remain a significant concern, often attributable to the disease's complexity and variations in access to specialized pathology or advanced reagents globally.[28] For instance, optical genome mapping has demonstrated success in analyzing sarcoma samples, identifying diagnostic-defining alterations in a substantial percentage of cases, thereby refining diagnoses and uncovering novel oncogenic and tumor suppressor gene alterations.[27] In light of these advancements, the integration of artificial intelligence and digital health platforms holds significant promise for synthesizing such vast and complex datasets, moving beyond isolated impacts toward a cohesive, data-driven strategy for personalized sarcoma care.[28] This convergence of artificial intelligence (AI) with precision medicine offers a breakthrough in biomarker research and disease diagnosis, addressing the inherent molecular heterogeneity of sarcomas where *one-size-fits-all* molecular targets are often ineffective.[28,29]

Therefore, comprehensive genomic profiling, including next-generation sequencing, is crucial for uncovering resistance mechanisms and guiding alternative treatment strategies in sarcoma patients.[25] Next-generation sequencing provides a comprehensive genomic profile, allowing for the identification of actionable genetic alterations that can inform personalized treatment strategies.[30] However, the clinical utility of next-generation sequencing in sarcoma remains contentious due to the low mutational burden and scarcity of recurrent targetable alterations across most histologic subtypes.[31]

Despite the *quieter* genomes in some sarcoma subtypes, structural variations are more common than previously recognized, with next-generation sequencing technologies proving highly impactful for characterizing these events and copy number variations clinically.[32] In these instances, *hot spot* or exome sequencing lacks the ability to discriminate structural genomic alterations.[33] Whole genome sequencing further expands upon this by detecting diagnostic and actionable genomic characteristics, as well as underlying hereditary conditions, thereby optimizing clinical care for sarcoma patients.[34] Whole genome sequencing has been shown to revise cancer diagnoses in a significant proportion of patients, leading to crucial changes in treatment plans.[34] This comprehensive genomic approach, encompassing whole genome sequencing, facilitates the identification of precise therapeutic targets and enhances prognostic accuracy, especially within the diverse landscape of soft tissue and bone sarcomas.

NF1 mutations are prevalent in soft tissue sarcomas and have implications for treatment response and prognosis. The NF1 gene can be altered in somatic fashion or through a germline hereditary cancer syndrome, such as NF1. The observed rates of actionable mutations in genomic profiling studies are high, particulalry with respect to NF1 mutations and RAS signaling.[25,35] MPNSTs, in particular, harbor NF1 mutationsin nearly 80% of cases, making this gene a critical focus for targeted therapeutic development and genetic counseling. Therapy resistance in MPNSTs is common, frequently attributed to mechanisms such as loss of CDKN2A and activation of receptor tyrosine kinase pathways, underscoring the necessity for combinatorial therapeutic strategies to overcome these intrinsic resistance mechanisms.[36,37]

Other mutations are also present in soft tissue sarcomas. For example, gastrointestinal stromal tumors commonly exhibit mutations in KIT or PDGFRA, with less frequent inactivation of the SDH or NF1 genes.[38] However, a broader analysis of various sarcoma subtypes reveals a diverse landscape of genomic alterations beyond these commonly recognized mutations, including alterations in cell cycle control genes, receptor tyrosine kinases/PI3K/RAS pathway components, and epigenetic regulators.[39] This genetic heterogeneity underscores the importance of comprehensive genomic profiling to identify subtype-specific alterations that may guide personalized therapeutic strategies. A table of relevant soft tissue sarcoma mutations is referenced as follows (**Table 1**).

Despite these advances, the clinical impact of genomic profiling in STS has not been prospectively investigated, and data regarding the efficacy of targeted treatments based on identified mutations remain scarce, particularly given the challenges in translating genomic findings into effective therapeutic strategies for many sarcoma subtypes. Consequently, despite the detailed reports on diverse gene mutations, fusions, or amplifications detected through various next generation sequencing (NGS) technologies, robust evidence supporting the clinical utility and efficacy of targeted treatments remains limited.[21] For instance, a multicenter, randomized phase III trial is currently underway to evaluate the feasibility of using molecular profiling by NGS-exome in clinical practice for advanced STS patients and to assess the efficacy of NGS-guided targeted therapies.[40] Such trials are essential to establish the prospective clinical utility of NGS in STS, given that, while genomic profiling can identify potential actionable alterations in up to 50% of advanced STS patients, the routine,

Table 1
Examples of chromosomal translocations and associated gene fusions most frequently detected in soft tissue sarcomas and mesenchymal tumors

Sarcoma Subtype	Translocation	Genes	Oncogenic Mechanism
Ewing sarcoma	t(11;22)(q24;q12); t(21;22)(q22;q12); t(16;21)(p11;q22)	EWSR1, FLI1; EWSR1, ERG; FUS, ERG	Transcription factor
DSRCT	t(11;22)(p13;q12)	EWSR1, WT1	Transcription factor
Alveolar rhabdomyosarcoma	t(2;13)(q35;q14); t(1;13)(p36;q14)	PAX3, FOXO1; PAX7, FOXO1	Transcription factor
Clear cell sarcoma	t(12;22)(q13;q12)	EWSR1, ATF1	Transcription factor
Extraskeletal myxoid chondrosarcoma	t(9;22)(q22;q12)	EWSR1, NR4A3	Transcription factor
Myxoid liposarcoma	t(12;16)(q13;p11)	FUS, CHOP	Transcription factor
Alveolar soft part sarcoma	t(X;17)(p11;q25)	ASPL, TFE3	Transcription factor
Low-grade fibromyxoid sarcoma	t(7;16)(q33;p11)	FUS, CREB3L2	Transcription factor
Sclerosing epithelioid fibrosarcoma	t(11;22)(p11;q11)	EWSR1, CREB3L1	Transcription factor
Low grade endometrial stromal tumor	t(7;17)(p15;q21)	JAZF1, SUZ12	Transcription factor
Synovial sarcoma	t(X;18)(p11;q11)	SYT, SSX1, SSX2, SSX4	Chromatin remodeling
Congenital fibrosarcoma	t(12;15)(p13;q25)	ETV6, NTRK3	Tyrosine kinase
Inflammatory myofibroblastic tumor	t(2;2)(p23;p13); t(1;2)(q22;p23)	TPM3, ALK; TPM4, ALK	Tyrosine kinase
Dermatofibrosarcoma protuberans	t(17;22)(q22;q13)	COL1A1, PDGFB	Growth factor
PVNS/TGCT	t(1;2)(p13;q37)	COL6A3, CSF1	Growth factor

Adapted from Vibert and Watson Cancers 2022.

nonselective use of NGS in sarcoma patients still lacks robust evidence. Moreover, the retrospective nature, small cohort sizes, and difficulties in capturing long-term treatment outcomes in many genomic studies on sarcomas present additional limitations to firmly establish the widespread clinical utility of NGS in guiding therapeutic decisions.

These limitations highlight the importance of multidisciplinary sarcoma-expert institutions in interpreting NGS results and guiding treatment recommendations, as evidenced by guidelines emphasizing expert review for complex genomic panels.[41] Further complicating the widespread implementation of NGS, barriers such as variable testing access, prolonged turnaround times, suboptimal specimen quality, and substantial costs impede its routine adoption. However, ongoing efforts to standardize protocols, reduce costs, and improve data interpretation through AI-driven analytics are critical for integrating these sophisticated diagnostic modalities into routine sarcoma management.[25] Overcoming these challenges is paramount for maximizing the impact of genomic insights on patient outcomes, particularly for advanced or refractory soft-tissue sarcomas where traditional treatment modalities like doxorubicin have reached their therapeutic ceiling.[42] This requires the exploration of alternative therapeutic strategies, including immunotherapy and targeted agents, particularly for patients with limited options.[43] Given the heterogeneity of STS and the modest improvements in overall survival with conventional chemotherapy, there is a pressing need to explore novel treatment avenues that capitalize on the unique molecular landscapes of individual tumors. This necessitates a paradigm shift toward personalized medicine, where treatment decisions are increasingly guided by comprehensive genomic profiling and a deeper understanding of tumor biology.

IMAGING

Imaging options for soft tissue sarcoma continue to evolve. Definitive characterization of a soft tissue sarcoma often requires advanced imaging modalities, such as MRI, which provides superior soft tissue contrast and detailed anatomic information for precise tumor delineation and local staging. Given that soft tissue sarcomas often present as large, painless masses with increasing volume, initial diagnostic evaluations can involve ultrasonography, which offers a cost-effective method with a high negative predictive value for ruling out soft tissue masses.[14] Multiparametric ultrasound, incorporating B-mode, Doppler, elastography, and contrast enhancement, has also emerged as a promising, noninvasive adjunct to MRI, offering comprehensive morphologic, vascular, and biomechanical insights to aid in differential diagnosis and potentially reduce unnecessary biopsies.[44] Other modalities, such as multiparametric magnetic resonance imaging (MRI) and positron emission tomography/computed tomography (PET/CT) with novel tracers, are crucial for improved tumor delineation, assessment of treatment response, and detection of subtle metastatic disease. Other imaging advances in soft tissue sarcoma include artificial intelligence-driven methodologies for enhanced diagnostic accuracy and prognostic stratification, moving toward noninvasive quantitative biomarkers for treatment monitoring.

MRI remains the gold standard for local staging due to its superior spatial resolution and tissue characterization capabilities,[45] enabling comprehensive assessment of tumor extent, involvement of adjacent structures, and neurovascular relationships.[46] The diagnostic utility of MRI extends beyond initial staging, playing a crucial role in detecting local recurrences posttreatment, often enhanced by contrast agents and sometimes integrated with PET imaging for improved specificity.[47] However, despite the advancements in MRI technology, a significant challenge remains in differentiating between benign and malignant lesions, particularly lipomas and well-differentiated liposarcomas, where radiomics—the extraction and analysis of high-throughput quantitative features from medical images—shows promise in augmenting diagnostic accuracy and improving differential diagnosis.[48] Moreover, the integration of multimodality imaging with clinical data and advanced computational techniques, such as radiomics and artificial intelligence, may further enhance the interpretability of imaging changes in patients undergoing neoadjuvant therapies.[49]

Beyond initial diagnosis, MRI is invaluable for monitoring treatment response and detecting disease recurrence, although ultrasonography is also a viable alternative in certain contexts. However, while ultrasound is highly accurate for identifying specific superficial lesions with typical features, it lacks specificity compared to MRI for diagnosing recurrence.[50] Despite these advantages, the choice between MRI and ultrasonography (USG) for surveillance depends on the clinical context, as USG offers benefits such as lower cost, portability, and shorter scan times, making it suitable for frequent follow-up and evaluation of regional lymph nodes. Conversely, PET/CT studies, while limited by small patient numbers and retrospective designs, offer metabolic information that complements anatomic imaging, with PET/MRI demonstrating improved accuracy for local recurrence detection compared to MRI alone.[15] The integration of advanced imaging techniques, particularly contrast-enhanced computed tomography, provides critical information regarding tumor location, stage, and post-treatment follow-up, offering enhanced delineation of nodular septa and differential enhancement patterns useful in distinguishing malignant from benign lesions.[51]

TREATMENT ADVANCES

Surgical resection, when possible, remains the cornerstone of sarcoma therapy. Complete tumor eradication, while preserving function, is paramount whenever possible. Unfortunately, curative surgical resection may be difficult to achieve in many patients. However, there have been several treatment breakthroughs in soft tissue sarcoma over the last decade. For instance, while progress in the overall treatment of bone and soft tissue sarcomas has been slow, molecular subgrouping through multigene next-generation sequencing is improving understanding of their genetic landscape leading to more informed precision medicine approaches.[52] Genomic approaches are confirming known genomic markers, such as the SYT::SSX fusion in synovial sarcoma, and providing deeper insights into the variability around known markers, as well as complex karyotypes that distinguish dedifferentiation from lower-grade lesions.[10] Such molecular insights are pivotal not only for refined diagnostic accuracy but also for identifying novel therapeutic targets and predicting treatment responses in a personalized medicine framework. Despite these advances, the rarity and heterogeneity of sarcomas continue to pose significant challenges to the development and regulatory approval of effective new therapies.[53]

Immunotherapy treatment options are emerging for soft tissue sarcoma. Specifically, immune checkpoint inhibitors, such as nivolumab in combination with ipilimumab, have demonstrated therapeutic activity in advanced STS subtypes like undifferentiated pleomorphic sarcoma, dedifferentiated liposarcoma, and synovial sarcoma, leading to their regulatory approval.[54] Beyond checkpoint blockade, other immunotherapeutic strategies are under investigation, including adoptive cell therapies like afami-cel for synovial sarcoma and tumor-agnostic therapies such as NTRK inhibitors for tumors with NTRK fusions.[55] The growing interest in immunotherapy for soft tissue sarcoma stems from its potential to offer new therapeutic avenues for this heterogeneous group of malignancies.[56] However, despite encouraging advancements, the response rates to anti-PD-1 monotherapies in STS remain modest, averaging approximately 15%, with notable variability across histotypes.[57] This underscores the critical need for identifying predictive biomarkers and developing combination strategies to enhance therapeutic efficacy and overcome primary or acquired resistance mechanisms within the diverse STS molecular landscape.[58]

Targeted therapy options are also emerging for soft tissue sarcoma. These therapies often focus on specific molecular aberrations identified through genomic profiling, such as inhibitors of IDH1, ATR, DNMT, HDACs, and BET, which are currently being investigated in early-phase trials.[59] Furthermore, drugs targeting BRAF, ALK, NTRK, ROS1, EZH1/2, RET, and KIT mutations in specific rare sarcoma subtypes have demonstrated relatively high response rates. While NTRK fusions are infrequent in sarcomas, they are nearly pathognomonic in certain pediatric tumors like infantile fibrosarcoma, highlighting the importance of comprehensive genomic profiling in identifying actionable alterations.[60] Similarly, RET fusions have also emerged as tissue-agnostic targets, with selective RET inhibitors showing promise in sarcomas harboring these fusions.[61] Moreover, several novel agents have recently gained regulatory approval, including tyrosine kinase inhibitors such as avapritinib and ripretinib for gastrointestinal stromal tumors, and the immune checkpoint inhibitor atezolizumab for alveolar soft part sarcomas. These advancements underscore the growing repertoire of targeted treatments, moving beyond conventional chemotherapy to more precise interventions based on individual tumor characteristics.

Combination therapy options are also emerging for soft tissue sarcoma. These regimens often combine immune checkpoint inhibitors with other therapeutic agents, such as nivolumab with gemcitabine/doxorubicin/docetaxel, or retifanlimab with gemcitabine/docetaxel, aiming to synergistically enhance antitumor responses.[58] Beyond chemotherapy combinations, other multi-modal strategies include the integration of immune checkpoint inhibitors with targeted therapies like cabozantinib[40] or radiation therapy to potentially overcome resistance mechanisms and improve clinical outcomes. The ongoing exploration of these multifaceted combination approaches, including those integrating oncolytic viruses or novel drug delivery systems, signifies a pivotal shift toward optimizing therapeutic regimens for the heterogeneous landscape of soft tissue sarcomas. The continuous evolution of therapeutic strategies underscores the critical role of robust preclinical models and comprehensive clinical trial designs to effectively evaluate the efficacy and safety of these complex regimens. However, despite these advancements, the inherent heterogeneity and rarity of sarcomas continue to present substantial challenges to the development and regulatory approval of broadly effective therapies.[53]

Sarcoma radiation therapy is also evolving with preclinical studies demonstrating the equivalent efficacy of photon and proton irradiation in sarcoma mouse models, offering promising avenues for optimizing radiation protocols.[62] Furthermore, innovative approaches combining radiotherapy with immunotherapeutic agents, such as pembrolizumab in neoadjuvant and adjuvant settings, have demonstrated transformative potential in high-grade sarcomas such as undifferentiated pleomorphic sarcoma and liposarcoma of the extremity.[63] Such combined modalities, particularly neoadjuvant immunotherapy, have shown encouraging preliminary results in phase 2 trials, with significant pathologic responses observed in specific STS subtypes.[64] Ongoing trials are further exploring the integration of immunotherapy with radiation therapy by investigating habitat-escalated adaptive therapy, which tailors RT doses to radioresistant intratumoral habitats based on genomic and radiomic profiles.[65,66]

GENETIC COUNSELING

Evaluation is recommended for individuals with a family history of sarcoma or related cancers, as genetic testing can aid in personalized cancer management and surveillance.

SUMMARY

Soft tissue sarcomas have been rigorously characterized from a genomics and transcriptomics standpoint. Precision medicine trials are emerging, focused on immune therapies and selected targeted therapies, which appear to hold promise. Therapy resistance remains a significant issue, particularly for metastatic disease.

CLINICS CARE POINTS

- The clinical management of sarcoma should be done in a center with dedicated, multispecialty sarcoma expertise.
- The diagnosis of sarcoma is becoming increasingly sophisticated. Molecular diagnostics are essential for accurate and timely treatment.
- It is important to stay abreast of rapidly changing diagnostic and therapeutic technologies in the care of sarcoma patients.

DISCLOSURE

None.

REFERENCES

1. Aljuhani W, Alanazi A, Alshehri E, et al. Descriptive analysis of incidence, demographic characteristics, and survival outcomes of soft-tissue sarcoma of the extremities in Saudi Arabia. Sci Rep 2024;14(1):29123.
2. Arifi S, Constantinidou A. Editorial: precision medicine in sarcomas: the road to an effective biomarker-driven-care strategy. Front Oncol 2023;13:1194593.
3. Arthur A, Johnston EW, Winfield J, et al. Virtual Biopsy in Soft Tissue Sarcoma. How Close Are We? [Review of *Virtual Biopsy in Soft Tissue Sarcoma. How Close Are We?*]. Front Oncol 2022;12:892620. Frontiers Media.
4. Berclaz LM, Burkhard-Meier A, Lange P, et al. Implementing precision oncology for sarcoma patients: the CCCLMUmolecular tumor board experience. J Cancer Res Clin Oncol 2023;149(15):13973.
5. Berenguer-Rubio A, Such E, Hernández NT, et al. Exploring the potential of optical genome mapping in the diagnosis and prognosis of soft tissue and bone tumors. Int J Mol Sci 2025;26(6):2820.
6. Blanchi J, Taleb S, Bayle A, et al. Clinical utility of circulating tumor DNA sequencing with a large panel in patients with advanced soft-tissue sarcomas. Cancer Commun 2023;43(9):1051. Wiley.
7. Cai Q, Que Y, Zhang X. Neoadjuvant immunotherapy in the evolving landscape of sarcoma treatment. J ImmunoTher Cancer 2024;12(11). https://doi.org/10.1136/jitc-2024-010074.
8. Chmiel P, Rutkowski P, Spałek M, et al. What is the Optimal Treatment Strategy after Sarcoma R2 Surgery? [Review of *What is the Optimal Treatment Strategy after Sarcoma R2 Surgery?*]. Curr Treat Options Oncol 2024;25(6):798. Springer Science+Business Media.
9. Choi JH, Ro JY. The Recent Advances in Molecular Diagnosis of Soft Tissue Tumors [Review of *The Recent Advances in Molecular Diagnosis of Soft Tissue Tumors*]. Int J Mol Sci 2023;24(6):5934. Multidisciplinary Digital Publishing Institute.
10. Cordier F, Ferdinande L, Hoorens A, et al. Soft tissue and bone tumor diagnostics: harnessing the power of molecular techniques. Genes 2023;14(12):2229.
11. Crombé A, Roulleau-Dugage M, Italiano A. The diagnosis, classification, and treatment of sarcoma in this era of artificial intelligence and immunotherapy. Cancer Commun 2022;42(12):1288.
12. D'Ambrosio L, Sbaraglia M, Merlini A, et al. Extended molecular profiling in mesenchymal tumors: a consensus paper from the Italian Sarcoma Group. Crit Rev Oncol Hematol 2025;216:104960.

13. Damerell V, Pepper MS, Prince S. Molecular mechanisms underpinning sarcomas and implications for current and future therapy [Review of *molecular mechanisms underpinning sarcomas and implications for current and future therapy*]. Signal Transduct Targeted Ther 2021;6(1). https://doi.org/10.1038/s41392-021-00647-8. Springer Nature.
14. Dapper H, Diehl C, Knebel C, et al. Outcome of patients with soft tissue sarcomas of the extremities and trunk treated by (neo)adjuvant intensity modulated radiation therapy with curative intent. Radiat Oncol 2023;18(1). https://doi.org/10.1186/s13014-023-02238-z.
15. Dugage MR, Nassif EF, Italiano A, et al. Improving immunotherapy efficacy in soft-tissue sarcomas: a biomarker driven and histotype tailored review. Front Immunol 2021;12:775761.
16. Ferré AJ, Álvarez R, Casado A, et al. SEOM clinical guideline of management of soft-tissue sarcoma (2020). Clin Transl Oncol 2021;23(5):922.
17. Frezza AM, Stacchiotti S, Gronchi A. Highlights in soft tissue sarcomas and gastrointestinal stromal tumours (GIST) trials reported at ASCO 2017 Annual Meeting. BMC Med 2017;15(1). https://doi.org/10.1186/s12916-017-0931-4.
18. Fuchs B, Studer G, Bode-Lesniewska B, et al. The next frontier in sarcoma care: Digital health, AI, and the quest for precision medicine. J Personalized Med 2023; 13(11):1530.
19. Gennaro N, Reijers SJM, Bruining A, et al. Imaging response evaluation after neoadjuvant treatment in soft tissue sarcomas: where do we stand? [Review of *imaging response evaluation after neoadjuvant treatment in soft tissue sarcomas: where do we stand?*]. Crit Rev Oncol Hematol 2021;160:103309. Elsevier BV.
20. Gómez-Puerto D, Cicala CM, Valverde C, et al. Emerging treatments for sarcoma: from 2024 onward. Expert Opin Emerg Drugs 2025;30(1):53.
21. Gonzalez MR, Méndez-Guerra C, Goh MH, et al. Principles of surgical treatment of soft tissue sarcomas. Cancers 2025;17(3):401.
22. Gounder MM, Agaram NP, Trabucco SE, et al. Clinical genomic profiling in the management of patients with soft tissue and bone sarcoma. Nat Commun 2022;13(1). https://doi.org/10.1038/s41467-022-30496-0.
23. Grit J, McGee LE, Tovar EA, et al. p53 modulates kinase inhibitor resistance and lineage plasticity in NF1-related MPNSTs. Oncogene 2024;43(19):1411.
24. Gündoğdu Y, Taşçı EŞ, Özer L, et al. Next-generation sequencing-based genomic profiling of advanced soft tissue and bone sarcomas. Front Oncol 2025;15. https://doi.org/10.3389/fonc.2025.1627452.
25. Hayes A, Nixon I, Strauß D, et al. UK guidelines for the management of soft tissue sarcomas [Review of *UK guidelines for the management of soft tissue sarcomas*]. Br J Cancer 2024. https://doi.org/10.1038/s41416-024-02674-y. Springer Nature.
26. Hong JY, Cho HJ, Yun K, et al. Comprehensive molecular characterization of soft tissue sarcoma for prediction of pazopanib-based treatment response. Cancer Res Treat 2022;55(2):671.
27. Jarroudi OA, Bairi KE, Brahmi SA, et al. MAPK-targeted therapies in non-gastrointestinal stromal tumor soft tissue sarcomas: current landscape and future directions [Review of *MAPK-targeted therapies in non-gastrointestinal stromal tumor soft tissue sarcomas: current landscape and future directions*]. Front Oncol 2025;15. https://doi.org/10.3389/fonc.2025.1418537. Frontiers Media.
28. Joo MW, Park C, Lee Y-S, et al. Are imaging evaluations of soft-tissue masses before referral to a specialized center being performed properly? A systematic review. Cancers 2024;16(23):3935.

29. Kerrison W, Lee ATJ, Thway K, et al. Current status and future directions of immunotherapies in soft tissue sarcomas. Biomedicines 2022;10(3):573.
30. Kinnersley B, Sud A, Everall A, et al. Analysis of 10,478 cancer genomes identifies candidate driver genes and opportunities for precision oncology. Nat Genet 2024;56(9):1868.
31. Kokkali S, Boukovinas I, de Bree E, et al. The impact of expert pathology review and molecular diagnostics on the management of sarcoma patients: a prospective study of the Hellenic group of sarcomas and rare cancers. Cancers 2024;16-(13):2314.
32. Kokkali S, Georgaki E, Mandrakis G, et al. Genomic profiling and clinical outcomes of targeted therapies in adult patients with soft tissue sarcomas. Cells 2023;12(22):2632.
33. Li G, Feng P, Lin Y, et al. Integrating radiomics, artificial intelligence, and molecular signatures in bone and soft tissue tumors: advances in diagnosis and prognostication [review of *integrating radiomics, artificial intelligence, and molecular signatures in bone and soft tissue tumors: advances in diagnosis and prognostication*]. Front Oncol 2025;15:1613133. Frontiers Media.
34. Mavroeidis L, Napolitano A, Huang PH, et al. Novel therapeutics in soft tissue sarcoma. Cancers 2024;17(1):10.
35. von Mehren M, Kane JM, Agulnik M, et al. Soft tissue sarcoma, version 2.2022, NCCN Clinical Practice Guidelines in oncology. J Natl Compr Cancer Netw 2022;20(7):815.
36. Moyers JT, Pestana RC, Roszik J, et al. Examining stripes on a herd of zebras: impact of genomic matching for ultrarare sarcomas in phase 1 clinical trials (SAMBA 102). Clin Cancer Res 2022;29(2):401.
37. Nacev BA, Sánchez-Vega F, Smith S, et al. Clinical sequencing of soft tissue and bone sarcomas delineates diverse genomic landscapes and potential therapeutic targets. Nat Commun 2022;13(1):3405.
38. Naghavi AO, Bryant JM, Kim Y, et al. Habitat escalated adaptive therapy (HEAT): a phase 2 trial utilizing radiomic habitat-directed and genomic-adjusted radiation dose (GARD) optimization for high-grade soft tissue sarcoma. BMC Cancer 2024;24(1). https://doi.org/10.1186/s12885-024-12151-7.
39. Nannini S, Penel N, Bompas E, et al. Shortening the time interval for the referral of patients with soft tissue sarcoma to expert centers using Mobile health: Retrospective study. JMIR mHealth uHealth 2022;10(11). https://doi.org/10.2196/40718.
40. Natella R, Varriano G, Brunese MC, et al. Increasing differential diagnosis between lipoma and liposarcoma through radiomics: a narrative review. Explor Target Antitumor Ther 2023;4(3):498.
41. Noebauer-Huhmann I-M, Vanhoenacker F, Vilanova JC, et al. Soft tissue tumor imaging in adults: European Society of Musculoskeletal Radiology-Guidelines 2023—overview, and primary local imaging: how and where? [Review of *soft tissue tumor imaging in adults: European Society of Musculoskeletal Radiology-Guidelines 2023—overview, and primary local imaging: how and where?*]. Eur Radiol 2023;34(7):4427. Springer Science+Business Media.
42. Panagi M, Pilavaki P, Constantinidou A, et al. Immunotherapy in soft tissue and bone sarcoma: unraveling the barriers to effectiveness [Review of *immunotherapy in soft tissue and bone sarcoma: unraveling the barriers to effectiveness*]. Theranostics 2022;12(14):6106. Ivyspring International Publisher.

43. Pang K, Guo X, Liu T, et al. The role of a multidisciplinary team in the diagnosis and treatment of bone and soft tissue sarcomas: a single-center experience. J Personalized Med 2022;12(12):2079.
44. Park HY, Chung HW, Yoon MA, et al. Enhancing local recurrence detection in patients with high-grade soft tissue sarcoma: value of short-term ultrasonography added to post-operative MRI surveillance. Cancer Imaging 2024;24(1).
45. Patrichi A, Gurzu S. Pathogenetic and molecular classifications of soft tissue and bone tumors: a 2024 update. Pathol Res Pract 2024;260:155406.
46. Paudel A, Chattopadhyay PK, Rose B, et al. Systemic treatment in soft tissue sarcomas: are we making a difference? Cancers 2025;17(5):889.
47. Rothermundt C, Andreou D, Blay J, et al, Writing Committee on Behalf of CSSS Panellists. Controversies in the management of patients with soft tissue sarcoma: recommendations of the Conference on State of Science in Sarcoma 2022. Eur J Cancer 2022;180:158.
48. Rugge M, Buja A, Tropea S, et al. Indicators of clinical performance in monitoring soft tissue sarcoma management: a population-based perspective. Front Med 2023;10. https://doi.org/10.3389/fmed.2023.1226090.
49. Runkel A, Braig D, Bogner B, et al. Non-invasive monitoring of neoadjuvant radiation therapy response in soft tissue sarcomas by multiparametric MRI and quantification of circulating tumor DNA—A study protocol. PLoS One 2023;18(11). https://doi.org/10.1371/journal.pone.0285580.
50. Schipper LJ, Monkhorst K, Samsom KG, et al. Clinical impact of prospective whole genome sequencing in sarcoma patients. Cancers 2022;14(2):436.
51. Sedaghat S, Sedaghat M, Meschede J, et al. Diagnostic value of MRI for detecting recurrent soft-tissue sarcoma in a long-term analysis at a multidisciplinary sarcoma center. BMC Cancer 2021;21(1):398.
52. Seong G, D'Angelo SP. New therapeutics for soft tissue sarcomas: overview of current immunotherapy and future directions of soft tissue sarcomas [Review of *new therapeutics for soft tissue sarcomas: overview of current immunotherapy and future directions of soft tissue sarcomas*]. Front Oncol 2023;13. https://doi.org/10.3389/fonc.2023.1150765. Frontiers Media.
53. Serrano C, Bauer S, Blay J, et al. Guidelines for next-generation sequencing in sarcoma diagnosis and treatment. JAMA Oncol 2025;11(12):1527.
54. Sobti A, Mowery YM. Priming the tumor microenvironment with pembrolizumab and radiotherapy for durable cures in high-risk localized undifferentiated pleomorphic sarcoma and pleomorphic/dedifferentiated liposarcoma. J ImmunoTher Cancer 2025;13(8). https://doi.org/10.1136/jitc-2025-012053.
55. Soupir AC, Ospina OE, Hampton O, et al. Genomic, transcriptomic, and immunogenomic landscape of over 1300 sarcomas of diverse histology subtypes. Nat Commun 2025;16(1):4206.
56. Stanton BZ, Pomella S. Epigenetic determinants of fusion-driven sarcomas: paradigms and challenges. Front Cell Dev Biol 2024;12. https://doi.org/10.3389/fcell.2024.1416946.
57. Termite F, Galasso L, Capece G, et al. Multiparametric ultrasound in the differential diagnosis of soft tissue tumors: a comprehensive review. Biomedicines 2025;13(7):1786.
58. Vita AD, Bongiovanni A, Blay J, et al. Editorial: new insights into the landscape of rare tumors: translational and clinical research perspective. Front Oncol 2020;10. https://doi.org/10.3389/fonc.2020.593785.
59. Wallander K, Öfverholm I, Boye K, et al. Sarcoma care in the era of precision medicine. J Intern Med 2023;294(6):690.

60. Wang L, Xie A, Ke L, et al. Undifferentiated pleomorphic sarcoma in the anterior mediastinum: a case report and literature review. Front Oncol 2024;14. https://doi.org/10.3389/fonc.2024.1445149.
61. Weetall M, Rance M, Ingham M, et al. Editorial: new therapeutics for soft tissue sarcomas. Front Oncol 2023;13. https://doi.org/10.3389/fonc.2023.1297215.
62. Wisdom AJ, Raut CP, Haddox CL, et al. Clinician's primer for soft tissue sarcomas: nuances of histologic subtypes. Cancer 2025;131(5). https://doi.org/10.1002/cncr.35772.
63. Xiao K-W, Yang K, Hirbe AC. A sequencing overview of malignant peripheral nerve sheath tumors: findings and implications for treatment. Cancers 2025;17(2):180.
64. Yang J, Xu Y, Chen Y, et al. Therapeutic perspectives for adult soft tissue sarcoma—updates from the 2022 ASCO annual meeting. Cancer Biol Med 2022;19(10):1496.
65. Zhou C, Chen X, Huang Y, et al. Nanomaterial Technology and Soft Tissue Sarcomas [Review of *Nanomaterial Technology and Soft Tissue Sarcomas*]. Front Oncol 2022;12. https://doi.org/10.3389/fonc.2022.921983. Frontiers Media.
66. Zou Q, Gan S, Li Y, et al. Case report: giant paratesticular liposarcoma was resected and refused radical orchiectomy. Front Oncol 2023;13. https://doi.org/10.3389/fonc.2023.1223081.

Pediatric Solid Tumors

Genetics and Screening, Prevention, and Treatment of the General Surgeon

Laritza Diaz, MD[a], Elisabeth T. Tracy, MD[b,c,*]

KEYWORDS

- Cancer predisposition syndromes • Pediatric solid tumors • Genetic screening
- DICER1 • SMARCB1 • Renal medullary carcinoma • Wilms tumor • Neuroblastoma

KEY POINTS

- Pediatric solid tumors are largely developmental in origin and have a higher contribution from germline mutations compared with adult cancers.
- Germline pathogenic variants are present in approximately 8.5% to 15% of pediatric cancer patients, influencing diagnosis, management, and family screening.
- Advances in genomics enable risk stratification, targeted therapies, and molecular tumor boards, improving personalized treatment approaches.
- A notable proportion (9%–17%) of Wilms tumors are linked to syndromes such as WT1-related disorders and Beckwith-Wiedemann syndrome, affecting surgical decisions and surveillance strategies.
- Pediatric renal, neuroblastoma, and liver tumors are often associated with specific genetic syndromes (eg, anaplastic lymphoma kinase in neuroblastoma, APC in hepatoblastoma), emphasizing the importance of genetic testing and structured surveillance protocols.

INTRODUCTION

Pediatric solid tumors differ from adult tumors. Pediatric tumors are often developmental, arising from embryonal, mesenchymal, and epithelial tissues with germline variants playing a proportionally larger role in their pathogenesis (as opposed to somatic mutations). Although childhood cancer is rare, accounting for fewer than 1% of all new cancer diagnoses annually, it remains a leading cause of disease-related mortality in children. Advances in genomic medicine over the past 2 decades have advanced our understanding of tumor biology in tumors. For example, the 2015

[a] Department of Surgery, University of North Carolina, Chapel Hill, NC, USA; [b] Division of Pediatric Surgery, UNC Children's Hospital, University of North Carolina, Chapel Hill, NC, USA; [c] UNC Lineberger Comprehensive Cancer Center, Chapel Hill, NC, USA
* Corresponding author. 170 Manning Drive, Chapel Hill, NC 27599-7223.
E-mail address: lisa_tracy@med.unc.edu

Surg Clin N Am 106 (2026) 633–645
https://doi.org/10.1016/j.suc.2026.04.003 **surgical.theclinics.com**
0039-6109/26/

Abbreviations	
AACR	American Association for Cancer Research
ACC	adrenocortical carcinoma
BWS	Beckwith-Wiedemann syndrome
CMMRD	constitutional mismatch repair deficiency
CMN	congenital mesoblastic nephroma
CPS	cancer predisposition syndrome
FAP	familial adenomatous polyposis
MEN2	Multiple Endocrine Neoplasia type 2
MPNST	malignant peripheral nerve sheath tumor
MTC	medullary thyroid carcinoma
NF1	neurofibromatosis type 1
PPB	pleuropulmonary blastoma
RMC	renal medullary carcinoma
RMS	Rhabdomyosarcoma

study by Zhang and colleagues in the New England Journal of Medicine demonstrated that germline pathogenic variants in known cancer predisposition genes were present in approximately 8.5% of pediatric cancer patients.[1] Subsequent studies using expanded gene panels have suggested the prevalence may be as high as 15%.[2,3]

Over the last 2 decades, the care of children with solid tumors has grown increasingly complex as more risk stratification based on tumor biology has been possible. Targeted therapy and molecular tumor boards are increasingly common in the care of childhood cancer. Identification of a childhood cancer predisposition syndrome (CPS) can directly influence the surgical approach, such as the decision to perform nephron-sparing surgery in a child with Wilms tumor and an underlying WT1 mutation. Also, it allows for genetic testing of family members and enrollment in surveillance protocols that can detect subsequent tumors at earlier, more treatable stages. The 2016, 2023, and 2024 American Association for Cancer Research (AACR) Childhood Cancer Predisposition Workshops and the Society of Pediatric Hematology and Oncology have provided an evolving framework of surveillance recommendations that are directly relevant to surgical practice.[4–8]

This review provides a practical guide for the general or pediatric surgeon with emphasis on the tumor biology and screening implications of the most common pediatric solid tumors.

RENAL TUMORS

Wilms tumor (nephroblastoma) is the most common renal malignancy of childhood, with approximately 500 new cases diagnosed annually in the United States. Although the overall survival for Favorable Histology Wilms Tumor is greater than 90%, management complexity increases substantially when an underlying predisposition syndrome is identified. Approximately 9% to 17% of Wilms tumors are associated with a recognized CPS (**Table 1**).[9–11]

The most well-characterized predisposition syndromes include those associated with WT1 mutations and 11p15 abnormalities. WAGR syndrome (Wilms tumor, aniridia, genitourinary anomalies, and a range of developmental delays) results from contiguous gene deletions on chromosome 11p13 involving both WT1 and PAX6. The Wilms tumor risk in WAGR syndrome is 45% to 60%, and affected children also face significant risk of progressive nephropathy.[12] Denys-Drash syndrome, caused by dominant-negative missense mutations in WT1, carries a Wilms tumor

Table 1
Cancer predisposition syndromes associated with pediatric solid tumors

Predisposition Syndrome	Gene(s)/ Mechanism	Associated Solid Tumors	Screening Recommendations
Beckwith-Wiedemann Syndrome	11p15 (ICR1/ ICR2), CDKN1C, H19, IGF2	Wilms tumor, hepatoblastoma, neuroblastoma, ACC, RMS	Abdominal US q3 mo until age 7–8 years; AFP q3 mo until age 4 years
WAGR Syndrome	WT1, PAX6 deletion (11p13)	Wilms tumor	Renal US q3 mo until age 8; nephropathy monitoring lifelong
Denys-Drash Syndrome	WT1 missense mutations	Wilms tumor, gonadoblastoma	Renal US q3 mo; consider early bilateral nephrectomy
Li-Fraumeni Syndrome	TP53	Osteosarcoma, STS, ACC, neuroblastoma	Toronto Protocol: annual WB-MRI; abdominal US q3–4 mo until age 5; brain MRI annually
Familial Adenomatous Polyposis	APC	CRC, hepatoblastoma, desmoid tumors, thyroid carcinoma	Colonoscopy starting age 10–15; AFP and abdominal US for hepatoblastoma
Lynch Syndrome (HNPCC)	MLH1, MSH2, MSH6, PMS2, EPCAM	CRC, endometrial and ovarian carcinoma	Colonoscopy q1–2 y starting age 20–25
CMMRD	Biallelic MLH1, MSH2, MSH6, PMS2	CRC, brain tumors, hematologic malignancies	Annual WB-MRI; colonoscopy q1–2 y from age 6; brain MRI q6–12 mo
DICER1 Syndrome	DICER1	PPB, Sertoli-Leydig cell tumor, cystic nephroma, thyroid carcinoma, cervical/vaginal RMS	CXR at birth, then q6 mo until age 8; thyroid US annually from age 8; pelvic US; renal US until age 8
Hereditary Neuroblastoma	ALK, PHOX2B	Neuroblastoma, ganglioneuroblastoma, ganglioneuroma	Abdominal US and urine catecholamines q3–6 mo; chest imaging if PHOX2B
Rhabdoid Tumor Predisposition	SMARCB1 (INI1) germline	MRT (renal, extrarenal), AT/RT	Brain/spine MRI q3 mo until age 5; abdominal US q3 mo
Costello Syndrome	HRAS	RMS, neuroblastoma, bladder carcinoma	Abdominal US q3–4 mo until age 8–10; urine catecholamines annually

(*continued on next page*)

Table 1
(*continued*)

Predisposition Syndrome	Gene(s)/ Mechanism	Associated Solid Tumors	Screening Recommendations
NF1	NF1	MPNST, optical pathway glioma, RMS, pheochromocytoma	Annual clinical examination; ophthalmologic examination annually until age 8; MRI if symptomatic
MEN2	RET	MTC, pheochromocytoma	Prophylactic thyroidectomy (age per mutation); annual calcitonin and metanephrines
Hereditary Retinoblastoma	RB1	Retinoblastoma, osteosarcoma, STS, melanoma	Fundoscopic examinations q1–3 mo in infancy; lifelong secondary malignancy monitoring
Gorlin Syndrome	PTCH1, SUFU	BCC, medulloblastoma, RMS, ovarian fibroma	Annual dermatologic examination; brain MRI in childhood; pelvic US
Perlman Syndrome	DIS3L2	Wilms tumor	Renal US q3 mo until age 7
Simpson-Golabi-Behmel	GPC3	Wilms tumor, hepatoblastoma, neuroblastoma	Abdominal US q3 mo until age 7; AFP until age 4
Fanconi Anemia	BRCA2/ FANCD1 and others	Wilms tumor, hepatoblastoma, medulloblastoma, AML	Abdominal US q3 mo; AFP; hematologic monitoring
Hereditary Pheo-Paraganglioma	SDHx	Pheochromocytoma, paraganglioma, GIST, RCC	Annual plasma metanephrines; WB-MRI q2 yr from age 6–10
MUTYH-Associated Polyposis	MUTYH (biallelic)	Colorectal carcinoma	Colonoscopy q1–2 y starting age 18–20

Abbreviations: ACC, adrenocortical carcinoma; AML, acute myeloid leukemia; AT/RT, atypical teratoid/rhabdoid tumor; BCC, basal cell carcinoma; CRC, colorectal carcinoma; GIST, gastrointestinal stromal tumor; JMML, juvenile myelomonocytic leukemia; MPNST, malignant peripheral nerve sheath tumor; MRT, malignant rhabdoid tumor; MTC, medullary thyroid carcinoma; PPB, pleuropulmonary blastoma; RCC, renal cell carcinoma; RMS, rhabdomyosarcoma; STS, soft tissue sarcoma; WB, whole-body.

risk of more than 90%. Frasier syndrome, also caused by WT1 splicing mutations, carries a lower but appreciable risk of Wilms tumor and gonadoblastoma.[13]

Gonadoblastoma, a rare gonadal neoplasm that arises in dysgenetic gonads, is particularly associated with WT1-related disorders of sex development. In Frasier syndrome, the risk of gonadoblastoma is high in 46,XY individuals with streak gonads, and prophylactic gonadectomy is recommended when gonadal dysgenesis is identified. Gonadoblastoma has also been reported in Denys-Drash syndrome, and the risk of malignant transformation to dysgerminoma or other germ cell tumors mandates close surveillance and early surgical intervention.[13,14]

Beckwith-Wiedemann syndrome (BWS) is the most common overgrowth syndrome associated with Wilms tumor, resulting from various genetic and epigenetic abnormalities at the 11p15 locus. The cancer risk in BWS varies by molecular subtype. Patients with gain of methylation at ICR1 carry the highest risk (approximately 20%–30% for embryonal tumors), while those with loss of methylation at ICR2 have a substantially lower risk. BWS-associated tumors include Wilms tumor, hepatoblastoma, neuroblastoma, and adrenocortical carcinoma (ACC). Current surveillance recommendations, updated in 2024 by the AACR, call for abdominal ultrasound every 3 months until age 7 to 8, with alpha-fetoprotein screening for hepatoblastoma risk in the appropriate molecular subtypes.[5]

Other renal tumors of importance to the general surgeon include malignant rhabdoid tumor of the kidney, driven by biallelic inactivation of SMARCB1/INI1, clear cell sarcoma of the kidney, and pediatric renal cell carcinoma. Cystic nephroma, a benign renal neoplasm, is increasingly recognized as part of the DICER1 tumor predisposition syndrome spectrum.

NEUROBLASTOMA AND RELATED TUMORS

Neuroblastoma is the most common extracranial solid tumor of childhood. Although the majority of cases are sporadic, approximately 1 to 2% are familial, and germline mutations have been identified in 2 principal genes. Activating mutations in anaplastic lymphoma kinase account for the majority of hereditary neuroblastoma cases and have also been identified as somatic mutations in approximately 7% to 10% of sporadic tumors.[15,16] Germline mutations in PHOX2B, a transcription factor critical to autonomic nervous system development, are found in families with neuroblastoma and associated with congenital central hypoventilation syndrome (Ondine curse).[17] The spectrum of neuroblastic tumors includes neuroblastoma, ganglioneuroblastoma, and ganglioneuroma, which represent a continuum from undifferentiated to fully mature. Li-Fraumeni syndrome (TP53 mutations), Noonan syndrome (PTPN11 and related RAS-MAPK pathway genes), Costello syndrome (HRAS), and BWS are also associated with an elevated, though lower, risk of neuroblastoma.

LIVER TUMORS

Hepatoblastoma is the most common primary hepatic malignancy of childhood, typically presenting before age 3. Several predisposition syndromes carry an elevated risk of hepatoblastoma, most notably BWS (particularly the ICR1 gain-of-methylation and UPD subtypes), familial adenomatous polyposis (FAP), and Simpson-Golabi-Behmel syndrome. The hepatoblastoma risk in FAP is only 1% to 2%, but tumors appear early enough that surveillance with serial alpha-fetoprotein and abdominal ultrasound is recommended from infancy. The APC gene also plays a central role in the Wnt signaling pathway, and somatic APC mutations or beta-catenin (CTNNB1) activating mutations are found in the majority of sporadic hepatoblastomas.

Hepatocellular carcinoma in the pediatric population is far less common than hepatoblastoma and is often associated with underlying liver disease, including tyrosinemia type I (FAH gene), glycogen storage disease, progressive familial intrahepatic cholestasis, and biliary atresia. The fibrolamellar variant of hepatocellular carcinoma, which occurs in adolescents and young adults without underlying liver disease, may be characterized by a recurrent DNAJB1-PRKACA gene fusion. Although there is growing interest in this fusion as a translational target, complete surgical resection remains the most effective therapy.

SOFT TISSUE SARCOMAS

Rhabdomyosarcoma (RMS) is the most common soft tissue sarcoma of childhood, accounting for approximately 3% of pediatric cancers. The 2 major histologic subtypes, embryonal and alveolar, have distinct molecular profiles. Alveolar RMS is characterized by PAX3-FOXO1 or PAX7-FOXO1 gene fusions, which are powerful drivers of oncogenesis and are associated with a poorer prognosis. Embryonal RMS frequently harbors loss of heterozygosity at 11p15, overlapping with the Beckwith-Wiedemann locus. Several CPS are associated with RMS, including Li-Fraumeni syndrome (TP53), Costello syndrome (HRAS), neurofibromatosis type 1 (NF1), DICER1 syndrome (cervical and vaginal embryonal RMS), and Noonan syndrome.[18]

Malignant peripheral nerve sheath tumors (MPNSTs) arise most commonly in the setting of NF1, caused by germline mutations in the NF1 tumor suppressor gene. The lifetime risk of MPNST in NF1 patients is approximately 8% to 13%. NF1 patients should undergo annual clinical examination with a low threshold for imaging of rapidly enlarging or painful neurofibromas (**Table 2**).

Other soft tissue sarcomas of note include synovial sarcoma, characterized by the SS18-SSX gene fusion, and epithelioid sarcoma, which demonstrates INI1/SMARCB1 loss, placing it within the broader family of SMARCB1-deficient tumors.[19,20]

BONE TUMORS

Osteosarcoma is the most common primary bone malignancy of childhood and adolescence, with a peak incidence during the pubertal growth spurt. The strongest known genetic predisposition is Li-Fraumeni syndrome, in which germline TP53 mutations confer a substantially elevated lifetime risk of osteosarcoma. Rothmund-Thomson syndrome (RECQL4), Werner syndrome (WRN), and Bloom syndrome (BLM) are rare autosomal recessive conditions associated with increased osteosarcoma risk.[21,22]

Ewing sarcoma, the second most common bone tumor of childhood, is characterized by EWSR1 gene fusions, most commonly EWSR1-FLI1, resulting from t(11;22)(q24;q12). While the vast majority of Ewing sarcoma cases are sporadic, rare familial clustering has been reported, and genome-wide association studies have identified susceptibility loci. Unlike osteosarcoma, Ewing sarcoma is not strongly associated with any single CPS.

THORACIC TUMORS AND DICER1 SYNDROME

Pleuropulmonary blastoma (PPB) is the most common primary pulmonary malignancy of childhood, with an estimated 70% of cases harboring a germline DICER1 mutation. DICER1 syndrome is an autosomal dominant tumor predisposition syndrome with a prevalence estimated at 1 in 6099 to 8416 individuals. The DICER1 gene encodes an RNase III endoribonuclease that is essential for microRNA processing. Germline loss-of-function mutations in 1 allele, followed by somatic mutations in the RNase IIIb domain of the second allele, drive tumorigenesis through a 2 hit mechanism.[23,24]

PPB is classified into 4 types based on morphology: type I (purely cystic), type Ir (regressed), type II (mixed cystic and solid), and type III (purely solid), representing a

Table 2
Screening and surveillance guidelines for common pediatric cancer predisposition syndromes

Screening Component	Modality	Frequency	Duration
Renal Tumor Predisposition (BWS, WAGR, DDS, Perlman, SGBS)			
Abdominal or renal US	Ultrasound	Every 3 mo	Until age 7–8
AFP (if hepatoblastoma risk)	Serum AFP	Every 2–3 mo	Until age 4
Li-Fraumeni Syndrome (TP53)			
Whole-body MRI (Toronto Protocol)	WB-MRI	Annually	From birth, lifelong
Brain MRI	MRI	Annually	From birth, lifelong
Abdominal US	Ultrasound	Every 3–4 mo	Until age 5
DICER1 Syndrome			
Chest X-ray (PPB)	CXR	At birth, then q6 mo	Until age 8
Thyroid US	Ultrasound	Annually	From age 8, lifelong
Pelvic US (females)	Ultrasound	Annually	From Dx through age 40
Renal US (cystic nephroma)	Ultrasound	Every 6 mo	Until age 8
SMARCB1/INI1 Rhabdoid Tumor Predisposition			
Brain and spine MRI	MRI	Every 3 mo	Until age 5
Abdominal US	Ultrasound	Every 3 mo	Until age 5
Hereditary Neuroblastoma (ALK, PHOX2B)			
Abdominal US	Ultrasound	Every 3–6 mo	Until age 6–10
Urine catecholamines	Urine biochemistry	Every 3–6 mo	Until age 6–10
MEN2/RET-Associated			
Prophylactic thyroidectomy	Surgery	Age-dependent	MEN2B: <1 y; High-risk MEN2A: by age 5
Serum calcitonin	Biochemistry	Annually	From infancy if surgery deferred
Plasma metanephrines	Biochemistry	Annually	From age 11–16
FAP/Lynch Syndrome/CMMRD			
Colonoscopy (FAP)	Endoscopy	Every 1–2 y	Starting age 10–15
Colonoscopy (Lynch)	Endoscopy	Every 1–2 y	Starting age 20–25
Colonoscopy + WB-MRI (CMMRD)	Endoscopy + MRI	q1–2 y + annual MRI	From age 6, lifelong
AFP + abdominal US (FAP)	US + AFP	Every 3 mo	Until age 5

(*continued on next page*)

Table 2
(*continued*)

Screening Component	Modality	Frequency	Duration
Hereditary Retinoblastoma (RB1)			
Fundoscopic examination	Clinical	Every 1–3 mo	From birth through age 3–5
Secondary malignancy monitoring	Clinical + imaging	Annually	Lifelong

Adapted from AACR Childhood Cancer Predisposition Workshop recommendations (2017, 2024), NCCN, ATA, and International PPB/DICER1 Registry guidelines.

progression from favorable to unfavorable histology. Five year overall survival ranges from 53% for type III to 89% for type I and nearly 100% for type Ir. Importantly, type I PPB may be initially diagnosed as the far more frequent congenital pulmonary airway malformation, underscoring the importance of pathologic examination and DICER1 testing for resected lung cysts in young children.[23,25]

Beyond PPB, DICER1 syndrome is associated with a diverse spectrum of tumors, including ovarian Sertoli-Leydig cell tumors, cystic nephroma, thyroid neoplasms (multinodular goiter and differentiated thyroid carcinoma), cervical and vaginal embryonal RMS, pituitary blastoma, pineoblastoma, and nasal chondromesenchymal hamartoma. Updated 2024 surveillance guidelines from the International PPB/DICER1 Registry recommend chest radiography at birth and every 6 months until age 8, thyroid ultrasound annually from age 8, pelvic ultrasound for females from the time of DICER1 diagnosis, and renal ultrasound every 6 months until age 8.[26]

ADRENOCORTICAL CARCINOMA AND MEDULLARY THYROID CARCINOMA

ACC in children is strongly associated with Li-Fraumeni syndrome. In certain populations, such as southern Brazil where the TP53 R337H founder mutation is prevalent, pediatric ACC incidence is markedly elevated.[27–29] Surveillance for ACC in LFS includes abdominal ultrasound every 3 to 4 months and, in some protocols, urine cortisol screening until age 5 to 6, which corresponds to the period of highest risk.[6]

Medullary thyroid carcinoma (MTC) is the hallmark malignancy of Multiple Endocrine Neoplasia type 2 (MEN2), caused by activating germline mutations in the RET proto-oncogene. MEN2 is subdivided into MEN2A and MEN2B based on genotype-phenotype correlations. The American Thyroid Association guidelines stratify RET mutations by risk level and recommend prophylactic thyroidectomy: within the first year of life for MEN2B (the highest-risk category), by age 5 for high-risk MEN2A mutations, and potentially later for moderate-risk mutations. Annual biochemical screening with serum calcitonin and plasma metanephrines for pheochromocytoma is also recommended.

COLORECTAL CANCER IN CHILDREN AND ADOLESCENTS

Colorectal carcinoma is rare in the pediatric population but carries a significant genetic component when it does occur. In a German retrospective study of 31 pediatric patients with colorectal carcinoma, 11 of 26 tested patients (42%) were found to have an underlying genetic predisposition syndrome: 8 with Lynch syndrome, 1 with FAP, and 2 with constitutional mismatch repair deficiency (CMMRD). Notably, patients with an identified predisposition syndrome presented with more localized disease and had superior outcomes compared with those without.[30]

FAP is caused by germline mutations in the APC gene and is characterized by the development of hundreds to thousands of colorectal adenomatous polyps, typically beginning in the teenage years. Without prophylactic colectomy, the lifetime risk of colorectal cancer approaches 100%. In addition to colorectal cancer, FAP is associated with hepatoblastoma, desmoid tumors, thyroid carcinoma, and duodenal adenomas. Screening colonoscopy is recommended starting at age 10 to 15.[31]

Lynch syndrome (hereditary nonpolyposis colorectal cancer) is caused by germline mutations in DNA mismatch repair genes (MLH1, MSH2, MSH6, PMS2) or deletions in EPCAM. It is the most common cause of inherited colorectal cancer in adults, accounting for 3 to 5% of all colorectal cancers. The lifetime colorectal cancer risk for mutation carriers is 50% to 80%, with tumors often presenting before age 50. While the risk of cancer during childhood is not clearly increased in Lynch syndrome families, awareness is important for long-term surgical planning and family counseling. Colonoscopy every 1 to 2 years beginning at age 20 to 25 (or 5 years before the youngest affected family member if diagnosed under age 30) is the standard of care.[32]

CMMRD, caused by biallelic mutations in MMR genes, represents a more severe phenotype with markedly earlier cancer onset, often in childhood. CMMRD-associated cancers include colorectal carcinoma, brain tumors, hematologic malignancies, and small bowel carcinoma. Surveillance for CMMRD is intensive and includes annual whole-body MRI, colonoscopy every 1 to 2 years starting at age 6, and brain MRI every 6 to 12 months.[7]

MUTYH-associated polyposis is an autosomal recessive condition caused by biallelic MUTYH mutations, presenting with an attenuated polyposis phenotype (typically 15–100 polyps) and an elevated colorectal cancer risk. Colonoscopy every 1 to 2 years beginning at age 18 to 20 is recommended.[31]

PEDIATRIC AND ADOLESCENT MELANOMA

Melanoma is uncommon in children but increases in incidence during adolescence. Predisposing genetic factors include germline mutations in CDKN2A (the most well-characterized familial melanoma gene), CDK4, BAP1, POT1, and MC1R variants. Hereditary retinoblastoma survivors also have an elevated risk. Giant congenital melanocytic nevi confer a risk of melanoma that may approach 5% to 10% over a lifetime. Xeroderma pigmentosum, caused by defects in nucleotide excision repair genes, confers a dramatically elevated risk of melanoma and other skin cancers.[33] Sentinel lymph node biopsy has been demonstrated to have prognostic value in pediatric melanoma, and surgical management has generally been extrapolated from adult guidelines, although, as more pediatric-specific studies emerge, age-specific recommendations are emerging.[33–35]

TUMORS OF INFANCY

Neonatal and infantile tumors represent a distinct group of malignancies with unique biological features. The most common solid tumors presenting in the first year of life include neuroblastoma, sacrococcygeal teratoma, infantile fibrosarcoma, congenital mesoblastic nephroma (CMN), hepatoblastoma, and malignant rhabdoid tumor.

Infantile fibrosarcoma (also termed congenital fibrosarcoma) is a fibroblastic tumor that typically presents as a rapidly enlarging extremity mass in children under 2 years of age. It is molecularly characterized by the ETV6-NTRK3 gene fusion resulting from t(12;15) (p13;q25), although variant fusions involving NTRK1, NTRK2, EML4-NTRK3, MET, RET, RAF1, and BRAF have been identified.[36] The identification of NTRK fusions has transformed management, as TRK inhibitors (larotrectinib and entrectinib) have demonstrated dramatic response rates and avoiding the morbidity of radical surgery in infants. Infants with these tumors should have upfront biopsy instead of an attempt at resection unless resection is feasible with minimal loss of function or minimal morbidity.[37]

CMN is the most common renal tumor of the first 3 months of life. The cellular variant of CMN is histologically identical to infantile fibrosarcoma and shares the ETV6-NTRK3 fusion. The classic variant and mixed type may harbor EGFR kinase domain duplications. Surgical resection is curative in the vast majority of cases, with a 5 year survival exceeding 95%.

Malignant rhabdoid tumor of the kidney typically presents in infants under 2 years and is driven by biallelic SMARCB1 inactivation. Germline SMARCB1 mutations define rhabdoid tumor predisposition syndrome, which carries a risk of renal, extrarenal, and central nervous system rhabdoid tumors. Sacrococcygeal teratoma, the most common tumor of the newborn, is typically sporadic and managed surgically; mature (benign) teratomas predominate in neonates, while immature and malignant germ cell tumors become more common with increasing age at diagnosis.

RENAL MEDULLARY CARCINOMA AND INI1/SMARCB1 LOSS TUMORS

Renal medullary carcinoma (RMC) is a rare, aggressive renal malignancy that occurs almost exclusively in adolescents and young adults of African descent with sickle cell trait or other sickle hemoglobinopathies. RMC was first described in 1995 as the "seventh nephropathy of sickle cell disease" and is defined molecularly by loss of SMARCB1/INI1, a core subunit of the SWI/SNF chromatin-remodeling complex. The median age at diagnosis in the pediatric population is 13 years, and most patients present with advanced or metastatic disease, resulting in a median survival of 19 to 22 months in more recent series.[38–40]

The SMARCB1/INI1 tumor suppressor gene, located on chromosome 22q11.2, is inactivated in RMC through balanced translocations disrupting 1 allele with concurrent loss or deletion of the second allele. Loss of INI1 expression, readily detected by immunohistochemistry, serves as a highly sensitive diagnostic marker. The mechanism linking sickle hemoglobinopathy to tumorigenesis is hypothesized to involve chronic medullary hypoxia, sickling-induced cellular damage, and replicative stress in the renal medulla, creating a permissive environment for SMARCB1 loss.[19]

RMC belongs to a broader family of SMARCB1/INI1-deficient tumors that share biological features and therapeutic vulnerabilities. This family includes malignant rhabdoid tumor of the kidney and extrarenal sites, atypical teratoid/rhabdoid tumor of the central nervous system, and epithelioid sarcoma. Recent translational research has identified potential therapeutic targets in SMARCB1-deficient cancers, including sensitivity to proteasome inhibitors (through synthetic lethal dependence on the ubiquitin-proteasome system), EZH2 inhibitors (exploiting the antagonistic relationship between SMARCB1 and the PRC2 complex), and immune checkpoint inhibitors.[38]

For the general surgeon, awareness of RMC is critical because patients with this aggressive tumor should receive multidisciplinary oncology care and enrollment in clinical trials and registries should be prioritized.

THE ROLE OF GENETIC COUNSELING AND TESTING

Genetic counseling should be offered to all pediatric patients in whom a predisposition syndrome is suspected, and referral to a specialized cancer predisposition program is recommended when available. Indications for genetic referral include: bilateral or multifocal tumors; unusually early age at presentation; specific tumor histologies known to be strongly associated with germline mutations (such as pleuropulmonary blastoma, ACC); family history of cancer (particularly childhood cancers or multiple cancers in a single family member); and the presence of congenital anomalies, dysmorphic features, or overgrowth.

The International Society of Pediatric Oncology Europe Host Genome Working Group has recommended that all children with cancer be clinically screened for predisposition syndromes, and that focused germline gene testing be considered when appropriate. Comprehensive germline gene panel testing for all children with cancer is being trialed in studies in multiple countries.

SUMMARY

As the understanding of tumor biology for most types of childhood cancer continues to grow, the role of genetic testing has become increasingly important in pediatric surgical oncology. CPS are associated a significant number pediatric solid tumors, and their identification has direct implications for surgical decision-making—such as nephron-sparing surgery in renal tumors, the timing of prophylactic thyroidectomy in MEN2, and the approach to resection of cystic CPAM lesions.

Also, identification of a predisposition syndrome may prompt genetic testing of family members, enrollment in evidence-based surveillance programs, and identification of at-risk siblings before they develop tumors. Children, adolescents, and young adults with possible predisposition syndromes should receive multidisciplinary oncology care.

CLINICS CARE POINTS

- Surgical decision-making should take into account predisposition syndromes. For example, a child with Wilms tumor and an underlying WT1 mutation (as in Denys-Drash or WAGR syndrome) carries a high risk of bilateral or metachronous disease, making nephron-sparing surgery the preferred approach rather than radical nephrectomy.
- Type I pleuropulmonary blastoma is radiographically and clinically indistinguishable from congenital pulmonary airway malformation. Because approximately 70 percent of PPB cases harbor a germline DICER1 mutation, all resected lung cysts in young children warrant DICER1 testing — the diagnosis of CPAM should not be assumed until malignancy has been excluded and genetic evaluation completed.
- Renal medullary carcinoma should be suspected in any child or adolescent with Sickle Cell Trait presenting with a renal mass. Sickle cell trait — not only disease — is the associated hemoglobinopathy, and this distinction is frequently overlooked; most patients present with advanced or metastatic disease, making early recognition and prompt referral to a multidisciplinary oncology team critical to optimizing outcomes.
- The presence of a cancer predisposition syndrome in a pediatric patient has immediate implications beyond the index tumor. Surgeons should recognize phenotypic clues — overgrowth, aniridia, genitourinary anomalies, dysmorphic features, bilateral or multifocal disease — as triggers for genetic referral, since identification of a syndrome initiates family cascade testing and enrollment in surveillance protocols that can detect future tumors at earlier, more treatable stages.

REFERENCES

1. Zhang J, Walsh MF, Wu G, et al. Germline mutations in predisposition genes in pediatric cancer. N Engl J Med 2015;373:2336–46.

2. Gröbner SN, Worst BC, Weischenfeldt J, et al. The landscape of genomic alterations across childhood cancers. Nature 2018;555:321–7.
3. Kratz CP, Jongmans MC, Cavé H, et al. Predisposition to cancer in children and adolescents. Lancet Child Adolesc Health 2021;5:142–54.
4. Kalish JM, Doros L, Helman LJ, et al. Surveillance recommendations for children with overgrowth syndromes and predisposition to Wilms tumors and hepatoblastoma. Clin Cancer Res 2017;23(13):e115–22.
5. MacFarland SP, Kalish JM, Schultz KAP, et al. Update on surveillance for Wilms tumor and hepatoblastoma in Beckwith-Wiedemann syndrome and other predisposition syndromes. Clin Cancer Res 2024;30(23):5260–70.
6. Hansford JR, Greer MLC. Update on cancer screening recommendations for Li-Fraumeni syndrome. Clin Cancer Res 2024;30(10):1831–40.
7. Greer MLC, States LJ, Malkin D, et al. Update on whole-body MRI surveillance for pediatric cancer predisposition syndromes. Clin Cancer Res 2024;30(22):5021–33.
8. Ripperger T, Bielack SS, Borkhardt A, et al. Childhood cancer predisposition syndromes-A concise review and recommendations by the Cancer Predisposition Working Group of the Society for Pediatric Oncology and Hematology. Am J Med Genet A 2017;173(4):1017–37.
9. Grant CN, Rhee D, Tracy ET, et al. Pediatric solid tumors and associated cancer predisposition syndromes: workup, management, and surveillance. A summary from the APSA cancer committee. J Pediatr Surg 2022;57(3):430–42.
10. Liu EK, Suson KD. Syndromic Wilms tumor: a review of predisposing conditions, surveillance and treatment. Transl Androl Urol 2020;9(5):2370–81.
11. Harris CJ, Waters AM, Tracy ET, et al. Precision oncology: a primer for pediatric surgeons from the APSA cancer committee. J Pediatr Surg 2020;55(9):1706–13.
12. Tracy ET, Leraas H, Olson L, et al. Wilms tumor characteristics, surgical management, outcomes, and chronic kidney disease in children with WAGR syndrome. Pediatr Blood Cancer 2024;71(9):e31172.
13. Lopez-Gonzalez M, Ariceta G. WT1-related disorders: more than Denys-Drash syndrome. Pediatr Nephrol 2024;39(9):2601–9.
14. Love JD, DeMartini SD, Coppola CP. Prophylactic bilateral salpingo-oopherectomy in a 17-year-old with Frasier syndrome reveals gonadoblastoma and seminoma: a case report. J Pediatr Surg 2006;41(11):e1–4.
15. Mossé YP, Laudenslager M, Longo L, et al. Identification of ALK as a major familial neuroblastoma predisposition gene. Nature 2008;455:930–5.
16. Bourdeaut F, Ferrand S, Brugières L, et al. ALK germline mutations in patients with neuroblastoma: a rare and weakly penetrant syndrome. Eur J Hum Genet 2012;20(3):291–7.
17. Mossé YP, Laudenslager M, Khazi D, et al. Germline PHOX2B mutation in hereditary neuroblastoma. Am J Hum Genet 2004;75:727–30.
18. Rhee DS, Rodeberg DA, Baertschiger RM, et al. Update on pediatric rhabdomyosarcoma: a report from the APSA Cancer Committee. J Pediatr Surg 2020;55(10):1987–95.
19. Agaimy A. SMARCB1(INI1)-deficient renal cell carcinoma: medullary and beyond. Pathologe 2021;42(Suppl 2):S164–75.
20. Hollmann TJ, Hornick JL. INI1-deficient tumors: diagnostic features and molecular genetics. Am J Surg Pathol 2011;35:e47–63.
21. Wang LL, Gannavarapu A, Kozinetz CA, et al. Association between osteosarcoma and deleterious mutations in the RECQL4 gene in Rothmund-Thomson syndrome. J Natl Cancer Inst 2003;95:669–74.

22. Kleinerman RA, Tucker MA, Tarone RE, et al. Risk of new cancers after radiotherapy in long-term survivors of retinoblastoma: an extended follow-up. J Clin Oncol 2005;23:2272–9.
23. González IA, Stewart DR, Schultz KAP, et al. DICER1 tumor predisposition syndrome: an evolving story initiated with the pleuropulmonary blastoma. Mod Pathol 2022;35(1):4–22.
24. Tracy ET, Vasconcelos-Castro S, Malogolowkin M, et al. Nephron sparing surgery and surgical management of intravascular extension of Wilms tumor. Pediatr Blood Cancer 2023;70(Suppl 2):e30338.
25. Messinger YH, Stewart DR, Priest JR, et al. Pleuropulmonary blastoma: a report on 350 central pathology-confirmed pleuropulmonary blastoma cases by the International Pleuropulmonary Blastoma Registry. Cancer 2015;121:276–85.
26. Schultz KAP, Stewart DR, Messinger YH, et al. DICER1-related tumor predisposition: identification of at-risk individuals and recommended surveillance strategies. Clin Cancer Res 2024;30(24):5681–92.
27. Gulack BC, Rialon KL, Englum BR, et al. Factors associated with survival in pediatric adrenocortical carcinoma. J Pediatr Surg 2016;51(1):172–7.
28. Van Arendonk KJ, Tracy ET, Ellison JS, et al. Interfacility transfer of children with time-sensitive surgical conditions, 2002-2017. JAMA Netw Open 2024;7(10): e2440251.
29. Talbot LJ, Lautz TB, Aldrink JH, et al. Implications of immunotherapy for pediatric malignancies: a summary from the APSA Cancer Committee. J Pediatr Surg 2023;58(11):2119–27.
30. Ripperger T, Beger C, Gadzicki D, et al. Childhood colorectal cancer and polyposis syndromes: a retrospective analysis. Pediatr Blood Cancer 2009;52(7): 812–6.
31. Kanth P, Grimmett J, Champine M, et al. Hereditary colorectal polyposis and cancer syndromes: a primer on diagnosis and management. Am J Gastroenterol 2017;112(10):1509–25.
32. Bhattacharya P, Leslie SW, McHugh TW. Lynch syndrome (hereditary nonpolyposis colorectal cancer). In: StatPearls. StatPearls Publishing; 2024.
33. Aldrink JH, Polites S, Lautz TB, et al. What's new in pediatric melanoma: an update from the APSA cancer committee. J Pediatr Surg 2020;55(9):1714–21.
34. Kim J, Sun Z, Gulack BC, et al. Sentinel lymph node biopsy is a prognostic measure in pediatric melanoma. J Pediatr Surg 2016;51(6):986–90.
35. Tracy ET, Aldrink JA. Pediatric melanoma. Semin Pediatr Surg 2016;25(5):290–8.
36. Church AJ, Calicchio ML, Nardi V, et al. Recurrent EML4-NTRK3 fusions in infantile fibrosarcoma and congenital mesoblastic nephroma suggest a revised testing strategy. Mod Pathol 2018;31(3):463–73.
37. Laetsch TW, DuBois SG, Mascarenhas L, et al. Larotrectinib for paediatric solid tumours harbouring NTRK gene fusions: phase 1 results from a multicentre, open-label, phase 1/2 study. Lancet Oncol 2018;19(5):705–14.
38. Hong AL, Tseng YY, Cowley GS, et al. Renal medullary carcinomas depend upon SMARCB1 loss and are sensitive to proteasome inhibition. eLife 2019;8:e44161.
39. Su Y, Hong AL. Recent advances in renal medullary carcinoma. Int J Mol Sci 2022;23(13):7097.
40. Ezekian B, Englum BR, Gilmore BF, et al. Renal medullary carcinoma: a national analysis of 159 patients. Pediatr Blood Cancer 2017;64(11):e26609.

9780443429477